Notes and Observations on the Ionian Islands and Malta

With Some Remarks on Constantinople and Turkey, and on the System of Quarantine as at Present Conducted

VOLUME 1

JOHN DAVY

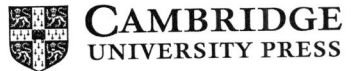

CAMBRIDGE
UNIVERSITY PRESS

CAMBRIDGE UNIVERSITY PRESS

Cambridge, New York, Melbourne, Madrid, Cape Town,
Singapore, São Paolo, Delhi, Tokyo, Mexico City

Published in the United States of America by Cambridge University Press, New York

www.cambridge.org
Information on this title: www.cambridge.org/9781108042352

© in this compilation Cambridge University Press 2012

This edition first published 1842
This digitally printed version 2012

ISBN 978-1-108-04235-2 Paperback

CAMBRIDGE LIBRARY COLLECTION

Books of enduring scholarly value

Travel and Exploration

The history of travel writing dates back to the Bible, Caesar, the Vikings and the Crusaders, and its many themes include war, trade, science and recreation. Explorers from Columbus to Cook charted lands not previously visited by Western travellers, and were followed by merchants, missionaries, and colonists, who wrote accounts of their experiences. The development of steam power in the nineteenth century provided opportunities for increasing numbers of 'ordinary' people to travel further, more economically, and more safely, and resulted in great enthusiasm for travel writing among the reading public. Works included in this series range from first-hand descriptions of previously unrecorded places, to literary accounts of the strange habits of foreigners, to examples of the burgeoning numbers of guidebooks produced to satisfy the needs of a new kind of traveller - the tourist.

Notes and Observations
on the Ionian Islands and Malta

The English doctor John Davy (1790–1868) was the younger brother of the chemist Sir Humphry Davy, of whom he wrote a memoir, also reissued in this series. After graduating from Edinburgh University, he entered the Army as a surgeon and was posted overseas. From 1824 to 1835 he was stationed in the Mediterranean, and later at Constantinople. Davy took detailed notes of the places he visited and the people he met, and turned some of these writings into books; his scientific observations led to him being made a Fellow of the Royal Society in 1834. Davy's account of his time in the Mediterranean was published in two volumes in 1842. Volume 1 begins with an overview of the respective histories of the Ionian Islands and Malta, and then discusses at length the geological and climatic aspects of the islands, examining their mineralogy, seasons, water temperature, and soil composition.

Cambridge University Press has long been a pioneer in the reissuing of out-of-print titles from its own backlist, producing digital reprints of books that are still sought after by scholars and students but could not be reprinted economically using traditional technology. The Cambridge Library Collection extends this activity to a wider range of books which are still of importance to researchers and professionals, either for the source material they contain, or as landmarks in the history of their academic discipline.

Drawing from the world-renowned collections in the Cambridge University Library, and guided by the advice of experts in each subject area, Cambridge University Press is using state-of-the-art scanning machines in its own Printing House to capture the content of each book selected for inclusion. The files are processed to give a consistently clear, crisp image, and the books finished to the high quality standard for which the Press is recognised around the world. The latest print-on-demand technology ensures that the books will remain available indefinitely, and that orders for single or multiple copies can quickly be supplied.

The Cambridge Library Collection brings back to life books of enduring scholarly value (including out-of-copyright works originally issued by other publishers) across a wide range of disciplines in the humanities and social sciences and in science and technology.

NOTES AND OBSERVATIONS

ON

THE IONIAN ISLANDS AND MALTA.

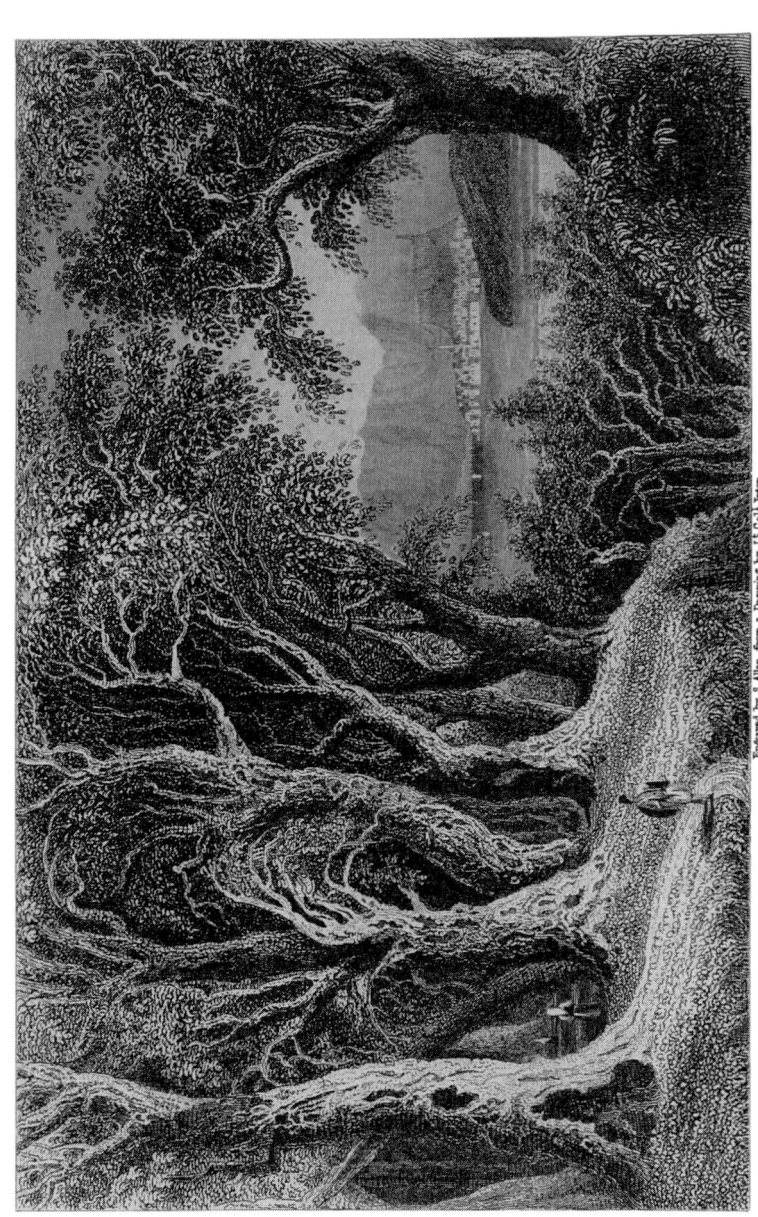

Engraved by S. Allen, from a Drawing by Lt. Col. Irton.

TOWN & CITADEL OF CORFU.

FROM AN ADJOINING OLIVE GROVE.

NOTES AND OBSERVATIONS

ON THE

IONIAN ISLANDS AND MALTA:

WITH SOME REMARKS ON

CONSTANTINOPLE AND TURKEY,

AND ON

THE SYSTEM OF QUARANTINE AS AT PRESENT CONDUCTED.

BY

JOHN DAVY, M.D., F.R.SS., L. & E.

INSPECTOR-GENERAL OF ARMY-HOSPITALS, L. R.

IN TWO VOLUMES.

VOL. I.

LONDON:

SMITH, ELDER & CO., 65, CORNHILL.

MDCCCXLII.

PREFACE.

Amongst the advantages enjoyed by the Medical Officers of the army, the opportunity which the service affords of visiting distant countries may justly be ranked as one of the most considerable, combining the pleasure and profit of travel with professional duties and culture, so that individuals, if intent on self-improvement, may derive at the same time a double benefit.

This advantage, I believe, has been duly appreciated and turned to good account: but too frequently it has happened that the individuals themselves only have profited.

During a period of twenty-six years of almost
universal peace, when many hundred well
educated and intelligent medical officers have
been employed in our extensive colonies,
how little has been contributed by them to
the general stock of knowledge, that is to
say, in proportion to their means and abilities.
This has always appeared to me a matter of
deep regret, especially as regards the extension of knowledge : the editor of a respectable and useful Medical Journal published in
India,* has judiciously chosen for his motto,

"Nihil est aliud magnum quam multa minuta."

If medical officers considered it a duty which
they owe to the public to communicate such
information, as they may have had it in their
power to collect, relative to the countries in
which they have been stationed, how many
doubtful points would have been cleared up,
—how many errors corrected,—how much

* Madras Quarterly Medical Journal.

more perfect would the histories of those countries have been rendered.

A persuasion of this kind has induced me to put together the notes and observations which I made during a period of eleven years that I was employed on the Medical Staff of the army in the Mediterranean, viz. from 1824 to 1835—with such additional information as I have since been able to procure.

The work resulting, is far more imperfect than I could wish; it has, indeed, required some resolution on my part to persevere in it, supported by a feeling of duty, such as that alluded to above ; and I shall be well pleased if it should be considered by others as not altogether a failure in the way of example. I may add, in justice to myself, that the greater part of it has been composed, not in the enjoyment of literary leisure, but in the midst of the pressure of business, and that al-

most uninterrupted, connected with the charge
of the General Hospital establishment at Fort
Pitt, which I held from May 1835 to October
1840, when I was sent by Her Majesty's
Government to Constantinople, on particular
service, under the Foreign Office, for the purpose of aiding to form a Medical Department
for the Turkish army, lamentably in want of
such a department, and to organize their
Military Hospitals, almost equally in want of
organization,—an occasion which enabled me
to collect the information given in the two
last chapters of the second volume.

The map attached to the work has been
formed expressly for it by Mr Arrowsmith:
parts of it are from actual survey, as Corfu,
and Zante, and Malta, and the whole of the
coast lines; and the remainder from different
plans and charts, either belonging to Mr
Arrowsmith, or to which he has been liberally
allowed access, especially by the Librarian

in the Colonial Office, Mr Mayer, to whom also I have to express my obligations for the facilities he has afforded me, in the kindest manner, of consulting many valuable documents respecting the Ionian Islands, deposited in his charge.

J. D.

MURRAYFIELD HOUSE, NEAR EDINBURGH,
June 4, 1842.

CONTENTS.

CHAPTER X.

ON THE SOILS, AND ON THE STATE OF AGRICULTURE AND HORTICULTURE IN THE IONIAN ISLANDS.

CHAPTER XI

ON THE SOILS, AND STATE OF AGRICULTURE AND HORTICULTURE IN MALTA.

Description of the principal varieties of Soil. Manner of bringing Ground into Cultivation, and forming " Campi artificiali." Proofs of extraordinary labour. Points of difference between the Agri-

LIST OF EMBELLISHMENTS.

VOL. I.

VOL. II.

NOTES AND OBSERVATIONS

ON

THE IONIAN ISLANDS AND MALTA.

CHAPTER I.

HISTORICAL NOTICES OF THE IONIAN ISLANDS AND MALTA.

Features of Difference between the Ionian Islands and Malta. Points of Resemblance in their History. Early flourishing Condition of the Ionian Islands in the Homeric Age. Their subsequent Fluctuations, and Subordination to Greece and Rome. Their further Degradation and Subjection in the Middle Ages. Form of Government when subject to Venice. Changes undergone before coming under the Protection of Great Britain. Obscurity of the Early, and imperfection of the Later, History of Malta, extending from the Fabulous Period to the 16th Century, when ceded to the Knights of St John. Condition of the Island under the Rule of the Order. Particulars in Illustration. Surrender of the Island to the French. Flourishing Condition under the Protection of Great Britain, as a great Commercial Entrepôt. The Plague of 1813. Its Consequences ; with the Opening of the Ports of Europe on the Cessation of War in 1814.

SITUATED in the same sea, distant from each other little more than three hundred miles, enjoying essentially the same climate,—it might, perhaps, be expected, that the Ionian Islands and Malta would be very similar, and that the history of the one would be very little different from that of the other; but the contrary of this is the case, and in a remarkable manner, and not even limited to the civil history of the two countries.

Although their solid geological structure and the incumbent soils are very analogous, yet the aspects presented in their scenery are very different, as are also their productions. The Ionian Islands generally are distinguished for beauty of landscape, for luxuriancy of vegetation. Malta is remarkable for apparent nakedness of surface, and an almost total absence of those features which constitute beauty. Where cultivation is neglected in the one,—the myrtle, the arbutus, the ilex, the cypress, commonly spring up, especially where most conspicuous, in the low grounds near the shore ; whilst, in the other, similarly circumstanced, in the place of such a rich and beautiful shrubbery, will be found only low plants, such as can exist in a shallow soil capable of bearing long continued drought, amongst which the thistle may be mentioned as most conspicuous. Nor are the products of cultivation (confining the attention to the more prominent, and, as it were, the staples) less strongly marked : these in Malta are chiefly annual crops, principally of grain and cotton ; whilst in the Ionian Islands, they are principally the olive and the vine,—one perdurable, the other of great durability.

Comparing the two countries, I apprehend it is not fanciful to say, that the one has more the European character, the other more the African : and, if their productions and aspect suggest this idea, it is greatly heightened by their population. The inhabitants of the Ionian Islands, it can hardly be questioned, are the descendants of the ancient Greeks; the antique beauty is common amongst them; they speak the same language, use the same written character, and, as far as regards person, may be considered a fine example of a European race. The Maltese speak a dialect of the Arabic, and are decidedly of Arabian descent,—with which their dark complexion accords, as well as many of their habits and manners.

The remains of antiquity, too, in the two countries, scanty as they are in both, point to the same difference. In the Ionian Islands, the most conspicuous are the old Greek walls, commonly called, from the magnitude of the blocks composing them, Cyclopian, —and tombs, formed as were the ancient Greek tombs, and containing similar relics.*

In Malta, including Gozo, the most remarkable are, the Giant's Tower in the latter, reminding one

* The only tombs I ever saw opened in the Ionian Islands, were some in the neighbourhood of the Cyclopian Walls of Samos in Cephalonia. They were in the form of oblong chests, about six feet long and three broad, and about the same depth, either made of four slabs of limestone, nicely fitting, or cut out of the limestone rock, and covered to the depth of about a foot with earth; their direction was commonly east and west; bones were found in most of them; in some, vases with ashes; in many, large quantities of bones, as if they were family vaults; the common accompaniments were a piece of money in the mouth, lamps arranged here and there, vases for wine and oil of elegant antique shapes.

at the same time of the Cyclopian architecture of Greece, and of the Druidical of Britain, supposed to be Phenician,*—and the tombs in the rocks, cut out of their solid substance.†

* This very singular structure is composed of two portions, parallel, adjoining and similar, one larger than the other, each containing three compartments, communicating. The walls (no roof is remaining, if there ever was one) are formed of large stones, mostly of irregular form; some of them of enormous dimensions, more than fifteen feet long, and hardly less in breadth, and, like the old Greek walls, not connected by cement. In the enclosed spaces, which are circular, or elliptical, there are the remains of altars, or what have been conjectured to be such. No inscriptions or coins have been discovered in the excavations hitherto made; and nothing throwing any satisfactory light on the age of the work, or even of the people by whom raised. It is pretty clear that it is neither Grecian nor Roman in character; the evidence that it is Phenician, I apprehend, is rather negative than positive. Similar remains, and on a more extensive scale, have recently been brought to light in Malta, close to the village of Krendi.

† Such tombs are common in Malta; the most remarkable, independent of the catacombs under Rabbato, are the excavations in the steep rocky side of the hill of Bengemma, in the wild, almost desert district about two miles to the north-west of Citta Vecchia. They are described and figured by Abela, but not very accurately;—he mentions and represents three rows in the face of the rock;—I found only two. The excavations are probably of a mixed nature, some designed for dwelling apartments, others as burying-places. The largest I saw might be 12 or 14 feet wide, about 24 feet long, and 12 high. There was a niche in the inner wall opposite the entrance, slightly hollowed, as if for holding water; and in the side walls, in several places, the rock was perforated, as if for the purpose of passing a cord through to fasten cattle. It is the smaller excavations that have the character of tombs. The catacombs just mentioned have also been described by Abela; but the plan he gives of them is too irregular; they are evidently a necropolis, and a very curious one.

But, though dissimilar in some respects,—in others, in their history they perfectly agree, especially in their dependency on foreign states, their successive occupancy by different dominant powers, the changes of government to which they have been subjected in consequence, and, as far as we can see, the inconsiderable effect which has been produced on either thereby. I allude, of course, to the mass of the people, and chiefly the lower ranks,—the inhabitants of the country and villages,—not the upper classes in the towns, the educated few, who are exposed to all the influences of the local government, with which they are commonly connected, and on which they are almost always dependent.

Of the Ionian Islands the earliest account we have we owe to Homer. Judging from his descriptions, which have much of the charm of verisimility, if not drawn from the life, these islands, at that early period, appear to have been well cultivated and populous, and in relation to the arts, in a more advanced state, perhaps, than at present. Take, for instance, the poet's description of the palace of Alcinoüs :—

> " Ulysses, then, toward the palace moved
> Of King Alcinoüs ; but immersed in thought
> Stood, first, and paused, ere with his foot he press'd
> The brazen threshold ; for a light he saw
> As of the sun, or moon, illuming clear
> The palace of Phæacia's mighty king.
> Walls plated bright with brass, on either side,
> Stretch'd from the portal to the interior house,

> With azure cornice crown'd ; the doors were gold,
> Which shut the palace fast ; silver the posts,
> Rear'd on a brazen threshold ; and above,
> The lintels, silver, architrav'd with gold.
> Mastiffs, in gold and silver, lined the approach
> On either side, by art celestial framed
> Of Vulcan, guardians of Alcinoüs' gate,
> For ever unobnoxious to decay." *

The abundance of gold and silver, of brass, and of ivory, at that time, judging from Homer's mention of their application to ordinary purposes, is very remarkable, and, with other circumstances, indicative of enterprise and success in commerce, much superior to its present languid state in these islands. And a similar remark, perhaps, applies to agriculture. Even of Ithaca he says :—

> " Rugged it is, not yielding level course
> To the swift steed ; and yet no barren spot,
> However small, but rich in wheat and wine ;
> Nor wants it rain or fertilizing dew,
> But pasture green to goats and beeves affords ;
> Trees of all kinds, and fountains never dry."

Forests, it is probable, then were not uncommon. Mount Neritos, in Ithaca, now a naked mountain, was then said to have been clothed with wood; and Zante, then, as afterwards by Virgil, was characterized as wooded. The diet of the people seems then to have been far more substantial than in the present time, and to have consisted almost entirely of animal food and bread, with wine for drink, and that old.

* Odyssey, B. vii., translated by Cowper.

The same fruits appear to have been common then as now, excepting the orange, and lemon, and pomegranate, which were long after introduced.* But the olive, probably, was not plentiful then, nor used ordinarily for the table ; it seems chiefly to have been cultivated for its oil, which was applied to the purpose of anointing after bathing. In viewing the favourable picture of these times and regions, as drawn by the poet, allowance must of course be made for the aiming at effect by poetical embellishment ; but all due allowance made, sufficient proof, I apprehend, is still afforded of what has been advanced above. In the notice of the garden of Alcinoüs, various kinds of fruit trees are described as always in fruit and flower,—the plum, the pear, the apple, and grape. That these fruits were the produce of the gardens of Corfu at that time, may perhaps be considered as fact ; and the perpetual flowering and bearing fruit, as the embellishment for heightening effect ; and so of other particulars. Then, as for many centuries after, in political condition the Ionian Islands seem to have been analogous to Continental Greece, and, at that very time, to have been under a mixed government, not, perhaps, unlike the government of Scotland, when an independent king-

* The orange, probably, has not been known in these islands above two centuries. Bishop Pratt, in his History of the Royal Society, published in 1667, noticing the beneficial effects of transplanting, and how they redound to the great advantage of the undertakers, adds, " The orange of China being of late brought into Portugal, has drawn a great revenue every year from London alone."

dom,—a monarchy, checked by an aristocracy in the lowlands, and by clanship in the mountains.

This early and poetical period of the history of the Ionian Islands, is by far the most brilliant and interesting, affording a remarkable proof of the power of genius in its hold of the human mind, especially when contrasted with that which followed, namely, of authentic history. From the remote Homeric time, down to the present time, with a very small number of exceptions, these islands have been little conspicuous in the page of history, whether from a want of prominent events, or of historians, or of both. They never appear to have taken any lead in the affairs of Greece, or, with the exception of one or two occasions, to have entered into rivalship with the influential states, or to have availed themselves of any of the many opportunities which offered, of earning honourable distinction. Whilst Greece was free, in its best times, the more important of these islands, as Corfu, Zante, and Cephalonia, appear to have enjoyed a certain degree of freedom, under republican forms of government,—sometimes, it may be inferred, independent, but more frequently in alliance, and under the influence and control either of Athens, or of Sparta, and never united in common league.

When Xerxes invaded Greece, these islands seem to have attained considerable power, especially Corfu; sixty triremes were prepared by the latter island on that emergency; and in the message of the Corcyrians to the Persian King, they described themselves as a naval power, second only to the Athenians, of which, in the occurrences that led to the first Peloponnesian war, they afforded demonstrative proof, in the great naval victory gained by them over the Corinthians, with the capture of fifteen ships. In the same war, Zante also gave proof of its strength and of its prowess. It afforded aid to Corfu of one thousand men; and when invaded by the Lacedemonians with a fleet of one hundred vessels and one thousand light-armed troops, the Zantiots successfully opposed, and expelled them. During the struggle of this terrible war, the courage of the Ionian people, as of the Greeks generally, appeared to more advantage than their morals. The great historian of the tragic events describes a thorough licentiousness to have prevailed; and speaking specially of Corfu, he says —" The whole order of human life was, for a season, confounded in that city." On the decline of Grecian liberty, these islands were alternately the prey of one or other conqueror, until they became, in common with Greece, an integral part of the Roman empire, included in the province which bore the name of Achaia. Under Roman rule, they appear to have remained undisturbed in ignoble tranquillity, like so many other parts of the Roman dominions, until the invasion of the Goths, A.D. 255, when Valerianus and Gallienus were emperors, and when they were cruelly devastated. Then it is supposed that the principal monuments of the ancient times were destroyed, and so unsparingly, by the barbarians, that hardly a vestige was left ; thus accounting for the remarkable deficiency of such remains now observable.

In the barren annals of the lower empire, few events of importance or interest are recorded of these islands. Ravaged and conquered by the Vandals, they were recovered by Belisarius. When the provinces of the empire underwent subdivision, shortly after, in the reign of Heraclius Libicus, the Ionian Islands were attached to the prefecture of Lombardy, and so continued, either united to Lombardy or Sicily, for the space of 250 years, until the time of Leo the Philosopher, who formed them into a province apart, under the title of Tema of Cephalonia. This arrangement lasted about 300 years, until the beginning of the thirteenth century, when the Greek empire was broken up by the conquests of the Franks. During the period that elapsed from this event to that of their coming under the Venetian rule, the history of the Ionian Islands is very confused. They appear to have been variously governed, principally by chiefs of Norman extraction, and by princes of the house of Valois. In 1386, Corfu was yielded up to Venice, on certain conditions, settled between the Republic and the Corcyrian delegates, not unfavourable, at first sight, to the interests of that island, and which were joyfully accepted by the people ; * and in

* This was after the death of Charles, the third king of Hungary, Jerusalem and Sicily, under whose protection the island had been.

a little less than another century, the other Ionian Islands came under the same government. During this period, they appear to have suffered much from piratical and hostile invasion, especially Cephalonia and Zante, which were more than once occupied and spoiled by the Turks. In 1485, after the purchase of the latter island from its conquerors, when almost deserted, a new colony was established there by the Venetians, formed chiefly of Greeks, collected from different parts of the Morea. Cephalonia came into their possession a few years later; they expelled the Turks by force of arms in 1499.

The form of government instituted by the Venetians on these islands was of a very mixed kind— little favourable to liberty—little conducive to their general and permanent improvement. Of its organization and influence, the reader may form a tolerable idea, from the sketch in the subjoined note, contributed by an enlightened individual, possessed of more than ordinary means of collecting correct information, and with which I was favoured from Corfu, in reply to some queries on the subject.*

In the treaty with Venice, the Corfuots describe themselves in a helpless state, " quasi assediata da Arabi e Turchi;" and that " niuno discrepante, hanno dato, costituti, ed ordinado in loro Deffensore, e Protettore, e Governatore, e Signor, il Venerabile Comúne di Venezia.'

* " The first representative of the Venetian Government in the Ionian Islands was styled the ' Provveditor General da Mar,' and his jurisdiction extended to all the Ionian Islands, great and small; and likewise to Prevesa, Parga, Vonizza, and Bucintro. Under his orders were placed the land and naval forces of the Republic stationed within these territories. For his approval were submitted all administra-

Venice maintained possession of the Ionian Islands until the extinction of the Republic in 1797. From

tive and judicial acts, and all appeals, previous to transmission to the Venetian Government.

" The Provveditor-General da Mar was usually chosen from the second class of Venetian nobles; he remained three years in office ; was responsible only to the Senate of Venice ; and in his person constituted what would now be considered the general government of these states.

" The city of Corfu was permitted to send an ambassador, or representative, who was styled Nuncio, to Venice. The duties of this functionary, who was elected by the Council of Nobles (Corfuots), were to watch over the interests of the city, and to present and sustain such appeals as might be made by its inhabitants against illegal acts on the part of the Venetian functionaries.

" The head of the local government of Corfu was styled ' Provveditor e Capitano all Isola di Corfu,' and likewise Prefect. His jurisdiction extended to cases relating to public servants, or employés; feudal property; the public revenue; church property, di jus patronato publico ; and sentences by the governor of Parga, whose jurisdiction was limited in pecuniary cases to thirty ducats. [See decree of Dominico Mocinigo, Capitan-General, dated 6th May 1691.] The individual holding the situation was always a Venetian, and usually selected from the Barnabotti, or poor class of Venetian nobles.

" Next followed ' Il Pótere Pretorio detto Reggimento,' which was composed of three individuals, the president being styled ' Bailo. These were likewise Barnabotti; and, in conjunction with a noble Corfuot, they elected annually the Council of Nobles.

" The causes of individuals not employed under government, and of the country people, were tried in this court, from whence appeals were carried directly to the Provveditor General da Mar. The individuals composing this court remained in office two years.

" In the courts styled Foro Pretorio and Prefetizio, the inhabitants of Paxo had their claims adjudged, as decreed by the Cavalier Bortolo Contarini, Provveditor General Inquisitor. Causes appertaining to the inhabitants of the continent were tried in the latter, and its jurisdiction extended over the property of banished individuals.

" There was likewise a court composed of three noble Corfuots,

that time, until the peace of Paris, when they were placed under the protection of Great Britain, their

elected annually by the Council of Nobles; of these, two were of the Greek rite, and one of the Latin. Before them were tried causes not exceeding in value fifty ducats, or twelve and a-half dollars. [Decree of Capitan-General Alessandro Molin, 27th February 1697.]

" There was a functionary styled Barone de' Cingani (Gypsies), which dignity appertained to the eldest son of the now extinct family of the Counts Rossalindi del Maggio ; and any sentences emanating from any other court, with respect to this race, were null and void.

" In the country, there was the jurisdiction of the Governor of St Angelo, who was a noble Corfuot. His authority extended over the villages in the vicinity of the castle, from Liapades to Coropiscopus, St Atanasio, and Spagus, with the villages near them. His jurisdiction was limited to the amount of nine ducats, or rather according to the authority granted him by the Provveditor e Capitano.

" The ' Magistrato alla Sanita,' or Sanitary Commission, was composed of three noble Corfuots, elected by the Council, and its power to fine transgressors was limited to fifteen ducats. It acted under the superintendence of the Provveditor e Capitano, who took part in its proceedings. If the offence merited a greater fine, the case was referred to the Potere Pretorio, who, together with the Sanitary Commission and the Provveditor e Capitano, judged the case; and, thus united, the power of this court extended to the infliction of capital punishments, as established by the Provveditor-General Filippo Pasqualego, 20th July 1606.

" Every year were elected four Syndics, or heads of the municipality, two of the Greek and two of the Latin rite. Their duty was to superintend and look after the municipal property, and the revenue arising therefrom ; to examine and approve of plans for the improvement of the city, and to carry them into execution. The operations of this body were subject to the approbation of the Provveditor-General; but they were at liberty to appeal, either to the Senate of Venice, to the Council of Ten, or to that of Forty, as the case might be.

" There were two Provveditori of the Monasteries; their duties, however, only consisted in maintaining those establishments in good order ; they had nothing to do with the revenues.

fortunes were most various.   They were, indeed, very
like the foot-ball of fortune.   First,—namely, in the

" There were two Censors who watched over the due observance of
the regulations by the Council of Nobili.

" There were three Provveditori, who, in conjunction with the Bailo,
Syndics, and Provveditor e Capitano, managed the grain administration.

" There were two Provveditori for the roads, and two for the management of the Orfanotrophia; but both magistrates being totally
unsupported by the government, were almost useless.   The Council
likewise elected a Proto Medico, who had a miserable salary.

" At the period when the Ionian Islands came under the Venetian
dominion, that state was already in its decline; and perfectly aware
of its own weakness, it adopted such a line of policy as seemed best
adapted to enrich and strengthen the mother country, though to the
infinite injury, both moral and financial, of the Ionians.   Venice introduced into these islands all the vices of its own domestic government, without even those few redeeming qualities which so long enabled it to hold together.   The Provveditori-Generali were, in many
instances, sent to these islands, principally with a view to repair their
shattered fortunes, or to amass money.   In this they seem to have
succeeded; for, although the stipend of Pro-General was almost nominal, instances have been known of individuals, while in that situation, having saved near L.50,000.   When such evident and unlimited
corruption was permitted in the head of the government, it is not
difficult to suppose that his example was sedulously followed by the
subaltern employés; nor could they, indeed, do otherwise, their
salaries, like that of the Provveditor-General, being merely nominal;
and it was, therefore, to their perquisites that they looked for remu-
neration for their services.   One mode of extracting money from the
nobili of these states will serve as an illustration of the means resorted to by the Provveditori-Generali for this purpose.   It was the custom
of the Provveditor-General to invite to dinner, twice in the year, the
principal and most wealthy of the inhabitants.   On such occasions, it
was expected that each guest should put under his plate a paper,
stating the number of barrels of oil he intended giving his host.   As
every individual from whom it was thought possible to extract any

year before mentioned, 1797,—they were occupied
by the French—a force detached from the army of

thing was invited ; as the number of barrels of oil offered could in no
case be less than two ; and as the most certain way of obtaining favour with the Provveditor was to make a generous offer, it is not
surprising that, at the expiration of his three years service, that functionary returned to Venice a rich man. The object of this exaction
was twofold : It enriched, in the first instance, the Venetian Provveditor, who, therefore, continued it; and, as it tended to impoverish
the Ionians, it was not discouraged by the Venetian Senate.

It was the policy of the Venetians to encourage feuds between the
order of society called Nobili, and the rest of the community ; and if
any individual became more powerful than was considered convenient,
to foment intrigues, &c., between him and some rival, until both
were reduced to a proper state of dependence.

" EDUCATION.—No people or government better understood the value
of the old adage, that knowledge is power, than the Venetians; and
the method they pursued to retain the Ionians in ignorance, was
strictly in conformity with the rest of their policy, and gives no bad
idea of the spirit in which they governed these islands.

" Such an establishment as a public school did not exist in the
islands ; and, in the very few private schools which were attended by
the children of the Nobili of the country, little beyond the first ru-
diments of education were taught.

" From the facilities afforded to Ionians to study at Padua, that was
the city resorted to by young Ionians, who went to Italy with a view
to study ; and, indeed, it was, in a certain degree, imperative that
they should study nowhere else. The professors of this University,
which was under the influence of Venice, were strictly prohibited
from teaching any thing tending to open the eyes of the Ionians to
their real condition ; and the studies and examinations were so conducted, that in three months, an Ionian could obtain his diploma as
doctor of medicine or law. It must, however, be observed, that this
did not entitle him to exercise his profession, either in Italy, nor yet
in Venice, but merely in the Venetian colonies in the East.

" In the citadel, and not far from the palace of the Provveditor-Generale,

Italy. Next, the following year, the French were expelled by the Turks and Russians, acting conjointly. Shortly after, in 1800, the Septinsular Republic was instituted, under the protection of these powers. It appears to have been rather an anarchy than a government, and was productive of a state of society not very dissimilar from that alluded to, a few pages back, described by Thucydides, as existing in the same island during the Peloponnesian war. A native writer, speaking of the condition of Zante at that time, remarks,—" It was torn by internal factions, the origin and series of which had better not be recorded." Again, in 1807, they were invaded, and taken possession of by the French, who, in turn, excepting from Corfu, were expelled by a British force. Zante was taken from them in September 1809; Cephalonia, Ithaca, and Cerigo, immediately after; and Santa Maura in the following spring. Corfu, which was occupied by a numerous garrison, held out till the abdication of Napoleon, in 1814, shortly after

was placed the marble head of a lion, into the mouth of which it was permitted to thrust secret accusations; and, on such, it was in the power of the Provveditor-Generale to seize the accused, and send him to Venice, where instances may be cited of his having been condemned and punished, without even knowing his accusers, and scarcely the nature of his offence.

" The Island of Corfu once produced corn in abundance; so much so, that it was enabled to supply other countries; but, as this was found to interfere with the interests of many of the Venetian nobles, who possessed grain estates on the continent, this branch of agriculture was indirectly prohibited."

which it surrendered conditionally to the arms of Great Britain.*

The early history of Malta is even more obscure than that of the Ionian Islands, and not less poetical, if it be supposed to be the Hyperia of the Odyssey, as has been maintained by some authors, and the Island of Calypso, of the same poem. De Bres, an able writer, who rejects the former opinion,† has arrived

* For the following note, showing the extent of the Ionian Islands, I am indebted to the Colonial Office :—

" The Ionian Islands consist of Corfu, Cephalonia, Zante, Santa Maura, Ithaca, Cerigo, and Paxo, and all the other islands, great and small, inhabited or uninhabited, situated opposite the Peloponnesus and Albania ; that is to say, all those which have been detached from the Republic of Venice.

" To the Island of Corfu belong Fanno, Merlere, Saseno, Samothracio, Sivota, and all the others in or out of the channel to Cape Formaggio.

" To Cephalonia belong Guardiani, Luca, Dia, and all the uninhabited ones round the island.

" To Zante belong Stivali, Marathonisi, Piluso, Trentenove, Prodono, Sapienza, Porto Schisa, Venitico, and all the others which are scattered upon the sea to Cape Gallo.

" To Santa Maura belong Meganisi, Chitios, and all the uninhabited ones in the channel of Santa Maura to the Port of Figlia.

" To Cerigo belong Cerigotto, Poro, Poretto, Dragoneres, Cervi, and all the others from Cape St Angelo to Coron.

" To Ithaca belong Kalemos, Castus, Arkudi, Atako, and all the others out of the channel to the rock Cazzolani inclusive.

" To Paxo belong Antipaxo, Cassionisi, San Nicolo, La Madonna, and all the others round the Island of Paxo, and along the neighbouring continent, from Cape Formaggio to the mouth of the channel of Prevesa."

† De Bres, in the opening of his " Malta Antica (Roma, 1816)," protests against the probability of Malta being inhabited by giants, in a manner somewhat more grave than useful.

at the conclusion, that Malta was first colonized by the Phenicians, and from Tyre, about 1400, B.C.,— at least, two centuries before the assigned period of the Trojan War,—and that it was used by that maritime people as a commercial station, for which it is so well fitted, by situation, and its excellent ports.

The Phenicians, it is supposed, retained undisputed possession of Malta until about 757, B.C., when it is conjectured that a Greek settlement, with a republican form of government,* was established,—colonies of that people, about the time mentioned, having been founded in Sicily.   Whether the Phenicians were expelled by the Greeks, or that they remained joint occupiers of the island, is a disputed point ; but the latter seems the more probable, and is supported by the circumstance, that Phenician coins have been found in Malta, bearing a Greek inscription.   How long the Greeks maintained their sway in Malta, like almost every thing else relating to the early history of the island, is matter of conjecture.   It is conjectured, as probable, that they were subdued by the Carthaginians about 402 years B.C.,—that is, after the conquest by these people of Sicily and Sardinia. The termination of their rule is less uncertain.

---

* That the Greek settlers in Malta lived under a republican form of government is proved by a *tessera hospitalis*, in bronze, now in the Museum of Naples, found in the island, and referred to by De Bres and Heeren, from the inscription on which it appears that the republic of Malta had its Senate, and three supreme magistrates—viz., the Pontiff, who was also president of the Senate, and two Archons.

It is recorded by Livy, that a Roman fleet, under the command of the Consul Titus Sempronius appeared before Malta about 216, B.C., and that the Carthagenian garrison submitted, the native people having refused to act with them on the defensive.

Under the Romans, the Maltese enjoyed many privileges. They are called by Cicero, *Socii;* and appear to have exercised very successfully those arts of manufacture which were probably introduced by the Phenicians and Carthagenians, especially weaving, and the making of fine cotton or linen cloth,— the *vestes melitenses,*—which incited and exercised the cupidity of Verres. Under the Emperors, even greater favour was shown to Malta than in the Republican period of Rome. The rights of citizenship were extended to its inhabitants ; and, from some inscriptions, it appears they were enrolled in one of the tribes of Roman citizens, and were entitled to vote in the election of magistrates, and might attain the rank of Roman knights, or any dignity or office in the state.

On the decline of the Roman power, and the invasion and dismemberment of the Empire, the fortunes of Malta were very like those of the Ionian Islands. At certain intervals, the island was invaded and made a conquest of by Vandals, Goths, and Saracens. The first invasion of the latter is referred to the year 870, A.D. ; and their second, and more successful one, to the beginning of the next century, when a ruthless severity, even to extermination, it is supposed, was exercised by them over the Greek part of the population, and was extended to the temples and public buildings; and to these devastations has been plausibly attributed the great scarcity of the remains of ancient art in the island.

This invasion must have refreshed the African blood of the inhabitants, especially as the Saracens retained their power for the space of about two hundred years, until overcome by the Norman conquerors of Sicily, in 1090.

Between this period and 1530, when Malta was ceded in sovereignty to the Knights Hospitallers of St John (the Baptist) of Jerusalem, by the Emperor Charles the Fifth, it was successively subject to the Emperors of Germany, to Charles of Anjou, in common with Sicily, and afterwards to the Kings of Aragon and Castile.

These were bad times for the Maltese, and they must have suffered severely. This may be inferred, considering their ancient condition, as it has been imagined, under the Carthagenians, when garrisoned by 2000 men,* the same force nearly as the British stationed there at present, and when, as now, it was an entrepôt of commerce, and comparing it with their state just about the time above referred to, as reported by the commissioners sent by the Grand-Master, L'Isle Adam, in 1525, expressly for the purpose of collecting information, when he was

* Livy, xxi. 51.

deliberating on the choice of a residence for the Order.*

Under the government of the Knights, Malta rapidly rose in importance. Only thirty-five years after their establishment—namely, in 1565—they baffled all the efforts of a powerful Turkish army, and stood a siege of nearly four months—a siege which has been considered one of the most memorable in military history,† and most glorious to the

* They stated " that the Island of Malta was merely a rock of soft sandstone, called *tufa*, about six or seven leagues long, and three or four broad; that the surface of the rock was scarcely covered with more than three or four feet of earth, which was stony, and very unfit to grow corn and other grain, though it produced abundance of figs, melons, and different fruits; that the principal trade of the island consisted in honey, cotton, and cummin, which the inhabitants exchanged for grain; that, except a few springs in the middle of the island, there was no running water, or even rills, the want of which the inhabitants supplied with cisterns; that wood was so scarce, as to be sold by the pound, which forced them either to use cow dung, dried in the sun, or wild thistles, for dressing food; that the island contained about 12,000 inhabitants, of both sexes, the greatest part of whom were poor and miserable, owing to the barrenness of the soil; and, in a word, that a residence in Malta appeared extremely disagreeable, almost insupportable, especially in summer. —VERTOT, vol. iii. p. 286, 8vo edition.

The Order landed at the Borgo, and took possession of Malta, October 26, 1530. On the 30th November following, the Grand Master went in procession to Citta Vecchia, accompanied, as we are informed, by Bossio, by a large company of the natives, five hundred of them riding on asses, with rich garniture. The Maltese are described as having long beards, and clad in short cotton vests, so thick as to resist an arrow, and even to turn a bullet.

† In this siege, it has been estimated that the Turks lost about 30,000 men; the Order nearly 300 knights, and about 7000 men.

defenders; and in the following year, the city of
Valetta was founded; on the 28th of March, the
first stone was laid by the heroical Grand-Master La
Valette,* from whence it derived its name, and who,
before its completion, died, and was interred in the
Chapel of " Vittoria," † which he himself had dedicated, and which was the first building erected within
the walls.

In little more than a century from this time,
Malta, probably, was in its most flourishing state
under the knights, and the order at the height of its
power, at least of its opulence. Possessed of rich
Commanderies in the different kingdoms of Europe,
their means were very ample; it has been estimated
that their expenditure amounted annually to nearly
half a million sterling, principally derived from fo-

---

* The ceremony is described as a very impressive and picturesque
one by Bossio, in his Istoria dell. Sac. Rel. The foundation-stone, it
may be presumed, was laid exactly at noon, as the chief engineer, the
gallant Laparelli, who planned the new city, is mentioned as standing by the Grand-Master with an astrolabe in his hand, in the midst
of the high officers of the order, and a great concourse of people. If
my information be correct, the first stone was laid on the highest part
of Mount *Sceb e Ras*, looking inland, where now is the bastion which
holds part of the remains of another chivalrous character, the Marquis
of Hastings. The fortifications were first attended to; 8000 men,
guarded by 18,000 soldiers, were employed on the works. Even after
the convent was removed within the walls, in 1571, the knights lived
in tents and rude huts.

† When the splendid Church of St John was completed, the remains of this great man were removed from the Church of Vittoria,
and deposited in a vault, possessed of great architectural beauty, constructed expressly for their reception.

reign sources. From the narrative of a French gentleman who visited the island in 1673, and who has given an interesting and animated account of what he witnessed, it appears that the total number of knights then belonging to the order, available for service, amounted to eighteen hundred, of whom four or five hundred were always resident; and that the population of the island was then about fifty thousand. He describes the Grand-Master, who was the second Cottonera, as living in great state;—his palace sumptuously furnished,—his word law to all around him,—never addressing a knight but *en maître*,—attended to chapel by four hundred knights, who ranged themselves in the hall whilst he dined, and did not move until he made the signal permitting them. He describes the place itself as a delightful residence,—the rendezvous of Christendom, where persons might meet in peace the subjects of hostile princes, and where the best intelligence was to be had of all that was passing in the adjoining kingdoms. The manner of living he dwells on as luxurious,— the markets well supplied,—fruits in abundance and of choice quality,—excellent meat,*—plenty of game, excellent wines,—and ice in common use. At this

---

* He speaks of the beef and mutton as " d'un goût merveilleux;" adding, " le veau et les poules s'y mangent en tout saisons quoy qu'il semble que la pasturage y soit fort rare; les perdrix, les pigeons, surtout les lapreaux, Grives et tous autres gibiers y sont plus gras qu'en aucun lieu de l'Europe." He mentions that two hundred fowls were used daily to make broth for the patients in the hospital.

time, although much luxury prevailed, the Order was respected,—the seven galleys of the Grand-Master were said to be more dreaded by the Turks than the whole navy of Venice.

The decline of their power, however, was not far distant;—their wealth and their luxury were their ruin;—both were contrary to their vows,*—and before another century had passed, the Order had more the character of a company of Sybarites, than of christian knights, and were feared (excepting, it is to be apprehended, as Corsairs) as little as they were respected. This clearly appears from the latter part of their history; and it is strongly indicated, in part, by a curious document, in manuscript, written by an individual of the name of Doublet, who was in the confidential service of the two last Grand-Masters, entitled " Memoires Historiques sur l'Invasion et l'Oc- cupation de Malte par une Armee Française, 1798," which was in possession of the late Sir Frederick Ponsonby. From his account, they appear then to have been, with a few exceptions, completely sunk

---

* The following words were addressed to a knight on his admis- sion into the Order, when the chain to which the cross was suspended was placed over his neck :—" Accipe jugum Domini quia suave et leve est, sub hoc invenies requiem animæ tuæ." To which were added :—" Non delicias tibi, sed panem et aquam et humilem vesti- tam tantum promittimus, atque participem facimus animam tuam tuorumque parentum et consanguineorum in bonis operibus nostri fratrumque nostrorum quæ per universum orbem fiunt et in futurum fient." To which the response of the " professus" was, " Amen, quasi dicat ite sit oro."

in profligacy and dissipation, and to have lost very much even the sense of shame; and, what I have heard related by old persons, who remembered their doings, was much in accordance. The caravans of the knights (as their cruises against the infidels were called) are described by Doublet as summer excursions of pleasure, in the direction of Sicily and Sardinia, passing from port to port; the knights boasting on their return only of the fêtes they had enjoyed, and of their sensual indulgences, varied, according to my informant, by an occasional act of piracy, the capture of some defenceless merchantman, or the sacking of some small town or village belonging to the Turks, for the sake of booty, and prisoners, who were sold as slaves.

The power of the Order ceased in June 1798, when Valetta was surrendered to the French under Buonaparte. The inglorious manner of the transaction is well known, and it is a strong proof of the degeneracy of the knights as a body. The subsequent events are few, though not unimportant.

The Maltese soon became dissatisfied with the French rule; they were subjected to the loss of many advantages they had before enjoyed, and to some privations, for which they found a nominal liberty, and certain republican forms—no adequate substitute; and their discontent was shortly ripened into insurrection by the exhortations of the clergy, whom the French made their determined enemies, by the want of respect which they showed both to religion, and to church property. This happened a few months after the expulsion of the knights; and, almost simultaneously, the French who were confined to Valetta, found themselves in a state of siege and blockade,—invested on the land side by the natives, headed by their priests,—and by sea, by a Portuguese squadron, and shortly by a more formidable English fleet. Although the garrison left by Buonaparte consisted only of 4000 men, it maintained the place, until compelled by starvation to surrender. The able and intrepid General Vaubois, who had the command, capitulated on the 3d September 1802, on honourable and favourable terms. From that time Malta has been under the protection or rule of Great Britain. By the treaty of Amiens, in the same year, the restoration of the Order, and its re-possession of the island, was guaranteed, the non-performance of which was one of the assigned causes on the part of Napoleon for the renewal of hostilities in 1803. During the remainder of the war, until the plague broke out, in 1813, the prosperity of the island was marvellous, and, perhaps, unparalleled in the records of history,—having become, in consequence of Napoleon's continental system, not only the entrepôt of our commerce for the Mediterranean, but also for the greater part of Europe,—every port of which was closed to our shipping from the Baltic to the Adriatic, and was accessible only to enterprise on its eastern shores, within the Turkish dominions. Baron de Piro, in his interesting little work on the plague,

as it appeared in the year above mentioned, gives an
animated picture, in a chapter apart, of this flourishing period ;—how the capacious harbours were crowded to excess with shipping,—the concourse of people
of different nations,—the increase of population by
some thousands,—the enormous influx of wealth,—
the bustle and activity of business by day,—the public amusements by night.*

* " Immune dagli enormi tributi, dalle coscrizioni, dal ferro e dal
fuoco che straziarano l'Europa, Malta vide ben presto concorrere, in
lei un numero prodigioso di ricchi negozianti, e di fuggiaschi con-
tinentali d'ogni condizione e fortuna, li quali aumentarono di molte
migliaja la sua popolazione, e l'affluenza del traffico la rese ben tosto
doviziosissima. Li suoi porti in quei tempi felici, sembravano pochi
ed angusti a tante navi, che a guisa d'una selva di pini ondeggianti
l'ingombravano da tutt' i lati, fra le quali venivano condotte prede di
ricchi carichi, che aumentavano tutto di la sua opulenza. E non
che il solo traffico, ma qualunque professione, arte, o mestiere, era
in quei giorni una continua sorgente di guadagno per tutti coloro
che l'esercitavano, mentre anche l'umile contadino ritraendo un con-
siderabile introito da' prodotti delle sue fatiche, sodisfaceva puntuale
al signore di cui tenea le terre, e rimaneagli assai più che abbisognasse
al suo frugale sostentamento. L'isola del Gozo, per la sua dipendenza
da Malta, participava egualmente della prosperità di questa, ricavando
anch' essa un lucro pinguissimo dall' esportazione delle sue abbon-
danti produzioni campestri.

" Era grato il vedere in quei giorni avventurosi la città e particolar-
mente la Valletta, ricolme d'un foltissimo popolo tutt' intento allo
sbrigamento di lavori, di negozi, e all' intrapresa di nuovi ; fra il cui
incessante movimento e generale bisbiglio udivansi idiomi, osserva-
vansi costumi gli uni dagli altri diversi, per li molti forastieri di varie
nazioni ivi congregati ; un continuo attraversare di carri, di giumenti,
di facchini con somne, per le vie, e le marine ; navi a deporre merci,
altre, a riceverne ; un perpetuo veleggiar ne' porti di chi arriva e di
chi parti ; e quindi cessando col giorno quell' attività, e quell' affac-

The appearance of this dreadful disease, the introduction of which is still unexplained in a satisfactory
manner, entirely changed and reversed the face of
things ; commerce ceased, business was suspended,
even the courts of justice and the churches were
closed ; in brief, a city a few weeks before so flourishing and gay,—the great mart of Europe,—assumed the
appearance of, and in fact was converted into, a
Lazaretto ; and nothing was to be seen in it or heard
but sights and sounds of woe.* During the seven

cendarsi generale, vedeansi di notte le botteghe, i caffè, il teatro, e
tutti i luoghi di ritrovo, rigurgitanti d'una popolazione contenta e
festiva. Felicitavasi il nazionale nel vender bandita ogni miseria
dalla sua patria, resa emporio d'ogni dovizia commerciale ; godea lo
straniero nel ritrovarvi ospitalità, e sicurezza, e pago il governo com-
piaceasi de' suoi pingui introiti, e della generale felicità degli abitauti."
    * The Baron di Piro, who witnessed the change, describes it for-
cibly. As a contagionist, and advocate for the present system of
quarantine, which he seems to consider almost perfect, it may not be
amiss to give in his own words his recollection of the horrors. After
noticing some of them, he proceeds :—" Qual orribile cambiamènto
non era quello per l'isola di Malta ! Ricovero prima d'ogni straniero,
era divenuta, nel breve corso di varj mesi, una terra di spavento e
d'orrore per qualunque naviglio estero ; i suoi propri legni rigettati,
e sottoposti a dure e penose leggi, in qualunque porto che approda-
vano. Al suo florido commercio era succeduta la suppressione d'ogni
affare ; alle dovizie la miseria, alla libertà la prigionia, alla gioja il
lutto. Oh stato veramente deplorabile ! L'uomo, per conservasi,
dovea sfuggir l'uomo, il vicino paventar del vicino, l'amico dell'
amico, e sovente, fin dentro le pareti d'un istessa casa, il figlio era
barbaramente costretto di evitare il genitore, e l'amorosa madre di
abbandonare il frutto delle sue viscere, per tema d'appestarlo. Le
vie della Valletta, già tanto rumorose, non presentavano in certe ore
del giorno che una lugubre solitudine, ed un cupo silenzio, solo inter-
rotto di quando in quando or dal calpestio di qualche picchetto di

months that the disease prevailed, namely, from the first week in May to the last in December, it proved fatal to 4572 persons; and in the following spring, to 96 in Gozo, out of a population in the one of about 100,000, and in the other of about 16,000. The plague was speedily followed by peace, in 1814, on the downfal of Buonaparte; which, by opening the ports of Europe, and restoring commerce to its natural channels, deprived Malta of the means and opportunity of recovering its prosperity;—few of the merchants who fled returned;—and ever since, with an excessive population, it has been struggling more or less under adverse circumstances; or rather, it may be said, in needy and indigent circumstances, from the withdrawal of foreign capital and enterprise, and the want of that native talent and activity of mind, which are the source of enterprise and of capital, without which no country can flourish, excepting, as in the instance of Malta, in a forced state, and as

milizie, or da lenti tocchi d'una campana, che annunziava il passaggio dell' ostia sacra, portata da un sacerdote con un solo assistante, i quali ivano sussurando sotto voce gl' inni divini, ed ora dal tristo cigolio de' carri mortuarj, ni quali sovente i figli co' genitori, l'amico coll' inimico, col cristiano l'incredulo, stavano l'un sopra l'altro confusamente accatastati. L'orrore però e lo spavento cresceano coll' ombre della notte. Quella stessa luna che mesi prima, col suo chiaro lume sembrava arridere propizia a' diporti, ed ai sollazzi degli abitanti, parea non scroprire gli oggetti che per renderli alla nostra vista vieppiù tetri e lugubri. Non più canti notturni, nè strumentali concerti, non più voci di giulive brigate, che faceano echeggiare le placide rive, ma s'udivano in vece pianti e lamenti di chi gemmea, misti alle invocazioni ed alle preghiere, che ad alta voce s'intonavano, onde placari l'ira Divina."

it were by accident, however fortunately situated (as this island eminently is), and however much favoured by government, and unoppressed by taxation. It might be well for the Maltese, when complaining of their superabundant population and poverty, to reflect on the population of any great commercial and manufacturing town, of London, or Liverpool, or Glasgow, and compare conditions in connexion with causes, and they could hardly fail to come to the conclusion, that their island might be infinitely more populous than it is, and proportionally prosperous, could its inhabitants make the same exertions as have been made in these cities; that is, were their mental powers and resources similar.

CHAPTER II.

ON THE GEOLOGY AND MINERALOGY OF THE IONIAN ISLANDS.

Prevailing Rocks. Their Connexion with Scenery. Remarkable Caverns. Basin-like Valleys. Peculiarities of Stratification. Uses of certain Rocks. Notice of the few Minerals hitherto discovered. Remarkable Mineralizing Process, as exhibited in Ancient Coins, &c.

Of the geology of these islands, interesting and varied as it is, and deserving of careful study, I shall attempt only a sketch, in connexion with their scenery, and in relation to climate and agriculture, and some other useful applications.

The prevailing rocks of which the Ionian Islands are composed belong to two classes—the secondary and the tertiary; those of the primary and transition class are rare; and those of the trap family are unknown—at least I was not able to detect their presence, or to discover any traces of them, after pretty extensive and careful search. And the same remark applies almost as generally (with one doubtful exception) to the products and traces of volcanoes.

Of the primitive rocks, gneiss and marble are the

only two species which have yet been discovered, and these only in one island, viz. Cerigo; and in one place, viz. the site of the elevated and inland village of Potamo. These rocks are there contiguous, very partially exposed; they rise only a few inches above the soil, and present rounded surfaces. The first mentioned rock, even in the very limited space of a few feet, in which it comes to light, varies in structure. Whilst its general aspect is that of gneiss, in some instances it approaches more to granite; and parts of it are neither distinctly granite or gneiss, consisting chiefly of felspar, with a little mica and quartz interspersed, and iron glance. The marble is probably a small bed. It is finely granular, and beautifully white, but not free from stains of a bluish hue. In texture it very much resembles Parian marble, and appears to be well adapted to purposes of sculpture and ornamental building.

Of the transition class of rocks, those which are well characterised, and belonging to known species, are the following—mica-slate, clay-slate, and greywacke. They, too, are confined to Cerigo, and to the northern side of that island; the hills between Potamo and Caravè are formed of them. Mica-slate is the predominant rock of the two; it is variously modified, and passes, by an almost insensible gradation, into clay-slate. The stratification is distinct; the strata are generally much inclined, and in some places almost vertical.

Of the class of secondary rocks, the well marked

species are very few. They are principally mountain limestone, calcareous slate, and conglomerate.

The mountain limestone abounds in Corfu, Cephalonia, Zante, and Ithaca, and in the smaller adjoining islands and islets. It constitutes very generally the mountainous and higher hilly regions. It is commonly of a light fawn colour, occasionally gray, passing into black, and, by calcination, is rendered white. Its colour, I believe, is principally owing to the presence of bituminous matter. In the gray varieties this is manifest, both from the action of fire and of acids; and that the light fawn-coloured owe their hue to the same cause may be inferred from the circumstance that, when heated, the stone first becomes gray; and when acted on by an acid (by muriatic, for instance), the carbonic acid disengaged has a distinct bituminous odour. It very commonly contains a little magnesia, and also a little silica. In some places, especially in Santa Maura, the magnesia is in such proportions as to alter the character of the rock, so that it may be called magnesian limestone. In one situation (the hill of Aito, in Ithaca) quartz occurs in it, in the form of vitreous granules; spots of clay are found in the same rock, with occasional impressions of shells. The stratification of this limestone is very various; sometimes distinct, at other times confused. The former is most common; the latter is most strikingly seen in the higher mountains of Cephalonia. The strata vary greatly in thickness, and also in inclination. In some places they are nearly vertical; in others not far removed from the horizontal. In the higher mountains they are most thrown out of the horizontal line; and commonly in these situations, too, they are most massive; occasionally they are tortuous.

This limestone in many places contains, dispersed through it, silicious nodules and layers, not unlike flint. And sometimes it alternates with layers of silicious stone, according in character with the petrosilex of the older mineralogists. More rarely, slate-clay is intermixed, alternating with calcareous and silicious layers. Organic remains in this limestone are of comparatively rare occurrence. In Santa Maura specimens of a species of asterias of very large size are occasionally found in the central hills of that island; also coral in masses. And I may mention a very remarkable fossil which I observed in the same island, lying on the surface in the neighbourhood of the limestone formation; it was a fragment of a cornu ammonis of great size, the mineralizing matter of which was silex, in the form of quartz, and that pure and colourless, and crystallized. Some of the crystals were at least a quarter of an inch long.

Calcareous slate is comparatively of rare occurrence. In Corfu it is found on the flank of the mountain of St Salvadore, close to the village of Signes. It is in thin strata of a bluish-gray colour, considerably inclined; pretty firm and hard; its cementing principle carbonate of lime. When acted on by an acid, as the cement dissolves, the aluminous residue

falls to powder In Zante another variety of slate
occurs, close to the village of Langadachia, at the foot
of the hills of mountain limestone. It is in very thin
layers, which are readily separated; very soft and
sectile ; of a grayish or brownish white ; harsh to the
feel. One specimen of it which I examined was of
specific gravity 2.13. From the experiments I made
on it, it appeared to be composed of

    45 parts carbonate of lime.
    46 ... silica.
    8.5 ... water.
    ·5 ... carbonate of magnesia, with a slight trace of alu-
             mina, sulphate of lime, and vegetable matter.

    ———
    100.0

The 8.5 per cent. water may be considered as hygrometrical. When immersed in water, this slate rapidly
absorbs it, and as much as 18 per cent.* It resists
the action of fire; and in consequence of this property it is in estimation amongst the natives of
Zante, by whom it is used as a door-stone for their
ovens.

Conglomerate rock is very abundant. It is found
in all the larger islands, and in many of the smaller
ones. It appears commonly skirting the mountain
limestone, and often in strata highly inclined ; or disjointed, in ruins, and of massive thickness. It consists principally of water-worn fragments of limestone

* The specimen, the specific gravity of which was ascertained, after
the trial and after the application of blotting-paper to it, weighed 76
grains ; after exposure to the air about twenty hours, it was reduced
in weight to 62 grains.

cemented by carbonate of lime, and very often contains also pebbles of flint and quartz.

Accumulations of red clay occasionally occur, and, like the conglomerate rock, are found contiguous to the mountain limestone. In two or three parts of Corfu, hillocks are formed of it, and these not of very limited extent. It is destitute of calcareous earth ; consists principally of alumine, and silex in a very finely divided state, and is coloured by red oxide of iron. Water-worn pebbles, all of a silicious kind, are found intermixed in it, seeming to point out its origin as the result of some great flood.

The tertiary rocks and deposits are principally different varieties of sandstone, gypsum, and marl.

The marl deposit is the most abundant and important. Extensive districts consist of it in Corfu, Zante, Cephalonia, Ithaca, Santa Maura, and Cerigo. Its colour is various ; gray, greenish, and light fawn colour are its predominant tints. It is composed principally of carbonate of lime, of alumina, and silica, and appears to be coloured by oxide of iron—the gray and greenish by the protoxide, and the fawn-coloured by the peroxide. A specimen from Zante, of a light greenish hue, which I examined, was found to consist of

56 Carbonate of lime, mixed with a little carbonate of magnesia, and a very small proportion of sulphate of soda.
39 Alumine mixed with some silica, a little sulphate of lime, and a minute quantity of protoxide of iron.
5 Hygrometrical water.
___
100

This clay may be considered as a species of marl. It absorbs water readily, and falls to powder in water. When examined by a powerful lens, it is found to be composed of extremely minute particles. It resembles the clay of the marl formations of Sicily and Calabria and other parts of Italy, and also the mud deposit of the Nile* and of some other great rivers. It is plastic; and, after exposure to a red heat, it is no longer liable to disintegrate from the action of water, though it is still permeable to water; in consequence it is well adapted for pottery, especially that kind which is so much in use in hot climates, for holding and cooling water. Exposed to a high temperature, for instance a white heat, it fuses, and gives rise to vesicular scoriæ, very much resembling the scoriæ of Etna and Vesuvius. A specimen of the clay of Zante, already referred to, after having been heated to redness, was of specific gravity 2.48.

As the clay of this formation in different places varies in colour, so I believe it does in some other respects, though not very materially in composition. It occasionally alternates with argillaceous limestone. It is occasionally connected with a kind of shale,

* A specimen of the mud of the Nile, which I have examined, consisted of

82 Impalpable silicious sand and clay.

9 Carbonate of lime.

4.5 Hygrometrical water, expelled at a temperature of 212°.

4.5 Vegetable matter and water expelled and decomposed at a higher temperature.

which occurs in thin layers, and contains a large proportion of carbonate of lime ; and indeed, in many
instances, it appears to pass into this shale by an almost insensible gradation.

In some situations it abounds in organic remains,
as in parts of Cephalonia and Cerigo ; in others, on
the contrary, such remains are very uncommon in it,
as in most parts of the clay formation of Zante and
of Corfu. Shells are found in great plenty in it, in
the two former islands ; impressions of fishes have
also been detected ; but I am not aware that any
bones of reptiles, or of animals of the higher orders,
have as yet been discovered in it.

Gypsum, in all the larger islands, is more or less
associated with the marl ; it commonly presents itself in beds or insulated masses in the clay, or resting
on it. In some places it is granular, in some slaty,
in others foliated and crystalline ; occasionally it is bituminous, or coloured black by carbonaceous inflammable matter. I am not aware that any organic remains have been discovered in it in the Ionian
Islands.

Sandstone is of almost as common occurrence as
marl ; indeed the one rarely appears without the
other. It very generally presents itself above the
marl, or alternating with marl, and most commonly
in horizontal strata. It consists of particles, evidently
water-worn, of limestone and shells, connected and
held together by a cement of carbonate of lime. A
specimen of that kind which is used in building in

Zante was of specific gravity 2.44. Occasionally silicious sand is mixed with the calcareous in its composition. Entire shells are not uncommon in it; in
Cerigo, in many places, they abound, and it occasionally contains lignite, and bears marks of the impressions of vegetables.

Conglomerate often connected with and passing
into sandstone occurs of various composition; its
cementing principle is always carbonate of lime;
limestone-pebbles, and pebbles of quartz and of
flint are its most common ingredients. Occasionally,
a conglomerate breccia is met with, the constituent
parts of which are black fétid limestone and flint in
angular fragments.

Two other conglomerates require to be mentioned.
One a bone-breccia; the other, at this very time in
the act of forming, being composed of the pebbles of
the sea-shore, cemented by carbonate of lime, deposited from the sea. The finest example of the latter
rock is at Santa Maura, on the shore, close to the
fort, where the waves break with great violence,
where the water is very pure, and the pebbles, by
continued attrition, are finely polished, and reduced
to a small size, commonly not exceeding sugar-plums.
I mention these circumstances, because I believe they
are connected in the relation of cause and effect. The
violent agitation of the water promotes the disengagement of carbonic acid gas, by which the carbonate
of lime in the water is dissolved, and consequently
the precipitation of the carbonate, which readily

adheres to the smooth surface of the pebbles, and, in adhering, cements them together. From the observations which I made when on the spot, I have been led to the conclusion that the cementing process goes on, not at the surface, but some inches below, where the precipitated carbonate of lime can rest undisturbed, defended by the superjacent gravel.

The bone-breccia is confined to the Island of Cerigo, where it has been discovered in three different places, viz. at Turko-vromi, in a cliff not far from the convent of Myrtea, and at Phoradomandra, near Vrulèa. Till very lately Turko-vromi only was known as the site of this curious rock. The second site was discovered a short time before I visited the island in the summer of 1827 ; and the third came to the knowledge of the resident, Captain (now Major) M'Phail, whilst I was there. With him I had the pleasure of visiting it, and I shall describe it, for it is the finest example of all.

The very spot where the breccia is, is known by the name of Bucolea. It is a small cavern, a few miles to the east of Kapsali, close to the sea, amongst rugged naked rocks of black limestone. The principal mass of breccia, which is exposed in the perpendicular side of the cavern, consists besides bones, of black and red limestone ; the latter of which appears to have acted the part of a cement. The mass is quite irregular in form and situation, as if it had been introduced in the state of a paste, into the crevices and fissures of the rock; where it is thickest, it may be about two feet thick. Black limestone, which burns white, lies over it, and in one place a layer of stalactitical limestone, and under it a conglomerate of limestone pebbles. This is succeeded by a smaller mass or layer of bone-breccia, and that by black limestone.—The stalactitical limestone in many places comes in contact with the breccia, and in one spot the limestone conglomerate does the same. It may be deserving of remark, that a pebble of limestone, evidently water-worn, was found included in a small portion of the bone-breccia, lying between two surfaces, or in a fissure, of the black limestone.

The character of the bone-breccia at this place, and also of that of Turko-vromi, is precisely the same, and the bones are very similar. They are principally jaw-bones, and the cylindrical bones of the extremities, and, judging from the teeth, of a ruminant animal,* probably the bullock. They are generally very much broken, so that it is difficult to find one complete. They exhibit no marks of attrition from water, and no mark of the action of fire. At Bucolea, I saw one or two teeth, which very closely resembled horses' teeth. The only other animal of which I found a

* The following are the dimensions of three teeth, the sides of which were well exposed, in the most perfect jaw that I ever saw taken from this breccia:—The *corona* of the anterior was .6$\frac{1}{10}$th of an inch long, that of the next .8$\frac{1}{10}$th, that of the last about the same; they are about the .4 of an inch above the jaw, and their fangs are fixed in the jaw. If these teeth were of a bullock, as I have conjectured, they belonged to a very young animal,—which the sharpness of the edge of the crown would seem also to indicate.

bone (and it was a solitary one), was of a bird, and it also was a long cylindrical bone.*

The fragments of the bones were all very similar in their characters. They are commonly yellowish white or grayish, and brittle, though not very easily broken. Before the blow-pipe, the remains of a very little animal matter is indicated, by the smell just perceptible, and by the slight grayish tinge produced; in muriatic acid, they effervesce pretty strongly, and dissolve entirely. The solution is very copiously precipitated by aqua ammoniæ, and by carbonate of ammonia, indicating the presence of phosphate of lime as the chief ingredient, and of carbonate of lime in a larger proportion than in recent bone. Some of the cylindrical bones have their cavities lined with crystalline calc-spar, and one that I examined had its cavity filled with the cementing red limestone.

I have compared specimens of this breccia with specimens of the bone-breccia of Ossola in the Adriatic, and of the rock of Gibraltar;—and they have appeared so very similar, that I should have supposed, had I not known the contrary, that they were all from the same spot.—This I mention with the belief that their history is the same,—that they are all involved in the same problem. What the solution of this pro-

* The late Mr Robert Jameson, whose untimely loss science has to deplore, in an interesting paper on Cerigo, published in the Edinburgh New Philosophical Journal, the number for October 1836, states that he observed in the bone-breccia " teeth and bones of oxen, deer, sheep, or goats, and birds ; also several bones, belonging apparently to the rodentia, but none of the order carnivora."

blem is, is yet doubtful ; the discussion of the question
I shall avoid. I may remark, however, that the two
situations in which I examined the bone-breccia in
Cerigo, seem incompatible with its having been
formed posterior to some great catastrophe, which
may have materially altered the face of the land, and
reduced it to its present form.—And the situation at
Gibraltar, where the same kind of breccia has been
found,—in a cave in the perpendicular side of the rock,
—at a great height above the sea, now approachable
only by means of ropes, supports the same opinion.*
Farther, I would remark, that the destruction of the
animal, or albuminous part of the bone, would seem
to indicate that the fragments of bone had been exposed to the decomposing influence of the atmosphere,
before they were included in the rock in which they
now occur; in such situations, for instance, as have
lately been discovered in the Morea ;—under-ground
passages through limestone rocks, communicating
with caverns in the rock, in which bones might be
washed and retained, and where, in long process of
time,—from slow deposition from the passing water,
the caverns might be filled up, and the breccia in
question formed.†

---

* Of this situation I was informed when at Gibraltar, and I was
shown specimens of the breccia in which are included the fragments
of bones decidedly of the larger mammalia.

† I have examined some fragments of bones not included in breccia, sent to the museum at Fort Pitt by the late Mr Robert Jameson,
found by him in a cavern in Cerigo, called the Cave of Nissachia.

On the comparative ages of the different rocks and deposits noticed, I shall not offer any remarks. To do the subject justice would require elaborate research, a copious collection of organic remains, and a careful study and determination of their species. The terms I have used, of primitive, secondary, and tertiary, I beg to observe, I have employed chiefly for convenience, with the belief that they are tolerably accurate, not with the idea that they are strictly so.

As regards external character, and the character which is imparted to the scenery, each kind of rock and deposit is well marked and distinct.

The tracts consisting principally of the mountain limestone, are commonly very rugged and barren, especially when the strata are highly inclined. According to the degree of inclination of the strata, the hills and mountains are either rounded and tame, which they most frequently are, or bold and cragged. The vallies amongst the hills of this limestone, are very often without outlets, closed more or less on all sides—complete basin-like hollows.

Where conglomerate is the prevailing rock,—skirting on the mountain limestone and adjoining, commonly rising above the marl district,—the scenery is generally wild and picturesque; the forms of rock are bold and diversified, often in a remarkable manner, embellished and heightened by luxuriant vegetation,

They were more brittle than the breccia-bone, and friable and soft, from being less impregnated with carbonate of lime ; the whole of their animal matter is decomposed.

common in such situations, even without the aid of cultivation.

The marl districts are very peculiar in their character.—When very unequal in surface, and hilly, they are, as it were, alpine regions in miniature, reminding one of a plan of Switzerland modelled in clay; and affording a striking illustration of the operations of water in giving form to the yielding materials, and producing every variety of feature which is witnessed in an alpine country. A very striking example of this occurs in Cephalonia, in the neighbourhood of Lixuri, where the clay hills, to a considerable extent, are uncultivated and naked, and indeed totally destitute of vegetation, presenting one of the most curious and extraordinary scenes imaginable. When, on the contrary, they are low, their character is chiefly dependent on their condition, as regards cultivation ; if neglected, their aspect is miserable,—a boggy morass, or a parched up, arid, fissured level; if reclaimed and subjected to careful culture, their aspect is in accordance, and in a very high degree pleasing.

The Ionian Islands are distinguished for beauty of scenery : no parts of the south of Europe in this respect surpass them, at least in their finest parts. Their beauty they owe partly to the great variety of ground;—partly to luxuriant vegetation;—partly to the boundary mountains and distant views,—and partly to the sea and sky ;—each, when seen at a favourable moment, admirable of its kind : The vegetation, the olive, the cypress, and the pine (I allude to the most striking scenes I have in recollection); with under-wood of myrtle, arbutus, and mastick, not to men-tion the orange groves and vineyards:—The mountains of continental Greece,—their summits great part of the year covered with snow, and in the morning and evening reflecting the glorious tints of the rising and setting sun:—The sea, that of the Mediterranean in perfection,—undefiled during the fine season by any turbid streams,—clear as crystal, and of the most per-fect blue,—rivalling the sky in its colour and purity.

I shall now notice some of the peculiarities in the geology of the Ionian Islands, which, whilst they are not without interest in themselves, may aid in illus-tration of the subject.

Caverns, in these islands, are principally confined to the limestone formation. In the limestone they are of pretty common occurrence; many of them are of large dimensions, and some of them are of curious forms, and picturesque appearance.—The most con-siderable occur in Cerigo, Cephalonia, Paxo, and Fanno. I shall mention some of them:

In Cerigo there are two of great size; one in the sea-cliff at the termination of the wild, and in some places beautiful, glen of Milopotamo, deriving its name from the stream which flows through it, and to mills which the stream works;* the other, known by

---

* The most picturesque part of this glen exhibits extraordinary luxuriancy of vegetation, depending on the perennial supply of water. The platanus, the chestnut, the myrtle, the tutsan, &c. overshadow

the name of the cavern of Sta Sophia, from a small chapel at its mouth, dedicated to this saint, and situated in the glen of the same name, about an hour and half's ride from Kapsali. The former cavern is said (for I did not visit it) to be three miles in length, but low, so that it is necessary to creep in many places on hands and knees to explore it, and winding and intricate in its passages. The latter, that of Sta Sophia, is a very remarkable one, and possesses singular beauty, which it chiefly owes to the enormous stalactites and stalagmites in which it abounds, formed of a cream-coloured marble, descending from the roof, and ascending from the floor,—some resembling columns, others altars, others buildings in ruins, and many resembling animals; the mimic forms, in brief, are of all kinds, and of the most fantastic shapes. I saw this cavern to great advantage, when it was illuminated in a rude manner, on the occasion of the Lord High Commissioner, Sir Frederick Adam, paying it a visit. The lurid light of the fires of brushwood kindled here and there, the volumes of smoke, the wild action and appearance of the natives, running to and fro with their fire-brands, added much to the picturesque effect. Considering the vast size of some of the stalactitical columns, many feet in circumference, and their highly crystalline prismatic structure, like

the stream, and indeed the glen, forming a dense shade and a cool retreat, very delightful in the sultry days of summer. The small stream is conducted by an artificial channel, and in a short space turns twenty-five little mills for grinding corn, of a very primitive and simple structure.

those of Antinaxos as described by Dr Clark,—one cannot reflect on their formation without a feeling of marvel, as regards the length of time their growth must have required, especially as there is only an inconsiderable dropping of water from the roof. The approach to this cave is hardly less remarkable than the cavern itself, and is worthy of the attention of the traveller. It is a glen of savage wildness, without any traces of culture, and only the slightest of vegetation; a chasm, between two rugged heights, of black limestone, perhaps 600 feet high.

In Cephalonia the number of caverns is small. The largest and the most remarkable one is that of Dracondispilo, in a perpendicular face of a lofty sea-cliff near the monastery of Taffeo, about three hours,[*] or ten miles from Lixuri. I had the pleasure of visiting it in company with Captain (now Lieutenant-Colonel) Ross. We were provided with wax tapers from the monastery, having been informed that the cave is of vast dimensions, but we found them unnecessary, the light of day penetrating to every part of it. Its height at the mouth was about thirty feet, its width as much, and its depth, perhaps, forty or fifty. The cliff and the walls of the cavern were of a light fawn-coloured limestone, the strata of which were much inclined. On entering the cavern one circumstance particularly struck me, which was its apparently high

* In the Ionian Islands, as in the south of Europe generally, distances are reckoned by time—the ordinary time required, travelling on the animals of the country, commonly mules.

temperature; it felt almost like an oven, it was so oppressively hot. This, perhaps, might have been in part fallacious, the external air being cold, for it was in the month of January, and the wind northerly and keen. I regret that we had not a thermometer to ascertain the actual temperature ; making due allowance, however, for being suddenly heated by the exertion of climbing, after a cold ride, and being suddenly immersed in a close atmosphere, I am of opinion that the temperature could not have been less than 70°. This high degree was perhaps partly, and chiefly, owing to the situation being sheltered from the north and exposed to the south, and partly to its being a place of shelter for large flocks of goats which take refuge in it in bad weather. Perhaps I dwell unnecessarily on this circumstance, but it has appeared to me not undeserving of attention in connexion with the temperature of springs, some of which may owe their excess of temperature, over the mean annual one of the spot, to some such local causes affecting the water that feeds them.*

The repute of the cavern of Dracondispilo amongst the natives of Cephalonia, as a natural curiosity, is overrated, on account, perhaps, of the difficulty and danger of approaching it; at least our expectations

---

* Since writing the above, I find that Mr Robert Jameson, in the paper on Cerigo already referred to, notices the temperature of the cave of Sᵗᵃ Sophia; when the open air was only 50°, he found it 70°, which he considers as about 5° above the mean annual temperature. I may add, that in this cave he found some bone-breccia.

of its wonders having been raised, we were disappointed on entering it. The dimensions I have noticed are very limited; the only feature belonging to it in anywise remarkable was a large stalactite that extended from the roof to the floor, perhaps ten feet in circumference, of an irregular columnar form.

Paxo, more than any other of the Ionian Islands, is distinguished for its caverns. All the caverns of note are on the west and south-west coast, and situated in the very lofty and perpendicular cliffs which form that coast; and, in consequence, they can only be approached by sea, and entered and explored in fine weather; indeed the calmest weather is desirable to visit them with satisfaction and pleasure. Such weather fortunately prevailed on the day I visited them, in company with Colonel Burrell, the then resident of Paxo, and the late Lieutenant-Colonel Harper of the Royal Engineers. It was on the 28th of August that we embarked at Gaja, the little capital of Paxo, in the resident's boat, with the double intent of going round the island and examining both its coast and its caverns.

The first cavern we visited was that of Grammattico, so called from the nearest village being of that name. This the favourable state of sky and sea permitted us to enter, though there was too much swell to allow of our reaching its extremity. It is considered one of the largest of the caverns of Paxo; I would say it is the largest, and, in all its circumstances, the finest. It is about 100 feet high at its mouth, the cliff being about triple that height; it is nearly as wide as it is high at its entrance, which capacious dimensions it retains some distance inward, and it may be between 300 and 400 feet deep. When we were about half way within, the view outward was very peculiar, and not without grandeur and a certain beauty, produced by a combination of circumstances, such as the great arched lofty roof, the vast perpendicular walls, the deep and transparent blue water beneath heaving up and down, the gigantic cliff skirting it on the outside, almost shutting out the sea and sky, the beautiful and vivid tints of the rock; the extraordinary play of light on the roof, and that clear-obscure which belongs to deep shade in a clear atmosphere under a bright sun.

The rock in which this cave is situated is in a stratum of limestone of extraordinary thickness, and rather of a loose texture, containing large nodules of flint, some of them of a fine bluish hue like chalcedony. The predominant colour is light brownish yellow. The varied and bright tints which had such a fine effect to the eye, were owing to vegetation partly, and partly to mineral incrustation. Where the sea reached or washed against the rock, the surface was purple from sea-weed and coral adhering. Above the reach of the wave, but where most exposed to the spray, a white polished surface was here and there conspicuous, like enamel, as if the effect of vitrification. A green tint was very generally diffused, imparted by some minute lichen or mucor; and was richly blended with bright green, dense black, and bright red and yellow. The bright green was produced by that elegant plant, Venus' hair, hanging in delicate fringes, growing in crevices where there was an exudation of fresh water; the dense black, by what may have been asphaltum, or perhaps a mucòr in a state of decomposition; and the bright red and yellow, by stains of the peroxide of iron.

The next cave we explored was one not very far distant,—one of many in a capacious cove, and the most considerable of them. From its conformation it might be called the Triple Cavern, there being three compartments, as it were, communicating. The largest, which we first entered, was but little inferior in magnitude and beauty to that already described. From it we passed into an intermediate cavern with which it was connected, having a circular aperture above, completely open to the sky, at the height of about two hundred feet, like an enormous telescope. This communicated with a third cavern, but the passage of communication was so low, and the cavern itself apparently so little inviting, that we did not think it worth while to explore it. From the comparative shallowness of the water underneath the circular opening in the roof of the middle cave, not exceeding twelve feet in depth, it may be inferred that the aperture was occasioned by the falling in of part of the superincumbent stratum.*

Near the Triple Cave is one which the resident

* This is an occurrence not uncommon in a limestone country. A

said he was wont to call Merlin's Cave, from a pecu- liar circumstance he witnessed there, not unlike a magical effect—it was a pigeon with outstretched wings, invisibly suspended at the mouth of the cavern. The bird was dead, but the minutest inspection could not detect the cause of its suspension. It was probably entangled in a spider's web, which, in the Ionian Islands, is often formed of very strong mate- rials, some of the cords being occasionally equal to fine silk thread in strength and thickness. This ca- vern we found comparatively small; it did not exceed fifty feet in height, and was not deep, but it was beautiful in its form, and elegantly arched, giving the idea of an artificial grotto; its lower part was lined with conglomerate rock, in grotesque masses, and ornamented with stalactites.

Of the many other caverns on this shore I shall make mention of only one more, the name of which, if it have one, I could not learn. Its relative situation is well marked by a very fine pyramidal rock, insulated in

very remarkable instance of it occurred about twenty-six years ago, on the mainland adjoining to Paxo, from whence the hollow formed in the side of the mountain is visible, and which I saw very distinctly, on account of its great magnitude, though perhaps five-and-twenty or thirty miles distant. It is situated in the side of a mountain, in the neighbourhood of Souli; its area is of many acres, and its depth has never been ascertained. According to Colonel Burrell, who informed me about it, and who collected his information from the Souliots them- selves, this great pit was of sudden formation; in the evening the de- clivity of the mountain was unbroken; in the morning the shepherds discovered this immense hollow. No earthquake had been felt during the night, and no noise heard.

the sea, just opposite to it, nearly two hundred feet high, and which is so near the cave that its shadow at noon almost reached it. In dimensions this cavern, too, was little inferior to that of Grammattico ; and the view from the interior of it, which we entered, was very striking; indeed it was extraordinary, owing to the pyramidal rock standing before it, hiding almost entirely the sea and sky, though not intercepting the light, and producing, by its break-water effect, a mirror-like smoothness of the water.

To the traveller interested in bold and picturesque scenery an excursion to the caverns of Paxo may be safely recommended. No cliff scenery in the Ionian Islands is more deserving of being seen,—none will probably afford greater gratification,—none is more easily and securely visited. The Island of Paxo being only about twenty-one miles in circumference, in one day it may be easily circumnavigated. In fine weather it is delightful rowing along shore under the great limestone cliffs, in deep blue water, owing to its depth and purity, almost like that of the ocean. And, besides the caverns, many other objects and peculiarities occur, well adapted to invite curiosity and afford amusement, especially the singular forms of rocks, many of them resembling architectural effects, and the very varied aspect of the cliffs, and the variety of the country here and there, and villages seen through the narrow gulleys and chasms opening on the sea. And, should the season of the year be spring, the traveller may have an opportunity of witnessing a singular species of angling, in which, I was informed, the natives indulge from the lofty cliffs, not in the sea beneath for fish, but in the air for birds—swallows—which then crowd about the cliffs, and which they catch with a fly, attached to a fine hook and line, thrown and managed very much in the same manner as in common fly-fishing.

In the little island of Fanno there is one cave of considerable magnitude, called by the natives " The Cave," and which, by the French, when they had possession of Corfu and its dependency Fanno, was named the Cave of Calypso. It is at the western end of the islet, on the shore, in the limestone cliff under the lofty hill Meraviglia. It is about three hundred feet deep, one hundred feet wide, and between twenty and thirty feet high. By land it is very difficult of approach, and also by sea, excepting in the finest weather ; and, in consequence, it has always been a favourite resort of robbers and pirates, for which, indeed, it is much better adapted than for the abode of a goddess. Of irregular form, and of savage appearance, its floor is the sea-beach, and, though dry in fine weather, in a storm it must be washed by the waves.

Another peculiarity is that already alluded to, the basin-like hollows or valleys without any apparent outlet, which belong chiefly to the limestone formation. Some of the principal of them I shall notice briefly.

In Cerigo there is only one of these valleys with

which I am acquainted.   It is amongst the hills of
gray limestone near the convent of Myrtea, and is
about a mile in circumference.

In the large Island of Cephalonia, too, there is only
one of any note.   It is the valley of San Jerasimo,
in which stands the convent of the same name.

In the Island of Zante there are several.   The following villages mark the site and number of the
principal ones, viz. Oxocora, Luca, Trapies, Ambelo.
That, in the upper part of which the village of Luca
stands, is about a mile long, and nearly a quarter of
a mile wide, where widest.   The other valleys are
smaller; and, besides those named, there are some
very small ones towards the summits of the mountains.

Santa Maura is more remarkable for these valleys
than any other of the Ionian Islands.   All the valleys
between the village Commiglio and Dragono are of
this description, and also between Dragono and Attanè; and there are two such in the neighbourhood
of Marandicori, and also two, but communicating,
between Alessandro and Vathkirri; and one below
the village of Sfachiotes; all of which are either partially bounded by, or are in the midst of limestone
hills, and all of them of considerable size.   The valley near Attanè is on one side bounded by a limestone
cliff, which is precipitous towards the sea, and scarped
towards the land,—a feature of ground of common
occurrence in these islands.

In Corfu there is only one well-marked hollow

valley with which I am acquainted—that of Stovis-tona, situated at a considerable elevation above the village Prinilla, bounded partly by lofty precipices of limestone, partly by conglomerate, and partly by hills of marl and freestone.

In the little Island of Fanno, also, there is one ; it is called Daphnè, from the village of that name, situated in it ; and it is an excellent example of the kind, —its limestone barriers on all sides completely shutting it in, and secluding it.

These valleys differ in their forms, which are very irregular ; some of them approach the circular in form ; but they do not convey the idea that they owe their origin to volcanic eruption. In their character they are very similar ; in all of them there is an alluvial deposit, which commonly consists of red clay, in most instances, without calcareous matter ;* all of them are, more or less, flooded in winter, when, in fact, they are shallow lakes, and all of them are dry in summer. These circumstances render them well adapted for cultivation ; and they are accordingly all cultivated ; and they are valuable to the inhabitants on account of the water which they collect. In some of them pits have been sunk, in which water is preserved during the whole of the dry season ; thus in that near Oxocora, in Zante, there are sixty cisterns ;

---

* The clay of Stovistona is the only exception I know of: it is brown, and effervesces with an acid, perhaps from some of the alluvium being derived from the marl hill adjoining.

in that of Luca fifty-five; and in that of Trapies several. What the depth of the clay deposit is I could not ascertain. The cisterns of Luca are from fifteen to twenty feet deep; and the limestone rock below has not been reached. As the water in them is retained by the clay, and they are apparently dried only by evaporation (so that in a more humid climate they would be perpetually lakes), it might be expected that their bottoms would be encrusted with saline matter. This, however, is not the case, which would seem to indicate that they are not of very great antiquity. However, this argument of the absence of saline matter is deprived of some of its force by the circumstance that the cisterns are commonly emptied for use every year before the commencement of the rainy season. This might prevent any notable accumulation of saline matter; yet, even with the aid of the effect of cultivation, it seems insufficient to account for there being no slight incrustation on the surface.

These valleys form very remarkable features in the scenery. Whether under water, or covered with Indian corn or wheat, the crops for which they are best adapted, they are very peculiar and pleasing, contrasted with the rugged and naked heights by which, excepting in Santa Maura, they are commonly surrounded. And when their declivities are cultivated and planted, as is the case in a few instances, they constitute scenes of great beauty and interest in their seclusion, like oases in a rocky desert. Daphnè, in

the Island of Fanno, is a happy example of this; and
the picturesque village in the side of the valley, and
scattered farm-houses, with their small olive groves
and patches of fruit trees, and sprinkling of the beautiful shrubbery of the country, heightens very much
the pleasing effect. That of Myrtea, in the Island
of Cerigo, is another striking example; but the impression which it makes is chiefly owing to contrast, the surrounding country being of the wildest
and most rugged kind—a bare surface, a desert of
rock. Another striking example is the valley of San
Jerasimo, in Cephalonia, one of the largest of these
valleys, its level or plain part being between two and
three miles in circumference, and well cultivated,
partly in currant plantations, and partly in grain—the
whole the property of the monastery of San Jerasimo, which stands in the middle of the plain, and is
the largest and richest in the Ionian Islands. As you
descend to this valley from Argostoli, by the new
road, its appearance is very beautiful;—from the regular cultivation; from numerous cypress trees, intermixed with olive trees, particularly in the narrow
approach from the northward; from the villages
scattered on the declivities of the hills; from the
striking appearance of the convent, standing alone
on a fertile plain, on every side shut in by hills, and
by the huge Black Mountain above all, its main
barrier, partially covered with dark pines;* its summit

---

* It is said that the whole of the forest of the Black Mountain was

and side white with snow, as it was in the month of February, the time of my visit.

Deep depressions, cavities, and perforations in the rocks, may be deserving of being noticed amongst the peculiarities of the Ionian Islands. They are not uncommon; but few of them are sufficiently remarkable to require a particular description: one only I shall notice specially. It is a natural excavation, near the monastery of Sta Andrea, in Cephalonia, a few miles from Argostoli, towards San Georgio. It is situated in the side of a hill, composed of white calcareous rock, very similar to chalk. Its mouth is about 100 feet in circumference; its bottom 200 or 300 feet; its walls shelving rapidly inwards, and very much overhanging; its depth about fifteen or twenty feet. I visited it, with a friend, who, by means of a rope, descended into it, and explored it. He found nothing deserving of notice, excepting numerous bones, and entire skeletons of animals, dogs,

destroyed by fire just before the Ionian Islands came under the protection of the British Government. This is not quite correct; parts of it escaped; the destruction of wood, however, was enormous; the heat from the conflagration is reported to have been so great, that while it lasted, the adjoining valleys were almost uninhabitable. The fire was kindled intentionally by the peasantry during a period of anarchy, for the purpose of clearing the ground for the cultivation of grain. Wheat sown in the spring following the summer of the conflagration, I was assured, yielded sixty-fold. The destruction of so much forest is believed to have had an injurious effect on the climate: the snows now disappear in May; before they remained on the mountain till August and September; the summers are considered hotter, the winters colder; and malaria more active.

PLATE I.

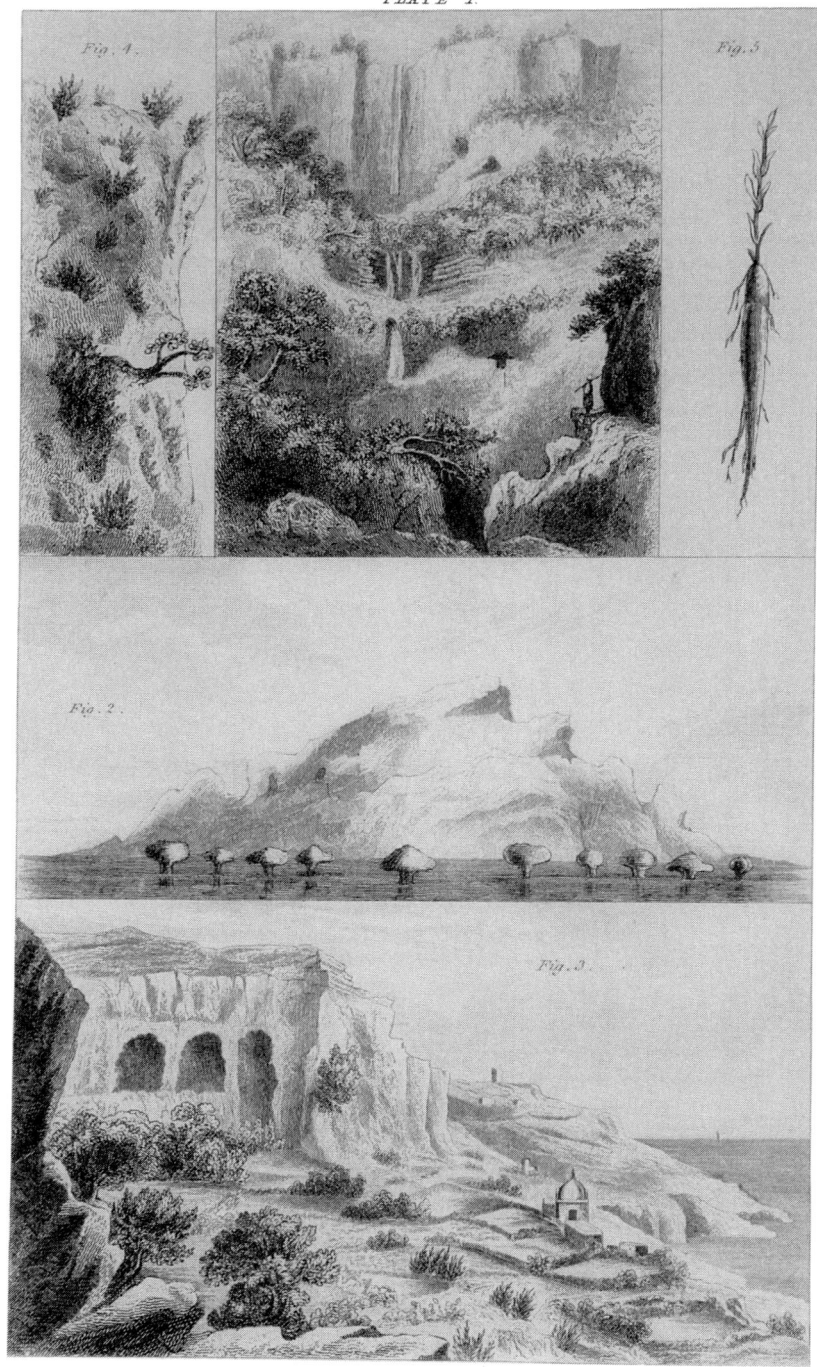

Fig. 4.   *Fig. 5.*

Fig. 2.

Fig. 3.

FOUNTAIN OF ARETHUSA, ITHACA; — ISLET OF DRAKEA, OFF THE COAST OF CORFU:
SAN GEORGIO, MALTA.

goats, and mules, and many of them in the innermost part of the cavity. The probability is, that they fell in, when grazing or prowling about by night, and being unable to get out, died there. Search was made, but in vain, for the bones of other animals; no diluvian remains could be detected. A priest who accompanied us, declared that there is an underground communication between this pit and the castle of San Georgio, on the hill above, and distant more than a mile; but this was not confirmed by examination; no passage could be found leading from it.

I shall now pass on to peculiarities of stratification. It may suffice to notice a few instances; were all described, even those only which I witnessed, they would fill a volume.

In Ithaca are some very interesting examples; one of them is the inland cliff, where there is a spring, called by the natives Parapapigadi, and which modern travellers have been pleased to name the fountain of Arethusa. The upper part of the mural precipice, which is perpendicular, and in part overhanging, shows no stratification; it is a mass of limestone about fifty feet thick. Below this, the cliff consists of layers of limestone, flint, and slate-clay, of from one to two or three inches thick, somewhat inclined.* Another instance occurs in the cliff of Port Skino, a small part of the great outer harbour of Vathi. There, in a height of between 80 and 100 feet, there may be between three or four hundred different strata of lime-

* Plate i. fig. 1.

stone and flint, both exceedingly various in appearance and thickness. In some parts of the cliff, the calcareous layers are most abundant; in some the silicious. In one or two places the former approaches to freestone. In some of the calcareous layers, the flint occurs in nodules. The strata, both calcareous and silicious, vary from half an inch in thickness to two or three feet; they are considerably inclined. The shore is difficult of approach by land; by water it is of easy access, and is best seen; and the traveller will be amply repaid in visiting it, rowing or sailing thence from Vathi, by the impressive nature and beauty of the surrounding scenery.

In the bold south-west coast of Corfu, there are excellent examples of marl, and its associated strata, as near Cape Sidari, and in the adjoining headland of Point Strachieri. There the cliff is nearly 100 feet high; its strata horizontal, dipping to the east-north-east, at different angles, in different places, consisting besides of marl containing shells and flint-pebbles, of layers of lignite, from an inch to a line in thickness, of argillaceous limestone and coarse loose sandstone in which lignite is included.

In the cliff of Crionero, in the Island of Zante, and close to the town of Zante, is a striking instance of variety of strata, of marl, sand, and sandstone, nearly horizontal (the two latter chiefly calcareous), topped by a layer of silicious sand and pebbles.

In the ravine, descending to Scala from Racli, in Cephalonia, the precipice is formed of limestone, conglomerate, and marl. The limestone, a thick stratum, is above the conglomerate, the conglomerate lies over the marl, and the marl is intersected by, or contains highly inclined layers of sandstone. In the populous, highly cultivated, and picturesque district of Levato, in Cephalonia, marl and sandstone are generally associated in strata, nearly horizontal. At the beautiful village of Metaxata, in this district, where Lord Byron resided, there is a good example, exposed to view, of the arrangement;—a stratum of marl appears there, between two strata of calcareous sandstone, which are connected by numerous stalactites, penetrating the marl in a very curious manner. It is worthy of note, that basin-like hollows, of very small dimensions, occur in this district, which, like the larger valleys, before alluded to, are covered with water in the rainy season; they are commonly planted with the currant-vine, which is benefited by winter irrigation.

Mount Scopo in the Island of Zante, the *mons nobilis* of Pliny,—a mountain 1509 feet high,* is in many respects peculiar, both in composition and in its stratification. The general appearance which it exhibits, gives the idea that it is but of very recent formation, and raised by volcanic or some analogous force. Where its strata are distinct, they are highly inclined; whilst those at some little distance, as the

* This is from the admeasurement of Commander Slater, R.N. The convent on this hill, according to him, is 1433 feet above the level of the sea.

clay, and marl, and freestone of Vasilico, like those of Crionero, are horizontal, or nearly so. It consists principally of sandstone, conglomerate, black limestone, and gypsum. Sandstone, containing a notable proportion of clay, and differing but little from marl, prevails on one side at its base ;—sandstone, coarse conglomerate, and gypsum in successive strata on the other ;—conglomerate, composed chiefly of dark gray limestone in angular masses, not apparently water-worn, cemented by whitish carbonate of lime, rises above the preceding ;—and above that, sandstone, and marl, and conglomerate, with masses of black limestone,* and beds of gypsum of the hydrous kind, some foliated and some granular ; and, above all, conglomerate, forming the summit of the mountain. This conglomerate is of small extent; it is confined to the hummock-like termination of Scopo, and consists of pebbles, of flint, of whitish limestone, and of crystalline marble ; the limestone pebbles rounded as if water-worn, the flint more frequently in sharp angular fragments. Where this rock is freely exposed to the influence of rain, its surface is rough, and studded with projecting fragments of flint ; it is worthy of remark, however, that none of these fragments project very much ; and farther, that there is little or no detritus of flint at its foot. These are circumstances which suggest the idea that the mountain is of recent origin ;

* This limestone contains some sulphur and carbon, and perhaps bitumen.

whilst the stratification, either confused or perpendicular, favours the opinion that it owes its origin to elevation from below. And a small basin-like hollow between its double summit, on the margin of which the convent of Scopo stands, may be adduced in support of its origin having been volcanic. Still, however, the indications are far from conclusive; they appear to me barely to warrant the conjecture that this mountain may have been of volcanic origin, and itself an extinct volcano.

In some parts of the Island of Santa Maura, and these its most beautiful parts, there is an extraordinary variety and intermixture of strata, but without any mark of volcanic eruption or elevation. The country in the neighbourhood of Vathkerri may be brought forward as an example. There, limestone, sandstone, conglomerate, flint, freestone, marl, occur in irregular succession, and of various degrees of thickness,—the strata generally highly inclined, but occasionally curved and undulating.

The vast quantity of marl-deposit in these islands, —the vast quantity of silicious deposit, not to mention the calcareous,—cannot fail to excite astonishment on reflection, considering them as marks of the degradation of more ancient rock-formations. But it is superfluous to dwell on this subject, as in most parts of the globe indications as clear, and of a similar kind, and often on a larger scale, present themselves, demonstrative of the change referred to.

The association of silicious deposits with calca-

reous, which is so common in these islands, might
lead to the conjecture that, under certain circumstances, one earth may act on the other, and that at
a certain temperature a soluble compound of the two
may be formed, which on a reduction of temperature
may undergo decomposition, and that separation and
precipitation in successive layers may be the consequence. And, somewhat in support of this idea,
and seeming to show that the circumstances of their
formation were peculiar and unfavourable to animal
life, it may be stated, that organic remains, if they
occur at all in the associated calcareous and silicious
strata (and I do not recollect having met with them),
are certainly very uncommon.

In connexion with usefulness and the arts, the
geology of these islands must be viewed as a topic of
increasing interest. Hitherto, comparatively, but little
use has been made of the rocks, and clays, and marls.
From the mountain limestone quick-lime is procured
by calcination; it is employed only as a cement; it
has not yet been applied to agriculture.* This limestone has also been used as a building-stone, for which,
in some respects, it is well adapted. Its hardness,
and the consequent difficulty in working it, is some

---

* That of Agala, in Zante, is prized, and may be deserving of mention. The rock is very white, and has the appearance of chalk, from
a white powder of carbonate of lime attached to it. When broken,
it exhibits a slight crystalline texture, and is found to contain impressions of shells, which are commonly confused. Calcined, it is
excellent lime.

objection, owing to which, probably, it is not very generally employed. Antipaxo is the only place where, for architectural purposes, it has been quarried to a considerable extent. The limestone of that island is of admirable quality for great public works; masses of almost any dimensions may be obtained, and though sufficiently hard and compact, it admits of being worked with tolerable ease. Antipaxo chiefly consists of this rock and of conglomerate; its strata vary greatly in thickness; they are commonly horizontal, but occasionally they are curiously tortuous.

Fine freestone is not uncommon in the Ionian Islands; but hitherto it has not been extensively employed. Not far from Lixuri, in Cephalonia, a quarry of it has been opened; and the new market-house, in the town just named, is constructed of it. It very much resembles the Malta stone; is of a fawn colour, soft and easily cut, and almost entirely calcareous. I had in my possession a specimen of it, in which was imbedded the tooth of a squalus. At Zante, specimens of fine freestone were sent to me by Count Paolo Marcati, one from Sosti, the other from Catastari, in that island. The former was of sp. gr. 1.93; the latter, 2.06; they were both calcareous and well fitted for building, especially such works as require strength and lightness combined; they are particularly well fitted for the town of Zante, where such qualities, on account of earthquakes, are peculiarly valuable.

The sandstone of the Ionian Islands has been more used in building than any other. Some of its varieties are excellent for the purpose, being light as regards specific gravity, easily quarried and cut, of good colour, and of great durability. Such is the sandstone of which almost the whole of the large town of Zante is built. It is brought from Vasilico, an adjoining promontory, where it occurs in horizontal beds incumbent on marl. It is calcareous, and contains comminuted fragments of shells. Such, also, is the sandstone of Drakea, one of the scattered islets between Corfu and Fanno. Drakea is about half a mile in circumference, and about seventy feet high. It is composed entirely of sandstone and conglomerate, in massive strata * and disjointed masses. Its appearance is very singular; and the singularity is increased by the mushroom-like rocks by which it is surrounded, rising out of the sea,—a form no doubt acquired by the action of the waves, the waste of the insulated rocks being greatest in that part which rises just above the surface of the water.† Many other localities might be pointed out, in the larger islands and also in many of the smaller ones, where good sandstone for building may be procured. I shall notice only one, which is in Cerigo, near San Nicholo, at a spot called Castri. It is a hill of calcareous sandstone, and contains an ancient quarry,

* The strata are twenty or thirty feet thick. The conglomerate is in small quantity, and contains pebbles of flint.

† Plate i. fig. 2.

still exhibiting the manner in which it was worked, —a manner the most precise and economical; for, from the marks remaining, the stone was evidently cut out in square blocks of convenient size; and Major M'Phail, the resident of the island when I visited it in 1827, showed me a chisel of antique bronze which had been found in the quarry, and which had probably been used in working it.

The conglomerate rock is very little used; that of Santa Maura, near the Bassa's fountain, and the site of the ancient city of Ellominos, is employed for mill-stones, which it is said are of good quality. It occurs nearly in vertical strata, and is composed of pebbles of limestone and flint, firmly connected by carbonate of lime; the flint of various colours, the limestone principally black.

The marl and clay are used for making coarse pottery and tiles. The pottery is principally porous water-jars, which are manufactured in large quantities in Zante; and glazed drinking-jugs and plates glazed with litharge; and enormous jars for holding oil. In Paxo, where fresh water is often so scarce that the inhabitants cannot afford to employ it in washing their clothes, and are compelled to substitute sea-water,—they use marl in place of soap.

Although gypsum is very abundant in the Ionian Islands, it has hitherto been scarcely at all employed, either in the fine arts, or in agriculture. The granular variety, constituting alabaster, occurs in large masses in the side of Scopo, and may be deserving of trial for ornamental purposes. Should there be a demand for gypsum, in large quantities, whether for agriculture or the common arts of life, it can be obtained, with the greatest facility, from situations most convenient, close to the sea-shore, in the majority of the larger islands. Near Sinarades, in Corfu, the lofty cliff, in some places, 200 feet high, to the extent of about a quarter of a mile, consists chiefly of this substance. This I mention in proof of its abundance. *

The fine quality of the primitive limestone of Cerigo, and its probable fitness for statuary purposes, has already been alluded to. A specimen of this marble, a large block, which, through the exertions of Major M'Phail, was sent to Corfu, was delivered over for trial to that able native artist, the Cavalier Prossalendi. His opinion of it, at the time, was favourable; but whether he attempted to work it, I have not been informed. Other varieties of limestone in the Ionian Islands are applicable to ornamental purposes, and may be deserving of being called marbles. There are several different kinds in Corfu ; the finest of them are depositions from water, in mode of formation analogous to stalactite. The marble of Spartilla, of this description, is one of much beauty ; its colours are various, chiefly red, brown, and gray, in concentric circles.

* The gypsum in this cliff is partly white and partly black. It is generally of a schistose structure, highly inclined. It is intermixed with swinestone, and a breccia of swinestone and gypsum, and is associated with marl and conglomerate.

The mineralogy of the Ionian Islands is very limited, and the notices of it may be brief.

Of the class of inflammable bodies, the following are the only ones, of the existence of which I was able to satisfy myself, namely, sulphur, asphaltum, lignite, coal, and mellite.

Sulphur I met with only at the base of Mount Scopo in Zante,* in the cliffs of that part of the shore called Vrondonero, opposite the little Island of Peluso ; there I found good specimens of it crystallized, imbedded in gypsum. The place is well marked by its repulsive and dismal appearance, a scene of ruin and sterility, cliffs tumbling down, rocks crumbling away, a scanty vegetation, parched by the sun, totally uncultivated, neglected, and desert. A cavern opens into the cliff close by, and penetrates some way, rapidly ascending. The superstitious natives consider it as an entrance to the infernal regions, and that the souls of the Nobili of the island here commence their journey to the other world. My authority for this scandal was a talkative merry young Greek, one of the crew of the

* Since the above was written, I have been informed that it has been found to occur in Corfu, near St Pantaleone, and I have been favoured with specimens of it, included in rock of a mixed nature, composed of carbonate and of sulphate of lime. In these specimens the mineral was not crystallized ; it was proportionally abundant, and if not very limited in quantity, it is probable it may be extracted with advantage, and may become a profitable article of commerce.

boat, in which I explored, in company with a friend,* this part of the coast.

Asphaltum is yielded in considerable quantity by the pitch springs in Zante, and occurs also as an exudation between the strata of limestone in several places in the cliffs of Antipaxo. It exudes in the liquid state of pitch, and slowly descends, gradually hardening by exposure to the air, until ceasing to flow, it becomes solid and brittle. The dark lines and patches of black pitch and asphaltum on the perpendicular face of the light-coloured rock have a singular appearance. When I come to notice the springs of the Ionian Islands, I shall give such observations as I was able to make on the asphaltum of the pitch springs of Zante.

Lignite is rather of common occurrence. It has been found in Cerigo, in Zante, and in Corfu, either imbedded in insulated masses, or included in layers or seams between sandstone or marl. At Cerigo, I saw a specimen of it, which had been found in the marl, just above Capsali, in sinking a shaft in search of water. Portions of it exhibited the woody texture, other portions of it differed very little from jet. In the same bed of marl, thin strata of sandstone occur, and gypsum. In Zante, I have seen it imbedded in sandstone at the base of Scopo, and pass-

* Mr Charanda of the Commissariat Department, to whose kind attentions, whilst I was quartered in Zante, I was under many obligations, which I have great pleasure in acknowledging.

ing into bituminous coal. In the cliff, opposite to the little Island of Maratonisi, in Kieri Bay, and close to the valley of the pitch spring, lignite is found in thin layers. In the specimens which I collected and examined, the woody texture was distinct; in some even the filaments of the bark retained their natural appearance. The thinness of the lignite gave the idea of great compression. The strata, of which the cliff is composed, are different varieties of calcareous marl, passing into sandstone and freestone, not containing shells.

In Corfu, on the shore close to the city, immediately under the rampart of Fort Raymond, is a layer or seam of coal, nearly a foot thick. It lies between sandstone and a bluish shale, and is considerably inclined. It consists partly of lignite, and partly of bituminous coal, or of lignite approximating to that coal in its character. In a specimen of it, I detected some minute crystals, which had the characteristic properties of mellite. Nowhere besides have I met with this mineral; and nowhere have I found coal so like the bituminous kind. Whether it might be worth while to explore this spot in quest of coal, with the hope of the seam increasing in size and improving in quality below the surface with increasing depth, I have not sufficient practical knowledge of the subject of coal-mining to venture to give an opinion. But the association with lignite is decidedly an unfavourable indication; and the layer being on the sea-shore, almost on a level with the sea, is a very unfavourable circumstance in relation to the working of it.

Of the class of earthy minerals, the species which are distinct are very few indeed, and entirely calcareous and silicious. Calc-spar is of common occurrence, especially in the mountain limestone. Crystals of gypsum are not uncommon. Arragonite is very rare; I met with it only once, and that was at the base of Scopo, in a mass of granular gypsum, accompanied with sulphur, in a low cliff opposite Peluso, and in the vicinity of Vrondonero, a spot already mentioned.

I may here notice a form of carbonate of lime, which is frequently to be seen on the sea-shore,— the nature and origin of which was to me for some time a problem. It is always encrusting, and has a shining enamel-like appearance; is sometimes gray, sometimes almost black, and in form resembling chalcedony. At first, I was disposed to think that its peculiar appearance might be owing to fusion, and that it might be an effect of lightning, striking on the exposed limestone rocks.* But this idea I was

* An appearance of fusion, referred to lightning, has been witnessed by many accurate observers, on rocks on the summits and ridges of mountains. One of the most striking effects of lightning that I have ever heard of, was related to me by the late Mr Allen of Edinburgh; it occurred in the north of England many years ago. A waggon loaded with barrels of iron nails, drawn by six or eight horses (I forget which), was struck by lightning; the drivers (I believe there were two) were killed on the spot and all the horses; the nails were found agglutinated, and, as it were, mineralized. Mr Allen showed

obliged to relinquish, when I found that it was not confined to rocks of this description,—that it occurred on conglomerate, and on the silicious pebbles as well as on the calcareous and cementing carbonate of lime. On the lofty islet of Coraconisi, not far from Porto Timoné, in Corfu, I witnessed what I have just described very distinctly, near the water's edge, on the conglomerate, of which that islet in part consists. The next supposition that I formed was, that it is a deposition, from sea-water conveyed in spray, which I believe is really the case. Its composition agrees with this view, and also with its mechanical structure. It is composed of concentric laminæ, as if so deposited ; and besides carbonate of lime, which is its main ingredient, it contains a little vegetable or animal matter, to which it owes its colour, and a trace of silicious earth. And, farther, in accordance with this idea of its formation, I may mention, that I have never met with it in situations not exposed to the spray of the sea, and that it occurs most abundantly on rugged rocks and exposed situations, where the water is most liable to be broken

me a specimen of some agglutinated masses, and gave me a portion of it, which is still in my possession. The nails are adhering together, and their forms are changed, more or less, evidently the effect of fusion. Their surface in many places is studded with minute crystals of black oxide of iron, and covered generally with a crystalline crust of this oxide. It is also partially encrusted with a light greenish crystalline earthy matter, chiefly silicious. The minute details of the accident were not known. Probably there was a succession of flashes, and the iron was exposed to the action of the lightning, after coming in contact with the silicious matter of the road.

into spray The agitation of the water must promote the escape of the carbonic acid, by means of which the carbonate of lime in sea-water is dissolved; and the warmth of the rocks acted on by the sun must conduce to the same effect.

Of the silicious minerals, chalcedony and quartz are the only two well characterised, and these are not common. In the Island of Fanno, between Ano and Castri, where marl predominates, there chalcedony is pretty abundant in freestone, which occurs in layers in the marl. Chalcedony also is found in Zante, between the villages Langadachia and Galaro, at the foot of the limestone hills, in veins or layers in the schistose rock, already noticed. Some specimens have the appearance of the common opal, and some exhibit the tints of the precious. Some are strongly absorbent of water, and when plunged into it make a hissing noise; and from being nearly opaque and of a bluish hue, which they are when dry, become, when saturated with water, colourless, and semi-transparent. In consequence of this avidity for water, they adhere firmly when applied to the moist surface of the lip or tongue. In the same veins minute crystals of quartz occur. Crystals of this mineral are occasionally found in cavities of flint, and of the silicious pebbles of which there is a great variety,—some approaching to agate, some to jasper and chalcedony, some to jade,—many of them not without beauty, and not unfitted for ring and seal stones.

Of the class of very compounded minerals, I recollect only one species,—it was of cubicite in minute crystals, encrusting a dark gray limestone in Ithaca.

Of the class of metallic minerals or ores, there is great scarcity in the Ionian Islands. Iron and manganese are, I believe, the only ones which have hitherto been found;—the latter in the state of black oxide, the former in that of protoxide, and peroxide, and of sulphuret. I have met with black oxide of manganese in two or three different places. Near the village of Galaro in Zante, it occurs in layers about an inch thick in marl. Between Samos and Sta Euphemia in Cephalonia, close to the road by the sea-side, the limestone is dendritic, and black oxide of manganese is the colouring matter of the arborescent forms. Near Argostoli in the same island, in a quarry close to the Lazaretto, I found this oxide. As the colouring matter of rocks, and clays, and soils, the oxides of iron are very common. The red and brown tints are chiefly owing to the red oxide, the gray to the protoxide; the purple (not an uncommon colour of soil), to the red oxide of iron, with which is mixed a very minute quantity of oxide of manganese. Ores of iron are exceeding rare; amongst my notes, I can find one instance only, and that is of the peroxide in small nodules, about the size of peas, which I observed in a limestone quarry near Vathi in Ithaca, about a mile from the town.* Near

* In Cerigo both the black and red iron ores occur in a massive form; I have seen specimens of them sent home by Mr Robert Jameson,

Argostoli, in a sandstone quarry, I have seen iron pyrites in minute crystals. I have likewise met with the carbonate of iron, and of manganese, in very minute quantities encrusting rocks, but the localities I do not recollect. It is asserted and believed by the inhabitants, that native gold and silver have been found in the islands, and spots have been pointed out to me, with the reputation of bearing one or other of these precious metals. I believe the natives may have mistaken silvery mica (which occasionally appears in the sandstone), for silver; and iron pyrites for gold; and have been so deceived. And perhaps, in some instances, the notion may have been formed, from the circumstance, that the teeth of sheep feeding on the sides of the mountains acquire, occasionally, an encrustation of a golden or silvery hue (most frequently the former), the exact nature of which remains to be ascertained; I believe it is a vegetable matter; I have satisfied myself that it is principally so, and that it is destroyed by fire.

and in the paper already referred to, he states that they occur in graywacke, and were observed in veins. He well remarks, alluding to the occurrence, " it is important to know that the rocks of the transition class are the repositories of the principal ore-mines, and roofing-slate quarries now worked, also of several mines in ancient times, such as those of silver on Mount Laurion, which Zenophon says yielded an annual income of 100 talents to the State," and he adds, " we are therefore entitled to infer, that some deposits of valuable ore may one day be discovered in Cerigo. If there was a market, various quarries might be opened in the clay slate, limestone, and graywacke-slate, not only from being easily worked, but also from their accessible nature and vicinity to the shore."

Of the saline class of minerals, there is very little variety in the Ionian Islands. The only salt which is common, is sulphate of soda; it is of frequent occurrence, and in considerable plenty in the marl districts. It is most conspicuous in very dry weather, when it appears as an efflorescence, and from its whiteness much resembles snow; viewing the clay hills thus covered, especially by moonlight, it is difficult to believe that snow has not fallen on them, and more than once, in winter, I have been completely deceived. Mixed with the sulphate of soda, there is commonly some sulphate of magnesia, and a little common salt. I expected to find nitrate of potash, or of lime, or of soda in the same situations, but did not; nor, indeed, could I find any of these salts in the Ionian Islands. Alum I found in two or three places, near the base of Scopo, in small quantity, probably derived from the decomposition of iron pyrites exposed to the air, mixed with clay, an origin which its ochery tinge would seem to indicate.

There is a subject connected with mineralogy, which may be deserving of notice here: it is the changes which take place in bodies, from the effects of time,—or, to speak more correctly, the changes which slowly occur, and which are only well expressed after a long lapse of time, from the operation of the natural causes to which they are exposed. Few countries are more favourable for this interesting inquiry than Greece, where the remains of ancient art are not uncommon ; and many of those remains, being metallic, are peculiarly fitted to exhibit the effects in question.

The first object I shall notice, as an example, and one of the most remarkable, was a bronze helmet of the antique Grecian form, which, whilst I was at Corfu, was found in the sea, near the shore of the village of Castrades, by a fisherman, where the water was about four feet deep. It was brought to the then Lord High Commissioner, Sir Frederick Adam, to whom I was indebted for permission to examine it Both internally and externally, it was partially encrusted with shells, and a deposit of carbonate of lime. Where free from this crust, it was of a variegated colour, mottled with spots of green, dirty white and red, and wherever the crust was broken and separated, the same appearance was found underneath.

On minute inspection, the red and green patches exhibited a crystalline structure, most distinct in the red ; and these, on examination with a lens, were found to be octohedrons of the red oxide of copper, intermixed with crystals of the same form, of metallic copper. Chemical analysis confirmed this, and showed that the green patches were composed principally of carbonate and submuriate of copper, and the dirty white chiefly of oxide of tin. The mineralizing process had penetrated very little into the substance of the helmet ; the encrustation and rust removed, the metal was found bright beneath,—in some places, considerably,—in others very slightly, corroded. On analysis, it was found to be an alloy of 81.5 copper, and 13.5 tin.

Other similar alloys, as an ancient nail, from a tomb in Ithaca, an ancient mirror* from a tomb at Samos, in Cephalonia, and many ancient coins of bronze, on careful examination and analysis, afforded similar results, indicating the operation, as it were, of a mineralizing process, and a separation, of the elements into new groups,—the tin in combination with oxygen, forming gray spots; the copper in combination, either with oxygen alone, and in the first degree of oxidation, forming the protoxide; and, in the second, the black peroxide; or, in conjunction with oxygen, combined with carbonic acid, or the muriatic, forming the insoluble carbonate or submuriate. The isolation of these new compounds, and their state of aggregation into little raised masses, as well as occasionally their distinct crystalline structure, was remarkable, and especially deserving of note.

Other examples of change may be mentioned, though not so manifest as the preceding.

In an ancient tomb at Samos, a silver ring was found,—externally incrusted with a greenish matter, a compound of copper,—the exact nature of which I had not an opportunity to examine. In handling the ring, it broke, owing to its brittleness; and its fractured surface was highly crystalline and untar-

---

* It was copper alloyed with about six per cent. of tin, and a very minute quantity of arsenic and zinc.

nished silver-white. As it is difficult to suppose that the intense brittleness it exhibited was its original property, considering the use for which it was intended, it is reasonable to infer that it depended on the crystalline structure, and that that structure was gradually acquired during the lapse of ages. This ring was the property of a friend, by whom it was found, and with whom I was in company at the time of finding it.

In opening a tomb in Santa Maura, a mass of litharge was discovered, which is now in my possession, remarkable for its highly crystalline structure. I am disposed to think that when deposited, it might have been metallic lead, and that it gradually became oxidated and crystalline, and the circumstance that it contained a little carbonate of lead is rather favourable to this idea.

Ancient glass is of pretty common occurrence in the old Greek tombs; it is almost invariably much altered in appearance, and has more or less a mineralized aspect. One specimen which I examined, taken from a tomb at Samos, was iridescent and scaly; some of its minute laminæ had very much the appearance and colour of *aurum mcsivum*. It owed its hues, I believe, chiefly to the presence of a little oxide of iron and manganese,—as both these metals were separated from it by digesting it in strong muriatic acid. After the action of the acid, the laminæ were white; and they fused before the blowpipe into a bead of colourless glass, indicating that though the structure was so much changed, the composition was little altered,—that the principal ingredients—the silica and alkali—remained in union.

On what causes, it is natural to inquire, are the changes just described dependent? Probably they are chiefly dependent on electro-chemical action, and take place independent of solution.* In the instances in which solution is concerned, there is little difficulty of explanation. The early experiments of my brother, Sir H. Davy,—the subsequent and very elaborate experiments of M. Becquerel and other inquirers,—prove, in the most satisfactory manner, how readily crystalline combinations, similar to mineral productions, may be effected by feeble electro-chemical means,—means probably inferior in power to those in operation in nature in mineral veins,—and in strata of different kinds in which are mineral springs.

Whether water is essential to the changes described, which are supposed to take place without solution, is a question not easily answered. I am disposed to think that it is,—as being essential to electro-

* In Dr Birch's History of the Royal Society (vol. iv. p. 179), a remarkable example is to be found of the effect of oxidation in the mechanical force exerted by the particles of iron in combining with oxygen ; it is incidentally mentioned " that Sir Christopher Wren had found a great cake of iron, which had insensibly grown from the decay of a bar of iron, that fastened some of the stones of a pinnacle upon Westminster Hall ; which cake was of so great solidity, as to raise several tons of stone out of their place, and thereby ruin the pinnacle."

chemical action. Generally the drier the localities, in the instances of ancient coins, the less they are altered. It is only when the ground is dry, that bronze coins are found retaining the impression of the die complete, smooth and polished, and exhibiting that beautiful patina which is the delight of the antiquary. I have a small arrow head of bronze, from Marathon, probably Persian, and coeval with the battle of Marathon, which is only slightly tarnished;* and I have seen and examined a ball of glass from Thebes, in Egypt, which, from the hieroglyphic characters on it, was inferred to have been engraved 1640 years before the Christian era, and which has undergone very little alteration.†

Other questions might be started in connexion with this mysterious subject of very slow change. It has sometimes occurred to me to ask,—reflecting on the state of the silver ring from Ithaca, and the mass of litharge from Santa Maura, and supposing that they had both become crystalline,—whether, in the majority of uncrystallized bodies, the particles may not be in slow but constant movement,—that all bodies capable of crystallizing are thus tending to assume crystalline arrangements, and that many have as-

* It weighs twenty-six grains, is triangular, three-fourths of an inch long, and one-fourth of an inch broad at its base.

† The glass ball belonged to Captain Hènvey, R.N.; it was of a greenish hue, very like light-green bottle glass roughened; it was nearly transparent; contained a very few minute air blebs; was of sp. gr. 2.523; scratched common glass, and was scratched by a file; it weighed 123.3 grains.

sumed them. And I am sometimes disposed to ask, whether many rocks have not thus acquired an imperfect crystalline character, and some minerals,—as the old red silicious sandstone, some secondary limestones, and old and large stalactites. The latter commonly, the older and larger they are, the more crystalline they are, showing often a prismatic structure, like arragonite, radiating from the axis of the stalactite, as well as a concentric lamellar one,—seeming to indicate that their particles, after deposition in the solid form, had not been inactive and motionless, but acting on each other, had assumed new arrangements.

I shall not dwell further on the subject at present; but I cannot quit it without expressing the hope, that it will be taken up and more fully investigated by men who have favourable opportunities for the inquiry, and can avail themselves, in public museums, of the accumulated riches of antiquarian collections.

CHAPTER III.

ON THE GEOLOGY OF MALTA AND GOZO.

Points of Difference in the Rock-Formations of these and of the
Ionian Islands. Prevailing Rocks. Connexion with Character
of Scenery and Vegetation. Peculiarities of Ground indicative
of a great Catastrophe, associated with traces of Human Art.
Effects of Vegetation on Calcareous Freestone. Uses of this
Stone. Paucity of Mineral Substances.

MALTA and Gozo, in their geological structure, differ
principally from the Ionian Islands, in containing no
primitive, transition, or secondary rocks: they consist,
I believe, entirely of tertiary formations.

Limestone, calcareous freestone, marl, and calcareous shale, are the prevailing rocks and deposits.
Limestone commonly occupies the higher situations,
marl the lowest, and freestone the intermediate.
Their strata are generally horizontal; deviation from
that direction is uncommon, even where there are
indications of violent disruption; indeed, the sea-
cliffs of both islands, which may be considered as so
many examples of disruption, display the finest instances of regular horizontal stratification.

The limestone, freestone, and marl, though in

many places distinct, frequently pass one into the other, as it were by insensible gradations, and, in consequence, it is sometimes difficult to determine the character, and say whether the mass is of limestone or freestone, of marl or of shale. The limestone and freestone frequently occur intermixed, and the latter with shale.

The higher the situation of the limestone is, as on and towards the summits of the hills, and the lofty cliffs, commonly the more distinct is its character. It is generally of a light grayish hue, with a slight admixture of brown or yellow, is of a foliated crystalline structure, has no earthy smell when breathed on, does not adhere in the slightest degree to the tongue, and is not absorbent of moisture, or pervious to water or moisture. Its specific gravity is about 2.5. The specimens of it which I have examined, have not varied much in their composition; they have been found to consist principally of carbonate of lime, with a trace of silica and alumina, and sometimes with a trace of magnesia, and to owe their colour to oxide of iron. The fine grained varieties of this limestone are very like travertine; and both these and the coarse varieties may be considered as marbles. This limestone does not contain silicious layers or nodules. Where it is hardest and crystalline, it is most free from organic remains; and there, too, its strata are thickest. Caverns are abundant in it.

The freestone is commonly of a fawn colour, of

different shades, the finest grained generally the lightest. It is very soft, easily cut, easily scratched, even with the nail. Breathed on, it has an earthy odour, which it imparts to water in which it has been immersed, an odour the water retains, even after filtration through bibulous paper. It adheres slightly to the tongue, is slowly permeable by, and is retentive of, water; a specimen of it which I tried, gained after immersion in water 11.3 per cent.,—weighed after having been wiped; and this water it retained many hours. The subject of the trial was a small fragment, which weighed only 156.3 grains. The water it absorbed was 17.8 grains; after exposure to the air for seven hours in a dry atmosphere, there was a loss of seven grains of water by evaporation; and after an exposure for twenty hours, the whole of the absorbed water was dissipated. Rendered impervious to water by a thin coating of varnish, its specific gravity was 1.96; saturated with water before it was weighed in air, its specific gravity was about the same, it was 1.98; weighed in air dry, and then in water, after it had ceased to give off air, its specific gravity was 2.23. Its texture is not in the slightest degree crystalline, but finely granular, much resembling chalk. It consists principally of carbonate of lime, and of a small portion of matter not soluble in muriatic or dilute-sulphuric acid,* coloured by oxide of iron, intermixed occasionally with a trace of vegetable

* This insoluble matter I have not analysed; it is probably chiefly alumine.

matter. The varieties of it are numerous, both in its passage into limestone, and through a kind of shale into marl; in the one instance the proportion of crystalline deposit of carbonate of lime increasing; in the other, of clay. Organic remains are not uncommon in it, and in some situations are abundant.

The marl is very similar to that of the Ionian Islands, both in appearance and properties, and composition.

Freestone and limestone prevail in Malta; marl is there of comparatively rare occurrence. In Gozo, marl is common, especially the central parts; and in the intermediate little Island of Comino, the surface is entirely of limestone, or of a freestone, differing but little from limestone.

Each kind of limestone, freestone, and marl, impart a peculiar character to the country, not to be mistaken even by the most careless observer.

Where the surface is of limestone, or of freestone, approaching it in hardness, it is commonly exceedingly naked and rugged; in fact, a bare surface of rock, interrupted only here and there by little patches and spots of red clay, collected either in the hollows of the rock or its fissures, and supporting a few wild plants such as the squill, thistle, heath, &c., and almost defying cultivation. A considerable tract of the north-west part of Malta, in the neighbourhood of Marfa, is of this description; so also is that elevated ridge on the southern and south-western coast of the island, which extends for several miles,—presenting

towards the sea a precipitous face or cliff,—a little way
within, and above the sea cliff, and in the contrary
direction towards the land, either a mural precipice,
or a shelving declivity. Of the same kind is that
elevated chain which nearly bisects the island, extending across from one coast to the other, separating
the thickly inhabited portion from the comparatively
deserted part,—a natural line of defence which has
been fortified by art, and the strongest part of which,
and best known, is called the Nasciar Lines.

Where the surface is of the softer freestone, or of
shale approximating to marl, there the hills are commonly rounded, the declivities, gentle slopes, and all
the lines of the landscape are unbroken and flowing.
The greater part of the eastern coast and side of
Malta, the cultivated and thickly populous portion
of the island, is of this description. Gozo presents
the best example of the marl formation. Where it
prevails, and it does generally in the cultivated part
of the island, the open country is tame, the slopes
undulating, the hills truncated cones, the narrow
vallies formed of steep sides, terminating above in
mural precipices. The hills are the most remarkable
feature in the view; they are very like volcanic
hills, but from a very different cause. Their truncated appearance is owing to the circumstance that
they are surmounted with sandstone or freestone,
lying horizontally; and the mural precipices bordering the narrow vallies are owing to the same
peculiarity.

I shall select for description a few localities, the most interesting with which I became acquainted.

Near Marfa, between it and the headland called Ras-el-Kammich, the coast is very bold, the cliffs lofty, the surface of the country naked and rocky. One spot on the shore is particularly deserving of notice, both on account of the succession of strata, and the organic remains in which they more or less abound. It is a cliff about 200 feet high, and perpendicular, or rather partially overhanging. Its basement is marl, which is succeeded by a layer of a dark gray hue, composed of comminuted shells, of marl, and of a greenish matter in rounded particles, very much resembling serpentine gravel, and of reddish particles all intermixed, and above this is limestone, which constitutes the principal part of the cliff, abounding in shells, excepting towards the surface. The beds or strata are horizontal. Both the marl and mixed stratum contain organic remains, and the latter most plentifully, especially shells, many of them identical with existing species, and commonly filled with the matter composing the stratum, or petrified by means of iron pyrites. On the beach at the foot of the cliff, other fossil remains have been found, as the vertebræ of fishes and of cetaceous animals. These, judging from the matter which adheres to them, were probably afforded by the mixed stratum, in process of disintegration, or falling down, partly from the action of water exuding from the land, and partly and principally from the action of the waves and their spray in tempestuous weather.

It is worthy of notice, that close to this spot there are marks of carriage-wheels, deep ruts worn in the solid rock, indicating an ancient road, which extend to the margin of the cliff, and have evidently been interrupted by some dislocation or great subsidence of land. The appearance is the more remarkable and mysterious, as even the existence of such a road in this part of the island is apparently without object, and unaccountable. As the island is now constituted, it could lead to no port or landing-place, or from any fertile district, or be of any appreciable use. Viewing it on the spot, it was difficult to resist the conclusion, that it is a vestige of a continental road, belonging to a most remote period, when Malta and Gozo might not have been islands, but integral parts either of Europe or Africa.

Near San Georgio, on the south coast of the island, is a striking example of the form of ground which prevails generally along that coast,—one cliff within another, with a declivity intermediate,—admitting of cultivation, and commonly well cultivated and highly productive. The sea cliff here is in many places above 200 feet high, and the inland cliff often exceeds 100 feet. The former is of soft freestone, the latter is of a harder freestone, towards the summit passing into limestone, and the intermediate declivity is principally of marl. At San Georgio, the declivity is of some extent, is well cultivated and planted, and forms a little district almost as remarkable for its beauty as its singularity.*

Close to the village of Krendi, in the south-west part of the island, is a pit, similar to that near San Georgio, in Cephalonia, but on a larger scale, known by the name of Maklouba, signifying overturned. It is about 100 feet deep, and above 400 feet in circumference. Its walls are nearly perpendicular, and its appearance altogether is such as to convey the idea, that it was formed by the falling in of the roof of a great cavern. And tradition is in accordance with this notion. The tradition amongst the natives is, that at a very remote period the spot, then continuous with the general surface of country, was the site of a village, the inhabitants of which were distinguishedly wicked, and that they and their dwellings were swallowed up, the earth opening and ingulfing them. There is a considerable depth of soil in the bottom, which is cultivated as a garden, and is very productive. It is worthy of remark, that the rain-water does not collect in the cavity, seeming to indicate that beneath it are fissures, probably communicating with caverns. It is also deserving of notice,—in favour of the tradition relative to its mode of formation,—that in a portion of a rock, there is, or was a part of a cistern. It is mentioned both by Dolomieu and Abela, and particularly described by them. It was not pointed out to me when I visited the place, but it is probably still to be seen

* Plate i. fig. 3.

there. The latter writer, who says he repeatedly saw
it, states that it was lined with bitumen,—a circumstance in itself supposed to indicate great antiquity.
Belonging to Gozo, I shall notice only one locality, partly on account of a peculiarity connected with
it, but chiefly as affording an example of the structure of a large portion of the island. It is the hill
close to the town of Rabato, opposite that on
which the castle stands, remarkable for its flat
summit, surrounded by mural precipices, and for its
scarped declivities. The summit and mural precipices,—like the summits of the hills generally in
Gozo and the precipices, including even the greater
part of the sea cliff,—are of shell-limestone, approaching more or less to freestone, and the declivities are
of marl. The peculiarity alluded to is an intermediate layer of loose sand and of sandstone, between
the superincumbent shell-limestone and subjacent
marl, containing very little calcareous matter. It is
a bed of no great thickness, and is best seen in ascending the hill, where there is a winding path. Both
the sand and sandstone are of an ochrey hue ; they
both consist chiefly of quartz-particles of different
colours and of particles of iron ore, either hematite
or clay iron ore, in minute smooth grains.* I found
no organic remains in it; but my search was very

* Gold and quicksilver, it is reported, have been found in this
hill ; if true, probably the locality was this intermediate layer of
loose sand and sandstone, which, from its composition, there can be
no hesitation in concluding, was brought from a distance by the
agency of some powerful flood or current.

limited and slight. It is probably of the same date as the bed near Marfa, similarly situated between the inferior marl and superior shell-limestone and freestone. And I may remark, that in other parts of Malta there is a layer somewhat analogous in composition, and precisely so in relative position. A good instance of it occurs in ascending the hill to the Fontana Grande, or Inquisitors' Palace; there, by the roadside, is a bed with freestone above and marl below, containing small nodules of ironstone, as if water-worn, and small rounded masses of gray limestone included in marl, containing a large proportion of silicious matter.

At the Pietà, close to the city of Valetta, there has been recently discovered a remarkable funnel-shaped cavity in the side of the hill, partially filled up with clay, in which were found embedded a portion of the radius of a ruminant, probably of a goat, accompanied with masses of chalk, and water-worn stones, and a hard stone, the form and appearance of which clearly indicated that it had been fashioned by the hand of man. I shall insert below a letter from Mr Frere, which he was pleased to address to me on the subject; it was first published in the Malta Gazette, with the intention of giving publicity to the facts, and of calling the attention of travellers to the spot. It is with the same view that I give it a place here, believing that the facts recorded by Mr Frere, and so well described by him, and brought forward in so interesting a point of view, are important, and probably in a very high degree, as tending to connect the human race with great changes in the physical condition of the surface of the globe. Perhaps further and more minute research may detect in Malta, more such traces; one may illustrate the other, and something satisfactory may be deduced, which may link them together, and afford an explanation of them. Malta and Gozo are remarkable for the remains which they possess of a very remote antiquity. How curious and interesting would it be, could it be proved that these remains, such as the Giant's Tower, in Gozo, and other vestiges of the like kind, belonged to the country before it became an island;— that it was inhabited by the human race before the catastrophe occurred by which it was separated from the continent. *

* Extract of a Letter† from the Right Hon. J. H. Frere, written from Malta to Dr Davy, on the subject of a Natural Phenomenon recently discovered in the neighbourhood of the Pietà :—" You may recollect my attempt at forming a kitchen-garden at the Pietà by levelling a piece of rocky ground at the top of the hill; it has led to a discovery which is very extraordinary, and which to every person who has visited it, appears unaccountable.

" Near the Carruba tree, which you may remember on your right hand, at the top of the new flight of steps, a piece of rock had been left untouched for fear of injury to the tree; at length, however, we ventured to remove this last remnant of rock. It was found to rest on a body of clay, about twenty-seven feet in length, and (at the surface) about fifteen in width. As a welcome addition to the scanty collection of soil which had served to cover the rocks and stones, one half of the length and the whole of the width was excavated to the depth of about twelve feet; but on doing this, stones (one or two of

† From the Malta Gazette, 26th July 1836.

The stony valley, as it is called by the English, close to the village of Mösta, and in which is situated

them as big as a man's head) were found imbedded in the clay, evidently rounded by the action of water ; others were found of a luminous texture, in which all the crevices and interstices were penetrated by the clay, showing that this same clay (though it had now become so hard, and dense, and heavy, as to be with difficulty broken up by a strong man working with a pick axe) must at one time have been in a fluid state, suspended probably in a body of turbid water.

" Moreover, the sides of the rock, forming a sort of irregular funnel, in which the clay was contained, exhibited on one side (the side which may be called concave, and which, as we descended, was found to be vaulted and overhanging) indications distinctly suggesting, even to an unpractised observer, the notion of their having been formed by a rotatory action of water ; and that this rotatory action had probably originated in the rush of water to some great cavity below, forming a sort of whirlpool. Indications different in appearance, but equally bearing witness to the violent action of water, were observable on the opposite, or what may be called the convex side, the form of which might be described as resembling a portion of an inclined cylinder, or of a cone ; striped, as it was found to be, from top to bottom with deep longitudinal furrows, showing that the direct downward rush of water must have taken place on this side, while on the opposite and concave side the rotatory action, resulting from the contraction of the lower part of the rocky funnel had left its traces in a series of horizontal furrows.

" It followed, therefore, as an obvious inference, that the funnel upon which we had entered, would be found to penetrate through the whole depth of the rock. The work, therefore, was continued, partly from curiosity, and partly for the chance of finding water, till it was brought down to the level of the sea, a depth of sixty-three feet from the surface ; when all further operations were stopped by the influx of water. But the existence of a continued cavity filled with clay, and extending in a downward direction below the surface of the water, was ascertained by the facility with which iron-bars could be thrust down into it, for the water was not found at first, but flowed in gradually as soon as the fissures of the rock were left unobstructed by the removal of the clay.

the hermitage of St Paul, is deserving of mention as a striking example of a class of vallies and ravines

" If my report had ended here, it would hardly have been worth while to trouble you with it; but the only organized substance which was discovered is a fragment of bone, which I send, in the hope that some of your scientific friends may be able to determine the genus or species of animal to which it belonged.* It was found (after we had been at work about three weeks) imbedded in the dense and tenacious clay. But a more singular discovery was made a day or two after; a piece of hard and very heavy stone, about four inches in length, and two and a half in width. It was irregularly fractured at the back and at the edges, but on the other and larger side reduced to what may be called a smooth surface; that is to say, smooth with the exception of the traces of the instrument which had been employed for the purpose of giving it an even surface; these traces are very distinctly observable upon it. This stone, like many others which were found imbedded in the same clay, was covered with a black fuliginous varnish,—a mark of authenticity which, if I had had any suspicion of the good faith of the workmen, would have been sufficient to remove it. It was entrusted to a lapidary, who has carefully polished one of the edges, the rest of the stone being left in the state in which it was found, with its varnish untouched. He declares it to be what they call a *pietra dura*, of the hardness of a jasper or hone.

" Stones exactly of the same quality have been procured for me by favour of the lapidary above mentioned. They were found near St Julian's, imbedded in a red earth. Having examined their natural fractures, none of them were found to bear any resemblance to the surface which I supposed to have been produced artificially.

" Chalk is nowhere to be traced in the existing strata of the island, but nodules of perfect chalk occurred frequently in the clay; it is singular, however, that no fragment of flint has been found to accompany it. Another circumstance worthy of remark is this—that a slip of the rock is distinctly perceptible, extending from top to bottom, at the extremity of the major axis of the whole cavity; the

* Mr Cliff was of opinion that it was the radius of a ruminating animal, perhaps a goat. Dr Buckland thought it might have belonged to a seal.

in Malta, which appear, as it were to have been scooped out of the rock, by the passage of water.

rock itself being unbroken and perfectly solid till we descend to the level of the sea, where we find it broken and disjoined to such a degree as to have occasioned great difficulty, and made many precautions necessary for the safety of the workmen : this disruption must have been anterior to, or at least cotemporary with, the rush of turbid water in which the clay was suspended, since in nearly all those places where the rock is discovered to be in a broken and shattered state, its interstices are found filled with this hard and tenacious clay. Another circumstance might be mentioned in confirmation of the former conclusion, that the whole of this clay had been suspended in a torrent of turbid water. It was found, that in lateral cavities (which would have escaped the general rush and pressure of such a torrent) the clay did not completely fill the whole of such cavities, and was taken out in a loose granulated state. There is one circumstance, which seems to imply a very long continued action of water, or, more properly speaking, the same action renewed after long intervals. The rounded stones above described, " one or two of them as large as a man's head," must have been brought there by a torrent of water; but it is impossible that they could have remained in the place which they were found to occupy, only twelve feet from the surface, unless the turbid water had, at the time when they were brought there, already deposited a mass of mud firm enough to afford them support, and to prevent them from being borne by their own weight to the bottom of the cavity.

" I now come to a circumstance which, except to an actual spectator, might make the statement and inferences above mentioned, appear wholly fallacious and incredible. Accordingly, even to an actual spectator, it has usually been the last I have pointed out. I have said ; ' You see immediately beneath your feet the straight furrows stretching downwards; you see the horizontal furrows on the side opposite; in neither of them are there any salient parts; but every angle, either in a downward or horizontal direction, is worn and rounded off : you see farther down little niches and cavities worn out by the rebound of the water, and becoming gradually deeper and more marked, as you descend to those parts where the rocky funnel is more

They commonly open towards the eastern side of the
island, and run in relation to each other, nearly

traitened, and where the resistance and reaction must have been
greatest : in short, all the undoubted traces of a rush of water pour-
ing down the cavity from the side on which we are standing. Now,
let us turn round, and look for the higher or equal level from which
this rush of water must have proceeded. It has ceased to exist; you
can see nothing behind you, but a declivity leading down to a branch
of the present harbour.'

" This, therefore, is one of the local enigmas which are of frequent
occurrence in geology, and which are usually (and in the present state
of science perhaps justly) overlooked by those observers whose attention is more properly directed to general and comprehensive facts.

" The single circumstance, however, of the discovery of the traces of
human workmanship in the situation above described, is sufficient to
place it in a distinct class. If the frozen elephant of Siberia had been
discovered two hundred years ago, it would have given rise to a number of vain and fanciful theories. It now finds its just and proper
place; being classed apart, as a separate and (in our present state of
knowledge), an unaccountable fact, awaiting its solution from such
future discoveries as chance or science may produce, and which it
may contribute to confirm or to illustrate. In the same manner the
discovery (which I have been endeavouring to describe), though not
immediately available for the solution of any question actually in discussion, or even likely to be discussed for some time to come, appears
to me so singular and unusual as to deserve at least to be distinctly
authenticated and recorded. With this view, wishing that scientific
strangers, who may happen to pass this way, should have an opportunity of visiting the spot while the traces of every thing are fresh and
distinct, I hope you will not think that I take an unwarrantable
liberty with your name, if what I have written is communicated to
this portion of the public in the easiest and most obvious way, being
printed with its Italian translation in the *Malta Gazette.*"

In a letter with which I have since been honoured by Mr Frere,
of the 28th November 1839, he thus reverts to the subject; and, on
account of its great interest, I am induced to give an extract, with the
same hope in regard to the liberty taken, as he himself has expressed

parallel, descending from the high grounds on the western coast, and in the hilly country just within that coast. This valley, like that near Casal Curmi, called also the stony valley, is of a very wild and dreary aspect, and well worthy of a visit as a scene of wildness, and rude grandeur. Its precipitous, shelving, and cavernous sides (epithets applicable to different parts of it), are of the hardest kind of free-stone.

These vallies are distinguished for their nakedness; generally the harder the rock, the more destitute it is of vegetation. The softer kinds of freestone often

above:—" Having before written to you in print, per *Malta Gazette*, of July 1836, it may seem time, though a little late, to add a postscript. You may remember that I first imagined the stone which was found (among others bearing the marks of having been rolled in a water-course), but which, from its harder quality, had suffered little from attrition, to have been brought from a distance; but, upon cutting an adit into the cavern, about half-way down, on the precipitous side (for the satisfaction of the curious, and in order to avoid the renewal of ladders or scaffoldings), I found to my surprise that the whole was of the same quality, a pietra dura, as they call it, a kind of jasper; but in the whole of this process (a very tedious one), I was more and more convinced that the *smooth surface* of the stone originally found, had been *artificially produced;* the *forcible fracture* of the rock hav-ing, in no instance, presented a *surface at all resembling it.* But this stone, whatever was its original locality, found in company with other worn and rounded stones, must, *as all the features of the cavern testify,* have been borne by a torrent passing over a high level, the subsi-dence of which has formed the present quarantine harbour; and we have thus a specimen of human labour anterior to that catastrophe. This is a fact which, single as it is, seems so singular, that it is wor thy of being recorded. Sir H. Bouverie is excavating, and has found some curious unaccountable things in the style of those at Gozo."

are covered with vegetation in a manner to excite surprise,—often when the rocks are highly inclined, and even perpendicular. In the neighbourhood of the Inquisitor's Palace, where the freestone rises above marl, there are many remarkable examples of precipices clothed with plants,—plants of various kinds, growing in the rock, in fissures, and cavities, such as the fig, caper, mastic, bramble, thyme, thistle, ivy, Venus' hair, and many more of small size. The larger plants commonly are rooted in little cavities, in which is collected a small quantity of dark mould. Most of them are stunted in their growth, and some of them very remarkably so; their leaves small, the branches few and short, the roots disproportionally large, as if designed to be reservoirs of moisture.*

I have examined many of these plants chemically, and have found them to contain a large proportion of carbonate of lime, which probably was derived from the rock. On this supposition, there is no difficulty in supposing that these plants are instrumental in making or enlarging cavities in the rocks. And it has occurred to me that many cavities, now empty, or containing some vegetable mould, may have thus originated,—the plants which conduced to form them dying and decaying; and that as they are often of a cylindrical or rather conical form, and resemble very much the cavities produced by boring salt-water mol-

* Plate i. fig. 4, represents a portion of perpendicular rock, clothed as above described. Fig. 5, a myrtle plant extracted from the rock, showing the vast size of its root in proportion to its branch.

lusca, it is possible that cavities which have been referred to the latter agents, may really have been produced by the former.

On the application of the rock formation of these islands to the purposes of art, a very few remarks will suffice. The hard crystalline limestone, besides being employed for making lime for use as a cement, (it has not yet been applied to agricultural use) is in request as a floor and paving-stone, for which it is exceedingly well adapted, as it is very durable, and does not absorb water, and does not require varnish. In consequence of its being more expensive than the soft freestone, its use is more limited than is desirable, and more even than just economy would require.

Of the freestone of Malta—that which is well known as Malta-stone—there are several qualities, varying in degree of hardness and fineness of grain. The harder varieties are most employed in the making of floors and stairs of houses ; but as they are absorbent of water, they require to be either painted or varnished. The softer kinds are employed in building, in the construction of the walls and roofs of houses, and in the making of gutters for conducting water.

The softest and finest grained varieties are selected for the purposes of sculpture, in the formation of vases, &c., after antique forms, for which there is a great demand, on account of their beauty and cheapness. They are largely imported to England, and the manufacture, the only one in Malta, which has received much encouragement from the English, is an increasing and flourishing one. The work-shops of the Dimecks, both of father and son, are well deserving of a visit from the traveller. Great credit is due to these spirited and talented artists for the skill and enterprise they have displayed. The finest forms of antiquity in the galleries of the Vatican, and in the saloons of the Studio at Naples, have been imitated by them, and their copies possess a good deal of the beauty of the originals, whilst being of a stone almost as easily cut as chalk, instead of hard marble or delicate earthenware,—in point of cost they are infinitely cheaper.

Besides the stones just mentioned, there is another deserving of notice, which is found in Gozo—the Gozo marble; it is a limestone which has been deposited from water, is of very fine grain and crystalline, exhibits a waved appearance or marking, and is of an excellent brownish hue. Very handsome tables and vases have been made of it. This marble is said to occur in detached masses in marl. I had not an opportunity of seeing it *in situ;* and am uncertain whether it is to be considered as a moved stone or a local deposit.

The minerals of Malta and Gozo are even fewer in number than those of the Ionian Islands. They are confined to a very few saline substances, in minute quantities,—to calc-spar and gypsum. Foliated and crystallized gypsum is occasionally met with imbedded in marl in Gozo; no beds of gypsum, that I am aware of, have yet been discovered. The calc-spar occurs in many places crystallized in cavities and fissures in limestone, and in the form of stalactites. The saline substances are common salt, nitrate of lime, and muriate of lime. These I have detected in very minute quantities, particularly the two latter, incrusting the walls of caverns, and overhanging calcareous rocks. The nitrate of lime I found most abundant in caverns which had been used as stables for cattle. But I also detected it very slightly impregnating the surface of a decomposing and crumbling overhanging rock of freestone, where it was difficult to suppose that its production could in any way be connected with the decomposition of animal matter; for cattle did not take shelter beneath it, and neither bats, nor even insects could attach themselves to it, from its powdery and crumbling state; nor could I detect any traces of animal matter in admixture with it. The conclusion, therefore, is, that the materials of the acid are derived from the atmosphere, acted on by a surface of decomposing or disintegrating calcareous rock, favourable from its state of mechanical division and humidity to promote the combination in question. In my work on the " Interior of Ceylon," published in 1821, I have given a remarkable example of the spontaneous production of nitre, without any apparent intervention of animal matter; and M. Longchamp, in his " Treatises on Nitre," has adduced others, and, as they appear to me, satisfactory instances of the same kind. Theoretically, then, I believe that nitrates may form, and do form, unaided by the decomposition of animal matter; but at the same time I am convinced, that where there is a favourable base, the production of the nitric combinations is greatly promoted by the presence of animal matter in process of decomposition, in accordance with the results of common experience

CHAPTER IV.

ON THE SPRINGS OF THE IONIAN ISLANDS.

Distribution of Springs, in connexion with Geological Structure.
Division into Common and Mineral. Examples of the Former.
Aqueducts. Jubilee in Corfu on opening the Aqueduct supply-
ing the Town. Cisterns. Quality of Water preserved in them.
Saline Springs. Sulphuretted Springs. That called the "Grease
Spring" in Zante described. Bituminous Springs. Description
of the Pitch Wells in Zante. Springs with Peculiar Qualities.
Anomalous Instances of Sea-Currents flowing into the Land.

THE subject of springs is intimately connected with
that of geology; the association is no where more
manifest than in the Ionian Islands: all the more
considerable tracts of country in the different islands,
which are peculiar as regards their geological structure, are peculiar also in relation to water.

In the districts of mountain-limestone springs are
of the greatest rareness, and perennial springs are
unknown. The inhabitants are dependent entirely
on cisterns cut out of the rock, into which rain water
is directed during the rainy season and collected
for use. The only springs that are met with, and
they are very few, are those which burst out at the
level of the sea, on the shore, or actually in the sea
at a little distance from the shore; and the only

streams are the torrents of winter, as brief as they are violent, immediately following the rains, and ceasing almost as soon. The greater part of the hilly region of Zante, the western portion of Cephalonia, especially the large district of Erisso and Potamiano,* the whole of the Island of Paxo, the south-west extremity of Corfu, including the greater part of the mountain of San Salvadore,—the greater part of Ithaca,—considerable portions of Santa Maura, —the whole of the adjoining islets, including the considerable Islet of Meganisi,—and a large portion of

* According to the Statistical Tables of Cephalonia, composed by the municipal officers in 1823, and published by Sir Charles Napier in his memoir on the roads of Cephalonia, the different parts of that island were supplied with water as follows:—

	Running Springs and Fountains.	Torrents.	Wells, Public and Private.	Cisterns.	Population.
Argostoli,......................	...	...	191	4	4114
Lixuri,........................	7	1	319	...	5608
Pertin^{ia} Livato,...........	3	1	371	394	9838
... Icossimia, ...	5	...	10	76	1057
... Leo,.	13	1	16	12	976
... Catoleo,..........	3	...	2	...	618
... Scala,..	3	1	5	1	739
... Coronus,..	3	...	2	...	483
... Heraclea,.	7	1	2	8	1063
... Pirgi,..	4	1	1	16	1104
... Omala,...........	...	...	41	152	1627
... Talamies,........	...	...	42	43	725
... Potamiana,......	...	...	...	447	3247
... Samos,.	12	...	2	95	2501
... Tinea,..	25	2	4	43	2474
... Pilaro,...........	13	...	7	202	3711
... Erisso,...........	...	...	15	492	6641
... Missocoria,.. ..	3	...	30	5	2002
... Catoi,............	1	...	192	...	1890
... Anoi,............	7	...	19	34	2609
	99	8	1770	2044	53,090

Cerigo,—are of the rock in question, and exhibit the peculiarities noticed. And their vegetation, too, is peculiar; no plants can be cultivated there with success, which require continued moisture; those only flourish which can bear a long drought, as the fig, the vine, the olive, and caruba. Where there are neither vineyards nor olive groves,—there the face of the country in the dry season has the most arid aspect of russet brown; and the flocks are under the necessity of feeding chiefly on the parched stubble and withered grass.

In the marl districts, springs are not common, and yet there is no deficiency of water; whenever a pit is dug, there water is usually found. They are almost as destitute of perennial streams as the limestone districts. Their winter torrents are of similar character, rapidly rising and falling. They are loaded with mud, and after heavy rains, the sea to a considerable distance from land, off the mouths of the streams, is rendered discoloured and turbid. Nothing can be more various than these districts are in appearance, whether cultivated or neglected. When cultivated, as already observed, they are often rich and beautiful, bearing some of the finest vegetable productions of the Levant, as the. luxuriant currant-vine, Indian corn, and tobacco. Where neglected, they are the most dreary wastes;—during great part of the year, if low, they are a quagmire or marsh;—if hilly, in the rainy season, they are slippery, crumbling surfaces, and in the dry season, parched, naked, and fissured.

The plain of Zante, the neighbourhood of Lixuri in Cephalonia, the district of Leftimo in Corfu, are striking examples. The different parts of the plain of Zante, and the adjoining marl-hills, are strongly illustrative of the effects of cultivation; it is to cultivation that this plain owes all the beauty for which it is celebrated; where neglected, as it is in some parts, there, instead of the currant vineyard, the orange grove, the garden and corn-field, the dreary waste just mentioned meets the eye.

In the districts of mixed deposits, where there are alternations of rock and marl, or where limestone or breccia rest on marl, these springs are most abundant, and there only perennial springs occur. In Corfu, in Santa Maura, in Cephalonia, and in Zante, there are examples of the kind, and they constitute some of the most beautiful parts of these islands. Water and fertility and luxuriancy of vegetation,—especially the fountain water, the living spring,—are intimately associated in these regions; where the spring bursts forth, there the circumstances are all most favourable to vegetation, and the soil commonly, as well as the moisture and the means of irrigation. Where there is a fountain, there is generally a garden, and if not a garden, or orange grove, there is either the stately platanus or wild shrubbery of the finest kind, the myrtle in profusion, with which is occasionally mixed the oleander, the laurel, and arbutus.*   That part of Cephalonia which

* Not only is the shrubbery about the springs of peculiar beauty

is least known, which extends between Pronos and Scala, at the foot of the Black Mountain, looking towards Ithaca, is a region of this kind. When I travelled through it, the noise of waters was even impressive ; and my companion, a native, resident on the other side of the island, and who never before saw running streams, expressed himself surprised and delighted; it was to him a perfectly novel scene ; nature appeared to him in a new aspect. Witnessing the impression produced on his mind, it was easy to imagine the feeling amongst the ancients which led them to the personification of these beneficent sources, and the assigning to them living and divine attributes.

and variety in the Ionian Islands, but also the minute vegetation, clothing, and dressing the moist banks, rocks, and stones, many of the plants aquatic, and in their natural place beneath, or on the surface of the clear water. Botta, in his interesting little work on Corfu, describing the fountain of Crissida, makes mention of eighteen different plants, thus situated, growing abundantly, exclusive of rarer ones. He enumerates the following :—Conferva fontinalis, potamogeton natans, Venus' hair, Mnium serpillifolium, Pteris aquilina, Parietaria officinalis, Scrophularia scorodonia, Geranium columbinum, molle, Robertianum, moschatum, Mercurialis annua, Ranunculus ficaria, Ficus carica, Asphenium ceteraci, Avena elatior, Cerastium vulgatum, Convolvulus sepium, Rosa canina. These, he says, "intrecciandosi fra di loro in vari modi, formano un' umile boscaglia e folta, la quale veste il suolo e le pareti di quell' antro, e rendono questo luogo fresco e vagamente ombroso ed ameno."* The nightingale is a rare bird in these islands; when heard, I have been informed, it is always in the cool cover of the fountain brake, and that there are particular spots regularly resorted to by these birds This I was told in Cephalonia and of that island ; but whether applicable to the other islands I am ignorant.

* Storia Nat. e Med. dell' Isola di Corfu di Carlo Botta, vol. i. p. 26.

These peculiarities in relation to water, thus briefly sketched in connexion with geological peculiarities of country, are such as might be expected *à priori*, are such as are perfectly accordant with the properties of the different strata and deposits,—as of the limestone strata, impervious to water, and if receiving it between its strata, directing it downwards to greater depths, if not intercepted by clay;—of porous freestone, absorbing it, and allowing it to penetrate through, and descend to any depth, if not impeded by clay;—and of marl and clay, absorbing hygrometically, and retaining it, when saturated, in a manner not a little mysterious, shutting it up,—preventing its natural downward course, and so occasioning its rise and overflow, or bursting forth in the form of a spring.*

The indications of water, in connexion with geological structure, are so distinct in the Ionian Islands, as to be almost infallible. The traveller can read them as he passes; and, if he make inquiry, the information he obtains from the inhabitants commonly accords with his expectations, often to the surprise of

* An instructive series of experiments is most easily made, by introducing different earths and powdered rocks into tubes, confined below by linen or bibulous paper. Whilst the water poured in above, will rapidly penetrate, and descend through lime, or magnesia, or silica, and through powdered freestone, limestone, sandstone, &c., it will be arrested by the marl and clay. A few lines of these substances, saturated with water, will bear a pressure of many inches of fluid. Its progress in descending is hardly perceptible. After several weeks, the descent may not exceed half an inch.

his guide, especially if only acquainted with the roads, and not possessed of minute knowledge of the country.

The springs of the Ionian Islands may be divided into common and mineral;—the former, including all those springs, fit for ordinary use; the latter all those too strongly impregnated with adventitious substances to be so employed.

Of the common springs, I have examined a considerable number, above thirty, in the different islands. The trials which I made of them were chiefly confined to the ascertaining of the specific gravity of the water; to the testing of it by re-agents; and to the evaporating, in some instances, a definite portion to dryness, and experimenting on the residue. They were all found to contain common salt, and either carbonate of lime, dissolved by carbonic acid, or sulphate of lime. In the proportions of these, there was considerable difference. There was some difference, too, in their other saline contents, and necessarily in their specific gravity, depending on their contents. It may be worth while to notice particularly a few of them as examples.

The spring which is considered by the natives of Zante to yield the best and purest water in the island, bursts out of the side of Scopo, about 180 feet below its summit, which, from barometrical measurement, appeared to be between 1200 and 1300 feet above the level of the sea. When I visited the mountain, in July 1824, its temperature was 59.5° of Fahrenheit. Its specific gravity was the same as that of dis-

tilled water. Tested by chemical re-agents, slight
traces only could be detected in it of common salt
and of sulphate of lime ; and no traces could be discovered in it, of carbonate of lime. These results
accord with the popular opinion,—no other water
which I had an opportunity of examining in Zante,
was found so pure ; and I may further remark, that it
was the only instance I met with, amongst the
springs of the Ionian Islands, of water entirely destitute of carbonate of lime. Its peculiarities, in relation to purity were, no doubt, connected with its
height ;—generally, I believe, it will be found that
the greater the elevation of springs, the greater is
their purity.

Remarkably contrasted with this spring, is the well
or pit-water of the city of Zante, which is found
every where, in the lower part of the town, on digging a few feet below the surface. The water of the
well, in the house which I inhabited, near the sea,
was of specific gravity 10049, and it contained a
notable proportion of common salt, sulphate of lime,
and carbonate of lime, with some magnesian salt, to
such an extent as to render it hard and unwholesome.

The water used in the city for drinking, and for
culinary purposes, was principally that of Crionero,
a spring situated at a little distance from the town,
at the foot of a cliff on the sea-shore. When I examined it, in the summer of 1824, its specific gravity was 10016. It contained the same foreign ingredients as the last mentioned ; but all of them,

with the exception of carbonate of lime, in very much smaller proportions. This water was then brought by carriers into the town, and was sold with as much regularity as the produce of the gardens or the fields. Since that time, iron pipes have been laid; and the water has been conducted into the city, affording an abundant supply;—a benefit for which the inhabitants are indebted to Sir Frederick Adam, when Lord High Commissioner.

On the hill above the spring of Crionero, there is another spring, in the garden of a little villa, called Agrotiri, of even purer quality, of specific gravity 10008, and which contained only just perceptible traces of saline matter. So much was this water esteemed, that the well was kept locked up by the proprietor, for his own use. The hill and cliff in which these springs are, consist of sandstone and marl, both slightly saline to the taste, a quality probably derived from sea-water, drawn up in minute quantity by capillary attraction. The different degrees of purity of the water, at different heights, is favourable to this conjecture; as is also the circumstance that the saline matters of each source, do not differ materially from those of the sea.

In the plain of Zante, water is abundant a few feet below the surface; wherever pits are sunk, it is found. The water of one pit or well which I examined was of specific gravity 10006, and contained a little common salt, and a minute quantity of carbonate and sulphate of lime, without any magnesian salt.

The spring of purest water of all those which I examined in Corfu, was one of some repute amongst the natives, on account of the qualities which they believe it possesses; these are indicated by its name, Acqua Aphrosidiaca. It is situated high up, amongst rocks in the steep side of a hill of difficult access, a few miles from the city. I found it to be of specific gravity 10005, and to contain only a very little carbonate of lime and common salt. The reputation which it has acquired, as a remedy for barrenness, if well-founded, is probably more owing to the effect of the exercise taken in visiting it, in promoting the general health, than to any specific virtue belonging to it.

The spring of Crissida, a short distance from the town of Corfu, is so copious as to turn a mill at its source. It rises from underneath a limestone rock. When I examined it in April 1825, it was of specific gravity 10016. It contained some carbonate of lime and of magnesia, a pretty large proportion of sulphate of lime, a little sulphate of magnesia, and a trace of common salt.*

The springs of San Nicolo above Benitza (about 460 feet above the level of the sea), are copious, like that of Crissida, and where they burst forth, they are employed in turning mills. Their water is remarkably clear and beautiful to the eye; it contains some

---

* The carbonate of lime and sulphate of magnesia, may appear incompatible; I find that they are not so, when the former is dissolved by means of carbonic acid.

carbonate of lime, a little sulphate of lime, and a very little common salt. From one of these springs the town of Corfu is now supplied with water. The distance is about seven miles; the water is conducted through iron pipes. The undertaking was one of considerable difficulty and expense; it is said to have cost about L.30,000. It was accomplished whilst Sir Frederick Adam was Lord High Commissioner, in 1831. The event was an occasion of jubilee to the inhabitants; it was hailed with the greatest rejoicing, as well might be, the introduction of an abundant supply of water into a town, the inhabitants of which had previously, like those of Zante, been under the necessity of purchasing the first necessary of life from water-carriers perambulating the streets.* At first, and for some time

* The following is a translation of the account of this event, published at the time in the Ionian Government Gazette, No. 33, for August 13, 1831. Its length seems to call for abridgement : but were it to be abridged, it would fail to be characteristic, first, of the grateful feeling described as having prevailed on the occasion for the great benefit conferred ; and, secondly, of the surprise and admiration expressed, arising out of a very slight acquaintance with the powers and resources of art. Moreover, the article is curious as an example of the Ionian style of writing, somewhat approaching to the oriental.

"There are some enterprises which, even when they are well advanced towards their termination, still keep the mind in some degree doubtful respecting them, till the very moment in which success becomes palpable. This uncertainty, this anxiety, arises either concerning things long believed, and declared to be of extreme difficulty, or concerning those which, by their nature, so concentrate on them the wishes and desires of a whole population, that it seems too much to hope for such happy results till they are beheld actually accomplished. All these various feelings were experienced up to the morning of Sunday last by the people of this island. From the time at

after the aqueduct was opened, it answered perfectly.
Lately, I regret to hear, that there is the strongest

which the laborious enterprise was commenced of bringing an ample
supply of water into the city, from so distant a part of the island, as
the one mentioned in our Gazette, No. 16, the importance of the object
made it to every one matter of opinion, and reflection, and doubtful
speculation; and the difficulties which had hindered all former
governors, not only from attempting, but even from thinking of such
an enterprise, rendered its success an event, with the majority, altogether unexpected.

" The spring of water which it was proposed to conduct into the
city, is situated on a mountain in the district of Benitza, distant from
hence six miles and a quarter, and at a height above the level of the
sea more than 178 feet, exceeding by about 84 feet the highest point
of the city itself.

" The water from the above mentioned spring flows through strong
iron pipes, nine inches in diameter, which have been conducted over
much irregular and hilly ground, and across a valley before they
reach the city. At intervals along their course they have been furnished with air-vents (Castelletti), and stop-cocks, for the purpose
of giving escape to the air, and of effecting a stoppage of the water
when any accident occurring to the pipes may render this necessary.

"Before the commencement of this work, the water of the above mentioned spring was subjected to full examination, by several persons of
science, both of our own and of foreign countries, and was pronounced
pure and salubrious. When the height from which it flows is considered, it may easily be supposed that the force of the impetus in its
descent must have required pipes of no less strength than those by
which the water is now made to rise to the top of our loftiest edifices,
and to any part of the fortifications.

" In a short space of time from the commencement of the work, these
pipes having been carried into the city, the cistern situated in the
piazza opposite the church of the Madonna dei Forastieri was chosen
as the place best fitted to exhibit the first gushing forth of the water.
A voluntary contribution from the citizens was eagerly furnished to
meet the expense requisite for duly solemnizing so auspicious an event.
Above the cistern was constructed a temporary erection, a temple in
the Doric style, in the midst of which, corresponding to the mouth of

apprehension of its failure, from the unlooked-for circumstance of the pipes becoming obstructed by the cistern, was raised an altar, immediately over the tube from whence the water was to flow. As the hour of noon approached, all the clergy of the island preceded by Monsignor Topotirità and the most excellent Regent, at the head of the public functionaries, made their appearance on the appointed scene, followed by an immense throng of people, such as the piazza and all the streets leading to it were scarce able to contain. The piazza was lined with scaffolding erected for the occasion. The spectacle was truly sublime, not only from the thronging multitude of both sexes and all ranks, mingled together for a common object, but from the general expectation being at that moment raised to a point of excitement which held all alike in breathless attendance on the result. The prelate gave forth the prayer; blessed the place; and then drew back some paces with his clergy. At that instant a column of water, more than twenty feet in height, rushed with a loud noise into the air, and converted the deep silence of the multitude into a general cry of exulting jubilee, making the place echo with the name of their august protector and his representative. No citizen of Corcyra for ages had experienced a joy so pure and true as on that day. Never were the effects of a truly paternal government so profoundly recognised; never had they so brightly shone forth; never had they obtained so signal a triumph over every sophism, and over all individual selfishness. Many were the tears shed in gratitude to that distinguished person, who had the boldness to conceive, the ability to design, and the perseverance to carry out a work so important to this city, but whose modesty, in this moment of universal exultation, deprived the rejoicing people of his so-much-desired presence.

" The clergy and the authorities, on quitting the piazza, immediately proceeded to the church of St Spiridion to offer the thanks and praises due to the Almighty. The Reverent Tipaldo, professor of theology, concluded by a discourse appropriate to the occasion. At one o'clock P.M. the municipal council, at the head of a deputation, repaired to the palace of St Michael and St George to lay before his excellency the Lord High Commissioner, as the principal and only promoter of the undertaking, the general desire expressed in a memorial subscribed by the citizens, that the new aqueduct should bear the name of Adam, in

the production and deposition within them of an ochery substance, consisting, as I have ascertained perpetual commemoration of the importance of the benefit, and of the grateful acceptance of it. in the island. His excellency gave a gracious reception to the municipal council, signified his acquiescence in their request, and expressed his thanks, not in words, but with marks of feeling which were evidently beyond his power to express, and which betokened at once his high gratification in the good he had effected, and his pleased acceptance of the gratitude it had called forth. The municipal council next proceeded to the most excellent senate with the proposition above mentioned, which having been at once acceded to, the senate added another testimony of public gratitude, by decreeing the erection of a public monument, which should attest the greatness of the benefit, and the gratitude of those who received it, towards its author, on the first of the many fountains which were soon to be constructed in various parts of the city. [A statue of Sir F Adam has since been erected on a pedestal designed by Chantry.]

" In the evening, the general rejoicing displayed itself in an illumination throughout the city. Never did this island behold so impressive a spectacle,—never did the same sentiment exist at once in so many hearts. The whole city shone forth from afar glittering in festive splendour. Every one in it sought to surpass his neighbour in demonstrations of gladness, The very atmosphere on this evening was propitious,—there was a perfect calm.

" Those illuminated parts, which deservedly drew most attention by their beauty, were—the temple over the cistern mentioned above. This had its pillars, its front and sides covered with variegated lamps, which, shedding their refracted light on the rising body of water, as it continued to pour forth its crystal stream, produced a magical effect. During the whole night, this point had its crowds of spectators. In the middle of the esplanade was erected a Chinese tent, about sixty feet in height, surmounted by a resplendent regal diadem, formed of coloured globe lamps, having at some distance, in the obscurity of night, the effect of jewels. Opposite to this, towards the south of the esplanade, shone the monument erected by the city in honour of Sir Thomas Maitland, and on the upper part of it was represented a volcano. In the peristyle were twenty-four burning altars. The rest of the edifice was brilliantly illuminated, so as to exhibit the outline of all its parts. On the other side, the grand

by the examination of some specimens sent to me, of
hydrated peroxide of iron, and of a minute proportion
of silica (the latter probably derived from the cast-
iron), very much resembling, in its general loose
spongy appearance, varieties of bog-iron ore. The
formation of this production from the iron of the pipes
is probably dependent on the atmospheric air contained in the water; and it is to be feared there is little
chance of any means, sufficiently simple and economical, being discovered to correct the evil. It affords

facade of the palace of St Michael and St George presented three long
and dazzling lines of light of continued splendour; and above the
lateral arches of the same building were exhibited flaming stars of
the order of St Michael and St George. The seminary, the church
of the Plàtitérra, and a great number of other edifices, suitably placed,
displayed beautiful effects. The music, the motion, the universal
cheerfulness, converted night into day, and lasted till the morning.

" The acquisition, in any place, of so essential a comfort of life,
must be the subject of general joy, and the precursor of much advantage; but to this city it is peculiarly precious. No one who remembers the straits to which our people were reduced, during the hot
season, by the scarcity, and sometimes by the actual failure of water,
—the expense which the poor, often depriving themselves of bread,
incurred to obtain it,—the filth, the sordid habits, and the train
of evils thence arising,—no one, who remembers all this, can fail to
find reason to bless the author of so precious an acquisition, and at
the same time to feel some surprise that former governments not only
did not set themselves to the work, but had not even boldness to
imagine it possible, or that the country contained the resources need-
ful to carry it into effect. It was reserved for our present government
to immortalize itself by having designed and executed this work; and
it is owing to the strictly economical and prudent administration of
our affairs, under the powerful protection of a great sovereign, and
under the guardianship of the constitution, that means have been provided to meet the expense of this gigantic enterprise, as well as many
others, the execution of which is still in contemplation."

a striking example of the importance of exact knowledge in the conducting of great public works; and of
the necessity, to avoid failure, of an acquaintance
with the properties of bodies as developed by chemical inquiry.

Since the preceding was written, I am informed
that the late Lord High Commissioner, Sir Howard
Douglas, has, it is believed, effectually overcome the
evil, by substituting to a considerable extent ($3\frac{1}{4}$
miles) an aqueduct of masonry, a brick barrelled
drain, two feet in diameter, guarded by filters at its
commencement, provided with air-holes and turrets
at intervals of 100 yards, and terminating in a reservoir, capable of holding a day's supply of water for
the town, with which it communicates by a second
line of iron pipes, nine inches in diameter, recently
laid. These important and judicious alterations will
probably be successful. Chemically considered, they
can hardly fail, as, from past experience, there is no
reason to apprehend any deposition from the water
itself, which the filters cannot separate.* I am told
that the supply of water to the town is much increased, and that it rises higher, ascending freely to
the citadel, and to Upper Fort Neuf.†

---

* In Malta I have seen a leaden tube which conveyed water from
the aqueduct, nearly filled up by a deposit resembling tufa, a sedi-
ment from the water, turbid after heavy rains, consisting chiefly of
particles of the common Malta-stone, or of shale, connected by carbonate of lime: it is a good instance of the manner in which the formation of calcareous tufa is effected.

† The consumption of water at present, is stated to be a little above

The spring of purest water in Cephalonia is, I believe, that which rises in the town of Lixuri, and by which the inhabitants are chiefly supplied with water. Its specific gravity, when I tried it, was that of distilled water. It contained, in very minute quantities, carbonate of lime and magnesia, muriate of lime, and common salt.

The best spring in Argostoli, situated on the outskirts of the town, is very similar to the preceding. It was of specific gravity 10003. Its saline contents were of the same kind ; and it contained a trace of vegetable matter ; 1090 grains of it evaporated, yielded .5 of a grain of solid residue. Of inferior quality is the water of a well in the resident's garden in the same town, about one hundred yards from the sea, and very little above the level of the sea. Its specific gravity was 10013. It contained carbonate of lime and magnesia, a little sulphate of lime, some common salt, and a trace of vegetable matter. 1090 grains of it evaporated to dryness, afforded 1.8 grain dry residue. Notwithstanding the quantity of saline matter may appear so small, it is sufficient to vitiate the water, which is considered unfit for use.

I shall not proceed further with a description of springs of common water; those I have noticed may be considered as specimens of the good and

600,000 gallons a day ; previous to the alteration, it was supposed not to exceed 100,000, and never to have been more than thrice that quantity.

bad, to which those in the other islands are analogous as well as in Zante, Cephalonia, and Corfu.

It has been mentioned that many parts of the Ionian Islands are dependent on tanks or cisterns for a supply of water. In a few instances I have examined the water thus collected, and have found it to vary but little in its qualities;—the slight variation depending, probably, chiefly on the surface on which the rain fell, or the channel by which it was conducted into the reservoir. In illustration, the water of the Theatre-cistern, in the town of Corfu, may be compared with the water of the Palace-cistern, or of the Temple-cistern on the Esplanade. The first is supplied with rain-water, falling on and washing a dirty surface in the neighbourhood ; it contains some common salt, a little carbonate of lime, and a trace of sulphate of lime, and also a little vegetable matter. The other two receive their supplies from comparatively clean surfaces, and their water is purer, containing only a trace of common salt and carbonate of lime Occasionally, where the tanks are situated in the neighbourhood of the sea, and are not carefully kept and repaired, the water becomes contaminated with salt water from percolation. In the Strofades there is an example of this, in a cistern at a spot called Prassa, the water of which is slightly brackish. I found it of specific gravity 10033, and containing minute quantities of the salts which exist in the water of the sea. Occasionally, too, tank-water is rendered hard by carbonate of lime and sulphate of lime.

taken up by the action of the fluid on the containing calcareous walls of the reservoir The best marked examples of this which I have met with have also been in the Strofades. Amongst the samples (nineteen in number) of water sent me from these curious islets of classical celebrity,* there were two of considerable age, one which had been collected in 1785, the other in 1795, after which the cisterns were closed, and their contents kept in store for use on emergency. Both these specimens of water contained more carbonate of lime than usual, dissolved by means of carbonic acid, and a distinct trace of sulphate of lime; and they were not otherwise adulterated. Generally,

---

* The present state of the Strofades does not at all accord with Virgil's poetical notice of them, being neither volcanic, emitting smoke, nor mountainous. A Greek priest, who had resided there forty years, favoured me with an account of them, written in modern Greek. He began his account, like a sincere lover of the spot to which he was attached, with observing, " that though he had read many books of travels, and visited many countries, yet, in all his reading, in all his wanderings, he had never become acquainted with any place on the face of the globe, to be compared with the Strivali (their modern name), either in beauty, fertility, the variety of productions, or the abundance and excellence of their springs." He then proceeds to describe them as two very low islets, the largest about three miles and a half in circumference, the property of the church of St Dionysius, in Zante, inhabited and cultivated by about forty priests, whose monastery and dwelling-place is a lofty tower, built in the reign of one of the Greek emperors. With much simplicity, he remarks, that there is a tradition extant amongst them, relative to the visit of Æneas; and he expresses his opinion that the story of the harpies may have originated in the circumstance of the smaller islet being frequented in the breeding season by a species of sea-fowl, very clamorous at night, and very fierce in defending their nests when attacked.

the tank-water, when carefully collected, is excellent for use, approaching to distilled water in purity, differing from it chiefly in containing a trace of saline matter and carbonate of lime,—the former probably brought down from the atmosphere, the latter derived from the earth. Amongst some people there is a prejudice against cistern-water, on the idea that it is impure,—that it has suffered from stagnation and keeping,—and that it is in consequence unwholesome. These are notions which are not borne out either by experience or accurate science. Science teaches us that water in itself is subject to no change from rest, and that pure water might stagnate for thousands and millions of years without becoming impure,—without undergoing any alteration. Science teaches that if it become impure, it is from the admixture of foreign matters ; and experience proves the same ; and further, that the tendency of water from keeping is rather to improve, and to become more pure than the contrary,—owing to the tendency of animal and vegetable matter to decompose and be converted either into elastic fluids, which ascend and pass off as gases, or into insoluble compounds abounding in carbon, which subside and find their resting-place at the bottom. The subject of cisterns is one of great importance,—in every country deserving of attention,—but which hitherto has been little considered, excepting in those regions from which other sources of supply have been excluded. Great Britain is pre-eminent for abundance of water ; yet even in this country there are spots where the water is either scarce or bad, and where, probably, great advantage might be derived from the construction of cisterns.

Of the mineral springs belonging to the Ionian Islands, three kinds may be specified, viz. the saline, the sulphuretted, and the bituminous.

Of the saline class, the only ones I am acquainted with, of an unmixed character, are some in Cephalonia, those which occur between Samos and San Euphemia, and some smaller ones, close to the sea, below the ancient Pronos. Three of the former springs pour forth considerable streams. The largest, when I passed in January 1825, our party had some hesitation in fording. It bursts out beneath a ledge of limestone rock, about thirty yards from the shore; is perennial, and constantly turns a mill at its source. Another large stream gushes from the limestone, close to the beach, and a third rises through the sand, on the very margin of the sea, and is sometimes overrun by the waves. And besides these, there are other smaller springs contiguous. All of them are similar, as are also the smaller ones of Pronos; they are slightly brackish, and their water does not apparently differ from sea-water, excepting in degree of saltness. But this opinion I offer merely conjecturally, founded on the taste, for I did not examine the water chemically.

Of the sulphuretted kind, there are several, some of which are also saline. I shall notice the most remarkable: they are confined to two islands—Cephalonia and Zante; at least I am not aware of the existence of a sulphuretted spring, excepting of extreme feebleness, in any of the others.

In Cephalonia, there are two sulphuretted springs, both of them in the neighbourhood of Lixuri; one is called the spring of Stoccludio, the other of Sta Lagussa.

The Stoccludio spring rises from a marl hill about two or three miles to the southward of the town just mentioned; it is very scanty. Its water I found of specific gravity 10008; from the experiments I made on it, it appeared to be very slightly impregnated with sulphuretted hydrogen and carbonic acid, and to contain a very little sulphate of lime, carbonate of lime, and carbonate of magnesia, a trace of vegetable matter, a little common salt, and a portion of sulphate of magnesia; the last mentioned salt is the predominant ingredient in this very dilute mineral water. This spring is esteemed by the natives, and is much used, especially after excesses in eating, to which the Greeks are not a little addicted at their feasts.

The spring of Sta Lagussa is nearly three miles to the northward of Lixuri, close to the ruins of an old church. It is situated in a marl hill, in which slaty gypsum occurs, in strata highly inclined. The spring is very small, the flow from it not perceptible; it is not more than two or three feet in circumference, nor more than three or four inches deep. When I visited it on the 15th of February 1825, it was perfectly tranquil; no bubbles of gas escaped; it was covered with a white pellicle of sulphur, and emitted a strong smell of sulphuretted hydrogen, and had a strong taste of this gas dissolved in water. Its colour was light yellow. Its temperature was 47°, clearly showing that it was not derived from a warm source. The specific gravity of its water I found to be 10063. From my experiments on it, it appears to contain a large proportion of sulphuretted hydrogen (about 17 cubic inches of the gas to the 100 cubic inches of water),—some carbonic acid,—some sulphate of magnesia and sulphate of lime, with a little common salt, carbonate of lime, and carbonate of magnesia, and a trace of vegetable matter, and of sulphur suspended in it, to which I believe its colour is owing. It is in much repute amongst the natives for the cure of cutaneous diseases; in proof of which I may mention, that on a small tree contiguous there was a profusion of pieces of white linen suspended, perhaps as votive offerings, which had been used in applying the water externally to the diseased parts. From the large quantity of sulphuretted hydrogen dissolved in this water, its remedial reputation, no doubt, is well founded. Were it enclosed in masonry, and covered over, its strength would be secured, especially in summer; and if the supply of it could be increased, it might be bottled and advantageously sent to a distance for use, without any loss of its virtues.

In Zante there are three sulphuretted springs, one

called Bromonero (fêtid water), in the village of Ge-
rachorio-basso; the other at the northern shore of the
bay of Catastari. The first mentioned spring was discovered in making an excavation in search of water
for agricultural purposes. It is situated in clay; the
quantity of water it affords is very small. In composition it resembles very much the water of the spring
of Lagussa, but it is much less strongly impregnated
with sulphuretted hydrogen. A minute quantity of
sulphur is suspended in it. This spring was discovered whilst I was in Zante, in the summer of
1824, by Count Paolo Meroati. I was informed that
formerly a similar spring existed in this village, and
that its water was used by the natives for curing
their cattle of scabies. It was filled up on account
of its offensive odour. St Sauveur, in his work on
the Ionian Islands, makes the same statement. It is
worthy of remark, that at Gerachorio, subterraneous
noises, resembling the report of artillery, are frequently heard; and that earthquakes there, are more
common than in any other part of the island. They
are very slight, and usually accompanied by the
sounds alluded to. This information also I obtained
from Count P. Mercati.

Of the two springs on the northern shore of the
bay of Catastari, one rises close to the sea, the other
in the sea issuing from beneath the water, in a cave
in the cliff.

The first is a copious one. To see it, it is necessary to quit the road leading to the mountain-villages,

and descend the side of a steep hill and shelving limestone rocks. The spring gushes from the rock into the sea, which almost enters its mouth, and must overflow it occasionally in tempestuous weather. The quantity of water it pours out is considerable, almost sufficient to turn a small mill, and it flows with some velocity. It is slightly saline; and smells pretty strongly of sulphuretted hydrogen; its temperature, on the 26th of August, was 69°. From the few experiments I made on it, its saline contents appeared to be similar to those of the sea; it contained, however, more carbonate and sulphate of lime. The proportion of sulphuretted hydrogen dissolved in it, was small. Where it mixed with the salt-water, the sea was slightly discoloured; it exhibited a faint milkiness. From an adjoining rock in the cliff, there is an oozing out of the same kind of water; and, in the cavities in which it flows, there is a deposition of a whitish gelatinous substance, which, on examination, was found to consist of sulphur and another substance resembling vegetable mucor.

The other spring, that which breaks out under water, is better known by name than the former; indeed it has acquired a name and reputation, and become an object of curiosity, under the appellation of "Grease Spring." As its nature, at present, is but little understood, I shall enter into some details respecting it, and give an account of an exploring visit which I made to it on the 12th August 1824. The morning was very favourable for the boating excursion, the sea but slightly ruffled by a very gentle north-west breeze. We embarked at the Salines, distant about two miles from the phenomenon we were in quest of. When we had approached within about a quarter of a mile of the cliff from whence the spring issues, we perceived the smell of sulphuretted hydrogen, and very soon after we saw white flakes and particles floating in the sea, which thickened so much in nearing the source, as to render the water quite white. The odour and the whiteness of the sea, guided us to the principal spring, which is situated in a small cave, formed by limestone cliffs of moderate height. The cave is skirted on each side by projecting perpendicular rocks ; its roof is shelving, pretty lofty at its mouth, but rapidly declining, so that a boat can enter only a few yards,—cannot reach its extremity, which may be about twenty-four yards. About the middle of the cavern, or rather, I should say, as far as the boat could enter, the depth of the water was about twelve feet. This was ascertained by letting down the anchor. The water felt very cold where we sounded ; its temperature was 62°, the sea at a distance was 78°, and the air, under the awning of the boat, 81°. To explore the innermost part of the cave, it was necessary to leave the boat, and have recourse to swimming. It proved a very disagreeable task, partly from the coldness of the water, and still more from its stench. I was induced to undertake it, with the hope of discovering something interesting, but my observations were chiefly negative. I could observe no appearance of air-bubbles ascending, and no distinct gush of water; and the temperature of the water inwards did not increase. It was fortunate, in this rash attempt, that the sulphuretted hydrogen was not more freely disengaged: if it had been, in all probability it would have proved fatal. As it was, I returned to the boat with very disagreeable sensations, and was presently seized with purging and vomiting, which I mention as a caution to others. The walls of the cavern were either covered with green sea-weed, or with a dead white incrustation; the latter predominant. The current of water proceeding from the cavern, was well marked by the outward movement of the flakes and particles of white matter suspended in it.

With some difficulty, owing to the specific gravity of the white matter differing very little from that of salt-water, I collected sufficient for examination. The following are the results of my experiments on it, made after my return to the town of Zante, and also on the incrustation on the rock, and on the water itself. These experiments were not so minute as I could have wished, owing to my limited means; the results, however, were very distinct. I shall commence with the matter which gives a peculiar character to the water, and which has been improperly considered as a kind of mineral grease.

It is nearly milk-white, tasteless, and, after exposure for a short time to the air, it loses the odour of sulphuretted hydrogen, and has no smell. It is of a gelatinous consistence; examined with a lens, it has the appearance of a delicate semi-transparent membrane, studded with white particles. It is heavier than water, as is indicated by its sinking readily, when perfectly quiet. It is, however, even more readily suspended, when agitated, showing that its specific gravity is not much greater. Exposed to the air till dry, it appears in the form of a thin light yellow pellicle, of some toughness. This pellicle, before the blowpipe, partially fuses; it burns with a blue flame, emitting a strong smell of sulphureous acid, and leaves a coal of its own form, which is easily reduced to an ash,—white, very small in quantity, and consisting chiefly of lime. Dilute acetic acid does not dissolve the peculiar matter : it renders it, however, more transparent. Strong nitric acid imparts to it a yellow tinge ; when heated, it dissolves it slowly, and sulphuric acid is formed. Concentrated sulphuric acid appears to dissolve it rapidly ; a little white powder remains, which is chiefly sulphur. A solution of acetate of lead renders it more opaque and heavier, judging from its sinking more rapidly in water. Subjected to heat in a retort, connected with a pneumatic apparatus, the products were a gas that had an offensive empyreumatic smell, unmixed with that of sulphuretted hydrogen, a yellowish fluid, in which sulphur was suspended, and a residual coal. The fluid had an empyreumatic smell, similar to that of the gas, and, tested by a strong solution of caustic soda, it afforded indications of the presence of ammonia.

From these results, it appears that the matter in question consists of two substances,—of sulphur and of another akin to animal mucus, or to animal albumen, and very analogous to Barégine, or that matter which exists in the sulphureous water of Barèges, which has been examined by M. Longchamp, by whom the name has been given. I have the more confidence in expressing this opinion, having, through the kindness of Professor Forbes, received a specimen of Barégine, collected by him at Barèges, which I have submitted to a few experiments, the results of which tolerably accord with the preceding.

The specimens of rock which I brought from the interior of the cave, were of two kinds—varieties of limestone, one resembling indurated chalk, the other crystalline, and more resembling marble. They were both composed of carbonate of lime, and contained a very minute portion of alumine. I could not detect in them any sulphur, nor did they emit any smell of sulphuretted hydrogen, when in the act of solution. These remarks do not apply to their surface; for they were superficially incrusted with a light yellowish matter, which, on examination, was found similar to the peculiar substance in the water;—the only difference noticed was, that when subjected to distillation, the gas disengaged was not free from the odour of sulphuretted hydrogen.

A specimen of water taken from the cave, was of

considerably less specific gravity than that of the water of the sea adjoining;—its specific gravity was 101103. Besides the animal-like matter and sulphur suspended in it, and the sulphuretted hydrogen dissolved in it, it contained pretty much carbonate and sulphate of lime. As the sulphureous spring rose in the sea, and its waters were mixed with those of the sea, it necessarily contained the common ingredients of sea-water.

Besides the cavern I have described, there are one or two more in the neighbourhood, similarly situated in the cliffs, yielding the same kind of water.

These springs have been long known to the inhabitants; and it is stated by St Sauveur, in his account of the Ionian Islands, that the natives of Zante are in the habit of collecting the peculiar product of them, when thrown up on the shore, and applying it as a remedy to the cutaneous diseases of their cattle. This was not confirmed by those I had an opportunity of questioning on the spot. If it has ever been collected, as St Sauveur states, it was probably in a moist state, and when entangled and suspended, as it were, in the froth and foam of the waves.

The origin of the animal-like substance is not a little mysterious. M. Longchamp, in his memoir on Barèges, read before the Academy of Sciences, in 1833, does not even offer a conjecture respecting it. Various conjectures, no doubt, may be entertained on the subject. To me it appears most probable, that it is of a vegetable nature, a species of mucor, or perhaps of tremella, somewhat analogous to those found in the sulphureous springs of Aix, in Savoy, and described by Saussure. They there grow on the basin and rocky channels of the waters; their mucous filaments are impregnated with sulphur, and are liable to be detached. Perhaps the Zante springs flow through concealed caverns, to which air may have access in sufficient quantity to allow of the growth of such plants; and they may be destitute of colour, from the exclusion of light; and, in favour of this notion, I may mention that, on the rocks in the neighbourhood, under water, I observed what appeared to be a species of tremella, growing abundantly. In my notes, taken at the time, I have called it a soft velvetty species of sea-weed, perhaps an ulva, to which adhered slightly, and might easily be detached, a kind of gelatinous matter, not unlike that accompanying the sulphur from the cavern. I collected a portion of it, with the intention of examining it, but neglected to do so. If the gelatinous matter just alluded to were found to afford azote or ammonia, and to have the principal properties of the animal-like substance in question, strong confirmation would be obtained that the origin of both is similar.*

Of springs of the bituminous kind, the only ones in the Ionian Islands are those of Zante,—the same which were described by Herodotus more than two

---

* Since the above was written, I perceive from the proceedings of the British Association of Science, held at Liverpool in 1837, that Dr Daubeney has arrived at the same conclusion relative to the origin of barégine or glairine,—the more worthy of confidence, as drawn from numerous observations.—*Athenæum*, No. 516.

thousand years ago,—and which, there is every reason to believe, have flowed ever since without interruption, though diminished, perhaps, in size and number.* They are situated towards the southern extremity of the island, in a little valley open to the sea, between barren rugged hills of limestone, offsets of the mountainous range. It is commonly called the valley of the pitch-springs. These springs at present do not exceed two in number. One of them rises in a morass which occupies nearly the middle of the valley; the other appears on the skirts of the marsh, on its southern side, just where the declivity of the boundary hill terminates. The first mentioned is of an irregular shape, where widest, not exceeding four feet. It is said to be unfathomable, but to me it did not appear to be more than from four or five feet deep, where deepest, sounding it with a long stick. Its water is brackish and almost stagnant; its mineral product floats on its surface. Close by, are three pits, into which the pitch is transferred by those who collect it, after the manner mentioned by Herodotus (though not with a myrtle branch), and where, as mentioned by him, it is left some time, probably to allow the watery part

* The size of the little lakes or pools in which the pitch rose, in the time of Herodotus, as described by him, might then have been larger than at present, in consequence of the drainage of the valley having been more imperfect, and its level lower. Were the small stream, which now flows through the valley into the sea, obstructed, a considerable portion of the valley would necessarily be flooded.

to separate, before it is put into barrels and carried into the city for use. These secondary artificial pits have so much the appearance of wells,—are so like the natural well, that they have occasionally been considered as such by travellers,—and, in consequence, the number of the springs sometimes has been incorrectly stated. The ground around, to the extent of a few yards, is impregnated with bitumen; it is a mixture of mud and bitumen, and is tremulous, though little yielding under the pressure of the foot. The air, too, and for a greater distance, is impregnated with bituminous effluvia; so that, on entering the valley, if the atmosphere is in a favourable state for conveying odours,—as it commonly is in the dewy coolness of the morning and evening,—the sense of smell is a sufficient guide to the spot. The spring or well on the southern side of the valley is nearly circular, about nine feet in diameter, and about three feet deep. Its surface is generally covered with a pellicle of liquid petroleum; and the same substance, of thicker consistence, covered its bottom to the depth of a few inches. The water of this spring is clear and fresh, and flows out in a pretty copious stream. I never witnessed any bubbling of gas in either well, except on stirring the bottom, when air rose in large bubbles. On my first visit, in July 1824, I collected a portion of this gas for examination, and also of the water of each spring and a portion of the tar. I shall briefly notice the results of my experiments on each of them.

The gas was not absorbed by water, and only very slightly diminished in volume by barytic water and by phosphorus; 35 measures of it were reduced to 33.5 by the former, and to 33 by the latter, indicating the presence of a little carbonic acid, and still less oxygen. It had a slight smell of tar, but not the slightest of sulphuretted hydrogen. A taper being applied, it burned with a light-bluish flame. Hence it may be inferred, that besides a little carbonic acid and oxygen, it contains carburetted hydrogen; it probably consists principally of light carburetted hydrogen and of azote. The results mentioned were obtained on the spot; I examined the gas immediately after collecting it.

The water of the brackish spring was slightly turbid, but after filtration clear, and of a just perceptible tint of brown; its odour was bituminous, its taste like that of sea-water, but less strong. It was of specific gravity 10060. From the results of my experiments on it, it appeared to differ principally from sea-water (omitting the smaller proportions of its saline ingredients), in containing a notable quantity of sulphate of lime.*

The water of the fresh-water spring, filtered to separate the pellicle of tar floating on its surface, was

---

* In the water of the spring which I examined, as in sea-water, I found some carbonate of lime and of magnesia, but I could not detect either of these in the water of the artificial pits; no doubt they had separated, on exposure to the air, from the escape of the carbonic acid.

of specific gravity 10011. It had a slight taste and smell of tar. Subjected to the same tests as the saline water, it exhibited the same results, only in a less degree; consequently it may be inferred to differ from that only in being more dilute.

The mineral tar of these springs consists, I believe, of three substances,—one easily volatile, at a low temperature, like naphtha, with an odour of rosemary; another volatile at a much higher temperature, the boiling point of which is about 600° Fahrenheit, and which is entirely soluble in sulphuric ether; the third, decomposable by heat but not volatile, and neither soluble in alcohol nor ether, but soluble in olive oil, when heated. The former substance is most analogous to petroleum, if not identical with it,—the latter to asphaltum or bitumen. By the application of different degrees of heat to the mineral tar in an open vessel, operating on a definite quantity,

30 parts per cent. were driven off at a comparatively low temperature, chiefly water, naphtha, or the very volatile fluid and petroleum;

43 by a high temperature, approaching a dull red heat, chiefly petroleum; and

27 remained, chiefly asphaltum or bitumen, of specific gravity 1.08.

The quantity of mineral tar yielded by these springs in the course of a year, varies from sixty to one hundred barrels. It is not in the same estimation now that it was formerly;—at present it is but little used, except for the paying of boats.

Herodotus mentions that bodies which fall into the

pitch-springs are carried by an under current, and emerge in the adjoining sea; and the same opinion is maintained by the natives now. Its correctness, however, is very questionable.

Another prevailing opinion is, that the springs are powerfully affected by earthquakes,—and that, under the influence of earthquakes, the flow or extrication of pitch is most abundant. Of the correctness of this notion, too, I am very doubtful. After a rapid succession of earthquakes, in the middle of November 1824, I visited the wells for the express purpose of endeavouring to ascertain their effect, and then, instead of more, there was in reality less tar than usual in the springs.*

Tar is occasionally observed on the surface of the sea, in the neighbourhood of the springs. In the month of October, I saw a considerable extent of sea between Maratonisi Island and Kieri Point, covered with an irridescent pellicle of petroleum, and streaked with lines of pitch. This was at the distance of about three miles from the shore of the valley of the pitch-springs. The water there was very black, as if the bottom were black (giving the idea of a stratum of pitch); the depth was considerable, exceeding twenty fathoms, but how much more I

---

* A gentleman, many years resident in the Ionian Islands, has informed me, that "whilst the earthquakes in Zante were going on in 1839 (many hundred shocks altogether), he sent out to the pitch-wells to ascertain whether there was any apparent sympathy or co-effect there, but none was observable."

had not the means of ascertaining. Similar pellicles of petroleum were seen on other parts of the sea, but not to the same extent. Whether they arise from springs in the bottom under water, or are derived from the land springs, conveyed by the little stream which flows from the valley into the sea, it is not easy to decide; the first seems most probable.

Relative to the origin of the mineral tar,—how it is formed,—whence it comes,—these are questions not easy of solution. That its source is some great subterraneous collection of vegetable matter, seems highly probable, undergoing change under considerable pressure; and, judging from the low temperature of the springs, undergoing change unaided by the operation of heat,—a change probably similar to that which is witnessed in the formation of peat. And the existence of layers of lignite in the adjoining cliffs, opposite Maratonisi Island, already mentioned, are favourable to this idea. By boring, probably much curious information might be obtained on the subject, and some useful discovery made; the tar, it is likely, would rise in greater quantity; and it is likely that either a bed of bitumen and asphaltum would be reached, or of coal,—the working of which might be of the greatest advantage to those concerned, and of the first importance in connexion with the interests of the Ionian Islands. The experiment of boring is so easily made, and at an expense so trifling, comparatively, that one is surprised it remains to be undertaken.

In connexion with the general subject under consideration, some peculiarities may now be noticed; the phenomena are of a miscellaneous character, and may be described without attention to order.

In Zante, about a quarter of a mile from the village of Musachi, at a spot called Paneocora, is a well, to which the natives attribute remarkable properties. According to them, it overflows when the wind is from the south or the south-east ; and then, they say, its waters emit an odour similar to that of the tar-springs. They believe that it communicates with the sea, about two miles and a half distant, and with the pitch-springs, at the distance of about four miles ; and assert that, in cleaning it out, sea-weed has been found in it. I visited the spot, and examined the water. The well is about fifteen feet deep, and affords a copious supply of water. It is situated in marl, at a little distance from the limestone-hills which skirt the plain. The water is well tasted and light, of the specific gravity of distilled water ; 800 grains of it, evaporated to dryness, yielded only one-tenth of a grain of solid matter, which consisted principally of carbonate of lime, and of magnesia and common salt, with a trace of sulphate of lime and of vegetable matter. These results are not favourable to the notion that it communicates with the sea. If sea-weed has been found in it, it may have been driven from the sea-shore by the wind, or may have been thrown into it. Its communication with the pitch-springs is most improbable ; if there is occasionally a smell of pitch from its waters, the more natural inference is, that mineral pitch exists beneath the surface in its neighbourhood. Relative to its extraordinary rise with southerly and south-easterly winds,—(admitting the fact, which it is difficult to question, it is so well authenticated),—the phenomenon may be owing to the moist character of these winds, and not to any distant communication with the sea. When these damp winds prevail, evaporation from the surface must diminish ; less water will be absorbed and drawn up by the marl, and the flow of water into the well from the adjoining ground may be consequently greater.

In the valley of San Jerasimo, close to the monastery of the same name, is a well to which a kind of miraculous property is ascribed by the people. It is said to rise and overflow on the approach of the relics of the saint. This is an annual ceremony, and is attended by a great concourse of people, the pressure of whose weight crowding round the well, on a yielding soil, may be the cause of the effect in question. I remember witnessing something of the kind at one of the sulphureous springs in the neighbourhood of Lixuri ; the ground close to it was spongy ; jumping on it gave motion to the water, and the well being quite full, made it run over.

In the upper part of the rich and picturesque valley of Samos, in Cephalonia, are two springs, one called Strofola, the other St Andrens. The first, in accordance with the springs of the Ionian Islands, is generally lowest in summer. The other, on the contrary, is largest in summer. I was assured on the spot, that in summer it is twice as large as in winter; that it begins to increase in May, that it continues increasing till about the first of September, when it is at its maximum, and that it afterwards diminishes. I did not examine chemically the water of either of these springs; the temperature of the former, in the month of February 1825, was 63°, that of the latter 61°; both appeared to be good spring-water. The cause of this peculiarity of the spring of St Andrens, is obscure ;—it is possible that it may be connected with the melting of the snow on the Black Mountain.

In a wild valley contiguous to that of Samos, at a higher level, is a small lake, known by the name of Abatho, signifying bottomless, which it is supposed to be by the natives. It is circular, about two hundred yards in circumference, and is surrounded by rugged hills, composed chiefly of clay, conglomerate, and sandstone. A small stream constantly flows from it, most copious in winter, which joins another small stream flowing from a similar little lake, separated by an intervening hill ; and these two streams joining, form the river of Racli, the principal perennial stream of Cephalonia.*

* This part of Cephalonia, which is little known, is very deserving of being visited ; few excursions in these islands are better fitted to gratify the traveller than that from ancient Samos to Pronos; there is much variety of scenery, and some beautiful scenery, and on the sites of the ancient cities some fine remains of Cyclopian walls. The upper part of the valley of Samos is a most pleasing specimen of cultivation ; it belongs to small proprietors—orchards, villages, vineyards, intermixed in agreeable confusion ; and in the vineyards, vines and fruit trees.

In Cerigo, in the bay of Capsali in deep water, there issues out from the limestone cliff, a copious spring of fresh water. It rises through the salt water; it is distinguishable by its different refractive power, and when the sea is perfectly calm, the fresh water may be collected tolerably pure. I visited it in the summer of 1827, in company with Mr Fletcher, civil engineer, who was examining the harbour,—employed by Government, at the recommendation of the then Lord High Commissioner, Sir Frederick Adam, with the hope of offering some plan for its improvement. If a secure harbour were formed in this bay, the spring which is now merely an object of curiosity, might become one of great utility; it might easily be made available for the purpose of watering ships.*

The valley above Pronos, and leading to it, is not unlike that of Roslin, combining beauty with a certain wildness and grandeur, walled in by mural precipices, luxuriantly wooded. And then how glorious the distant views of some of the most interesting regions of Greece which open through the vallies, or are commanded from the higher hills, looking over the lower parts of Ithaca! When I passed through the country in the beginning of February, spring had hardly commenced; the mountains of the Morea, and the more distant range of Pindus were covered with snow, as was also Mount Enos (the Black Mountain), immediately above,—the winter aspect of the heights beautifully contrasted with the verdure of the low grounds, suffused with the bright bloom of the almond tree, which here abounds.

* Owing to the great depth of water in the bay of Capsali, the result of the examination was very unfavourable to the object in view. The idea then occurred to me, which may be worth repeating, now that floating break-waters are considered practicable, that shelter might be procured,—a useful harbour formed, by a chain of large deep boats or vessels properly stationed and secured.

At Samos in Cephalonia, in the summer of 1827, the sea rose about ten feet in perpendicular height, and raised on the shore some large masses of stone, brought there for the purpose of forming a new mole on the site of the ancient mole. The weather, at the time was fine and serene, indeed so calm, that the people of the place, alarmed by the rising of the water, came into the open air with lamps in their hands; it was at night. The phenomenon was without apparent cause; nothing unusual preceded or followed,—no motion of the earth,—not the slightest shock of an earthquake was perceived. It might have been occasioned by a large quantity of subterraneous water suddenly rising in the sea. As the adjoining hills abound in caverns, and the natural drainage of the hills takes place chiefly under ground, this explanation is not improbable, especially considering that the phenomenon was entirely local, and confined to the shore of Samos. However it may be accounted for, I have thought the fact deserving of notice, and worthy of being recorded. There is much that is mysterious in the physical history of these islands, especially in connexion with the distribution of water, and too many facts on the subject cannot be collected ; one may help to illustrate another, and, ultimately, some satisfactory explanation may be afforded.

The next phenomenon I have to mention is very extraordinary, and apparently contrary to the order of nature ; it is the flowing of the water of the sea into the land, in currents or rivulets which descend and are lost in the bowels of the earth. This phenomenon occurs in Cephalonia, about a mile and a half from the town of Argostoli, near the entrance of the harbour, where the shore is composed of freestone, and is low and cavernous, from the action of the waves.

The descending streams of salt water are four in number; they flow with such rapidity, that an enterprising gentlemen, an Englishman, has erected a grist mill on one of them, with great success. I have been informed that it produces him L.300 a-year. The flow is constant, unless the mouths, through which the water enters, are obstructed by sea-weed. No noise is produced by the descent of the sea-water, and rarely is any air disengaged: the streams have been watched during earthquakes, and have not been found affected by them. It is stated that fresh water is perpetually flowing through fissures in the rock from the land into the trench which has been dug for the reception of the mill-wheel, and that when the sea-water is prevented rushing in, then the water in the trench rises higher by several inches than usual, and is brackish to the taste. The phenomenon has been long known to the natives; familiar with it, it has excited no interest in their minds, they appear hardly to have given it a thought. It is only recently that it has been brought to the knowledge of the English, within the last five or six years, and it is now become a subject of curious inquiry and speculation. The little information I have obtained respecting these extraordinary currents, I owe to my friend Dr White, surgeon of the second battalion of the Rifle Brigade; it was collected by him when stationed in the Ionian Islands, several years after my departure from them. Probably, they will soon be fully described; till then, and till they have been minutely investigated, conjectures only can be made respecting their cause.

CHAPTER V.

ON THE SPRINGS OF MALTA.

ituation of Springs. Scanty Supply of Spring Water. Dependence of most parts of the Island on Tanks, even for Agricultural Purposes. How Made and Managed. Aqueduct Supplying the Town of Valetta. Notice of its Opening. Saline Spring of Missida. Incidental Notice of the Medicinal Waters of Alexandria Troas.

MOST of the general remarks which I have made on the springs of the Ionian Islands, are applicable to those of Malta and Gozo, both in relation to geological locality, and to chemical composition.

The only parts of Malta in which springs are tolerably abundant, are those of very limited extent, where the freestone rests on marl, and which are confined chiefly to the western side of the island. In Gozo, where marl is more prevalent, there, too, springs are more widely scattered, and water is easily found by sinking pits.

Owing to the comparatively few springs in Malta, and their situation, remote from the most populous and best cultivated districts, the inhabitants, with the exception of those of the city, are principally

dependent on tanks for a supply of water, and this not
only for their own use, but even for agricultural purposes. The vast number, and the great size of the
tanks in different parts of the country, in the city, in
the villages, in the fields, is astonishing, and one of
the wonders of the island. Almost every house is
provided with a capacious tank, and a very large
number of fields are similarly provided. The tanks
are commonly in the first instance quarries. Often
the building of the house and the formation of the
cistern are simultaneous ; there is merely a transfer
of stone ; the stone cut out, beneath the surface, is
employed, not only in the construction of the walls,
but even of the roof, floor, and stairs. Covered with
a thin layer of stucco, the house is complete ; beams,
doors, and window-frames constitute the only wood-
work ; and, covered with a layer of pozzolano, the
cistern also is complete. It is a curious sight, on a
day of heavy rain, after the termination of the dry
summer, to witness, in going from one village to
another, the innumerable little embankments made
for the conducting of the water from the flooded road
into the cisterns. beneath the adjoining houses and
fields; and it is the more remarkable as the mouths
of many of the pipes and gutters leading to them, are
in the road itself, covered commonly with a stone,
which at this time is removed. I know no circumstance in detail so well adapted as this to convey
an idea of the great antiquity of Malta, as an inhabited spot, and of the vast labour that has been ex-

pended in making it habitable, in cultivating it, and
adapting it for its crowded population. Its fortifications are more impressive to the eye in their gigantic
dimensions ; but the system of tanks impresses more
the mind, reflecting that the latter are the result of
ordinary industry and foresight to meet common
wants, not of extraordinary and forced exertion on a
pressing occasion and purpose, in which all Europe
was interested.

A minute account of the manner in which Malta
is supplied with water would be curious, interesting,
and instructive ; it would show how much can be
effected by persevering industry, how much by well
directed art and science, and how these can triumph
over the greatest difficulties. The city of Valetta is
the finest example. Its site is a rocky hill, a promontory, almost a peninsula projecting into the sea,
totally destitute of springs, and in a state of nature
perfectly arid : now it abounds with water, there are
fountains in the streets, one or more cisterns under
every house, and enormous tanks belonging to the
hospitals and barracks, deriving their supply chiefly
from springs in the distant hills, conveyed by an aqueduct, many miles in length. So ample and well
managed is this supply, that the rain water which
falls on the roofs of the houses, and which might be
conducted into the cisterns, is commonly directed
into the sewers for the purpose of keeping them clean.
No one who has not been in a hot climate, and who
has not experienced the evils and misery connected

with a scarcity of water, can duly appreciate the advantages, the blessings, a plenty of it confers.*
Relative to the varieties of water in Malta, a short notice may suffice.
The springs, generally, so far as I had an opportunity of examining their water, are very uniform in composition ; such as might be expected in a calcareous country. The water of the principal aqueduct may be taken as an example. Its specific gravity, when I examined it, in July 1829, fresh from a pipe in the lower part of the town, was of specific gravity 1008, with the temperature of 73°. 100 measures of it contained four measures of air : and this air consisted of ten carbonic acid gas, sixty-two azote,

---

* The following notice of the ceremonies observed, and of the festivities on the completion of the aqueduct, and the first bringing it into use, conveys a good idea of the feeling above referred to :—

" Fu principiata l'opera come si e detto, col favor del cielo l'anno 1610 ; e continuato da un gran numero di operai, che alle volte erano più di seicento ; nè fu compiuta prima del 1615, il dì 21 d'Aprile, e terza delle sante feste di Pasqua di Resurrezione ; nel qual giorno appunto, cominciò a scorrere l'acqua nella fonte di palazzo, previa la solenne benedizione, data dal Priore della maggior chiesa conventuale di S. Giovanni, allora Monsignore Camarasa ; il quale vestito d'abiti pontificali erasi quivi portato col suo insigne Clero, procedendo colla solita sagra ordinanza, e coll'assistenza del Gran Maestro (giuliva e contento in veder compiuta felicemente l'opera da lui intrapresa) e coll' intervento de'cavalieri della Sagra Religione, e con tanto concorso di popolo, che non avea luogo bastevole in quella piazza quantunque grande. Seguirono poi molte dimostrazioni d'allegrezza con bellissime macchine di fuochi artificiale, con diversi giuochi, e corse dilettevoli, collo spargersi dal Gran Maestro varie monete alla plebe colà concorsa.—*Abela. Malta Illustrata*, lib. not. ix. p. 333.

twenty-eight oxygen.* Its saline and earthy contents were very inconsiderable, not quite $\frac{1}{5000}$ part, and consisted chiefly of carbonate of lime dissolved by carbonic acid, and of common salt, with a very little lime and magnesia, and fixed alkali, in combination with the sulphuric and muriatic acids.

The best cistern water, that which has been carefully collected from prepared surfaces of rock, or the clean terrace-roofs of houses, is necessarily very pure. Its principal foreign ingredient is carbonate of lime, derived chiefly from the surfaces on which the rain falls, and from the walls of the cisterns. Further, it is deserving of mention, that it has the freshness of spring-water,—not that peculiar insipidity which commonly belongs to rain-water, and in a higher degree to distilled water. It owes this quality, no doubt, to the air it absorbs both in its passage into, and after it has entered, the cistern. And, moreover, it has the advantage of coolness ; the principal quantity of rain falling in winter, it enters the cistern comparatively cold, at a temperature below the mean annual, and it remains cool, from the manner in which it is confined, shut up in excavations made in the solid rock.

Both Malta and Gozo are entirely destitute of sul-

---

* The air was examined by means of lime-water and phosphorus. According to the experiments of Gay Lussac and Humboldt, the air expelled from rain-water by boiling, contains thirty-two per cent. of oxygen : which may account for the large proportion of this gas in water, like that of the aqueduct mentioned above.

phureous springs. The only mineral springs I am acquainted with in the former (and I know of none in the latter), are two of a saline brackish character, near the sea, and very little above its level; one in the neighbourhood of Valetta, at Missida; the other at St Julian's, about two miles distant, to the northwest. The former is a very copious spring, perfectly clear; it gushes out, unmixed with air, and immediately forms a rivulet, the largest perennial stream in the island. On the 27th October 1833, when its temperature was 69°, its specific gravity was 1008. It contains a little less than one per cent. of saline matter; 365.2 grains of it, carefully evaporated to dryness, at a heat a little below the boiling point, yielded 3.3 grains of saline matter; 100 parts of this saline matter (procured by the evaporation of a large quantity of water) consisted of 28 parts soluble in alcohol, and of 72 insoluble. The saline ingredients were common salt, sulphate of lime, sulphate of magnesia, muriate of magnesia, hypo-sulphate of magnesia, with a trace of iodine. The water of the spring at St Julian's is nearly of the same specific gravity as the preceding, and its saline contents are very similar. The only difference I detected was the absence of hypo-sulphate of magnesia. Neither of these springs has yet been employed medicinally. Considering their composition, they are likely to possess medicinal virtues, and they may be deserving of trial in many complaints, especially in those of a scrofulous character. Hitherto the only use made of them has been in washing. The Missida spring is the great resort of washerwomen. Under the shade of a roof, supported by arches, which has been built over it, of sufficiently ample dimensions, they follow their employment by beating the clothes in the running stream; and they afterwards bleach them by exposure to the sun on the adjoining rocks. The water is considered excellent for its whitening quality, which it probably owes to its saline contents,—the deliquescent salts, and particularly to the hypo-sulphate. The former may act by retaining that degree of moisture in the clothes to be bleached, favourable to the operation; whilst the latter may have effect more directly as a chemical agent.

I may here incidentally mention, that, whilst I was at Malta, I had an opportunity of examining the water of the warm mineral spring at Alexandria Troas, through the kindness of Captain the late Sir Fleming Senhouse, R. N., and of Dr Irvine, who furnished me with specimens of it. I shall notice briefly the results of the trials I made to ascertain its composition, not aware that it has yet been submitted to experiment. The spring has considerable reputation amongst the inhabitants of that part of Asia Minor, and is much resorted to for its medicinal virtues.

Sir Fleming Senhouse found its temperature to be 150° of Fahrenheit. The specific gravity of that which I examined, was 1017. The following ingredients were detected in it, viz. common salt, muriate of lime, muriate of magnesia, carbonate of lime, carbonic acid gas, proto-carbonate of iron, silica, and a trace of manganese, bromine, and iodine. Two quarts of the water yielded about two grains of silica. The proportions of the other ingredients I did not attempt to ascertain.

These ingredients, I may remark, are in favour of the medicinal repute it has acquired. As mineral springs of the same character are rare, if they exist at all, in the upper part of the Mediterranean, it may be deserving of having public attention called to it; and now that there is some hope of a better order of things being established in the Levant, * its usefulness may be less limited, it may prove a benefit to all the surrounding countries. In complaints of debility, and in scrofulous diseases, it is likely to be efficacious, taken internally, as well as in rheumatic complaints, of a chronic character, and in some others employed as a bath.

* The above was written before visiting Constantinople; a better acquaintance with the Turkish government has diminished that hope.

CHAPTER VI.

ON THE EARTHQUAKES OF THE IONIAN ISLANDS.

Great Obscurity of the Subject. The Different Islands, and Parts of the same Island unequally affected by Earthquakes. Apparent Relation between Liability to Shocks and Geological Structure. Irregularity of Occurrence Illustrated by the Record of Observations, Phenomena, and Effects of Earthquakes. Notice of some Remarkable Shocks. Consideration of some of the Causes on which they have been supposed to depend. Conjectures on the Subject.

It is with some hesitation that I enter on this subject, being fully sensible of the obscurity in which it is involved, and of the difficulty of treating it in a useful manner. The principal object I shall keep in view will be the relation of facts, to which speculation should always be subordinate, but more especially in an inquiry such as the present, in which almost everything is uncertain, excepting the most obvious effects.

From the earliest times, it would appear that the Ionian Islands have been the scene of earthquakes, in common with a considerable extent of the adjoining continent, especially the Morea, and the low country skirting the range of Pindus, included in modern Albania.

All the islands are not equally subject to them, nor indeed is the whole of any one island. Zante and Santa Maura are the two in which they have occurred most frequently, and in which their operation has been most severely felt. Next in point of degree, as to frequency and severity, Cephalonia may be mentioned ; and after it, Corfu and Cerigo, and last of all, Paxo and Ithaca.

Of the same island, those districts appear most liable to be affected in which marl and clay abound ; as the plain of Zante, and the adjoining low hills ; the towns of Argostoli and Lixuri, and their neighbourhood, in Cephalonia, the Fort of Santa Maura, the adjoining town of Amaxaki, and the larger number of its villages, and in Corfu the district of Leftimo. On the contrary, where there is no clay or marl formation, in those districts composed of solid rock, there the phenomena of earthquakes are either unknown, or witnessed only in a very slight degree. This is remarkably the case in the mountainous tracts of Zante, Cephalonia, Ithaca, and Corfu ; tracts composed, as we have seen, of secondary limestone, and in the mountainous parts of Cerigo, composed of primary and transition rocks. This information, I believe, may be depended on. I travelled through all these islands, and visited different parts of them, and every where made inquiry on the subject; and what has just been stated was the result.

Relative to the season of the year, it would not appear that they are confined to any one in particular; —they are said, indeed, to be most common in the height of summer, and in the depth of winter, but this even is not certain, as a general rule.* The following Tables show the number of times they have been observed for a certain period, in Zante, Santa Maura, Cephalonia, and Corfu.

TABLE showing the Number of Days in each Month in which Earthquakes were perceived at Santa Maura, during the period of six years.

	1820.	1821.	1822.	1823.	1824.	1825.
January, .	...	1	2	2	...	1†
February, ⎱	...	2	1	...	1	...
March, . ⎰ ‡	...	3	...	...	1	...
April, . ⎰	...	1	...	...	...	...
May, . .	2	...	...	...	...	...
June, . .	...	...	1	1	...	...
July, . .	...	...	5	...	...	...
August, .	...	2	2	...	...	1
September,	...	1	1	1	...	...
October, .	...	...	...	...	1	...
November,	...	1	...	2	...	...
December,	1	1	...	...	...	...

This Table is formed from the meteorological jour-

* The irregularity of occurrence of earthquakes in Greece, is strongly indicated by the popular opinion respecting them ;—anciently, they were considered judgments from the gods :—in Zante, I have known an unusual frequency of them at one time, attributed to the presence of a party of French jugglers,—at another, to the absence of the Bishop.

† On the 19th of January a destructive earthquake was experienced, which laid in ruins the town of Amaxiki, and the majority of the villages of Santa Maura.

‡ In these three months there were almost continual shocks.

nal kept by the late Major Temple. The numbers,
I should remark, do not express the total number of
shocks, but the days in which an earthquake was felt;
occasionally, on the same day, several shocks, it is
stated, were experienced.

The next Table gives similar information relative
to Zante, and is formed from the meteorological
journal kept in the town of Zante by Captain Cranfield, late of the 90th regiment.

	1823.	1824.	1825.
January, .	3	1	1
February,.	2	1	1
March, .	1	1	...
April, . .	...	5	...
May, . .	...	4	...
June, .	...	1	...
July. .	...	3	...
August, .	...	11	...
September,	1	3	...
October, .	3	8	1
November,	1	13	...
December,	1	7	...

The next Table relates to the town of Corfu, and
to Argostoli in Cephalonia, and is formed from the
observations contained in the meteorological journal
appended by Mr Goodisson to his work on the Ionian

They began in February. On the 12th of that month there was
nearly a continual shaking to the 2d of April, when they de-
creased very much. Much injury was done to the soldiers' barracks
in the fortress: the troops were under the necessity of encamping in
the barrack square.

Islands, commencing 21st June, 1818, and ending 23d December, 1820.

	1818.		1819.		1820.	
	Corfu.	Cephalonia.	Corfu.	Cephalonia.	Corfu.	Cephalonia.
January,	...	...	...	1	...	...
February,	...	...	...	...	...	2
March, .	...	...	...	...	...	2
April, .	...	...	...	...	...	2
May, .	...	...	1	2	...	2
June, .	...	1	...	...	...	2
July, .	...	...	...	...	...	4
August,	...	1	...	...	...	...
September,	...	1	...	1	...	1
October,	...	...	...	1	...	...
November,	...	1	...	...	...	3
December,	...	1	...	3	...	...

The following Table shows the general results, contained in the preceding, exclusive of the year 1820, in Santa Maura, which was rather an extraordinary than an ordinary year,—especially the early part of it.

	Jan.	Feb.	Mar.	Apr.	May.	June.	July.	Aug.	Sep.	Oct.	Nov.	Dec.
Stᵃ Maura,	6	4	4	1	2	2	5	5	3	1	3	2
Zante,	5	4	2	5	4	1	3	11	4	12	14	8
Cephalonia,	1	2	2	2	5	3	4	1	3	1	4	4
Total,	12	10	8	8	11	6	12	17	10	14	21	14

Relative to the time of day,—the direction of the wind,—the kind of weather,—the pressure of the atmosphere, as indicated by the barometer,—the electrical state of the atmosphere,—not to mention other circumstances,—it appears to me very doubtful that any connexion between them and the occurrence of earthquakes can be traced in a satisfactory manner.

Aristotle was of opinion that earthquakes were more frequent by night than by day, and more severe. The following Table, drawn up with the intention of seeing how the facts accord with the opinion, is not in favour of its accuracy. It is formed from the observations contained in the meteorological journals already alluded to, in which the exact time of the occurrence of the shock, in a large number of instances, is specified.

Hour.	Shocks.	Hour.	Shocks.
6 A.M.	8	6 P.M.	1
7 ...	3	7 ...	4
8 ...	4	8 ...	5
9 ...	3	9 ...	4
10 ...	4	10 ...	5
11 ...	3	11 ...	2
12 ...	1	12 ...	4
1 P.M.	7	1 A.M.	2
2 ...	5	2 ...	4
3 ...	6	3 ...	1
4 ...	3	4 ...	4
5 ...	5	5 ...	7
12	52	12	43

Aristotle was also of opinion that when earthquakes occurred by day they were most frequent at noon, which, too, is not in accordance with the above facts.

Further, he was of opinion that they prevail most when the sky is serene. The following table contains the results of the observations bearing on this point, from which it appears, taking into consideration that the number of serene days is much the largest,—the notion does not hold good, at least in the earthquakes of the Ionian Islands,—placing against the days of serene weather those of rain or clouds, thunder and lightning, or strong wind :—

Weather.	No. of Shocks.
Serene,	34
Rain,	15 ⎫
Cloudy,	6 ⎬ 35
Strong Wind,	5 ⎪
Thunder and Lightning,	9 ⎭

By many, especially natives of the Ionian Islands, it is believed that southerly winds, particularly the sirocco, conduce to earthquakes. The following Table shows the results of observation, in connexion with the winds, which are not in accordance with the popular notion alluded to, nor favourable to the idea that the phenomena are, either directly or indirectly, associated with the course of the wind.

Number of Shocks of Earthquakes observed in Santa Maura and Zante, with different Winds, extracted from the Journals of Major Temple and Captain Cranfield.

	S.	S.E.	S.W	N.	N.E.	N.W.	E.	W.
Santa Maura, .	1	10	29	6	21	9	1	10
Zante, ...	3	6	...	7	1	2	...	...
	4	16	29	13	22	11	1	10

On the degree of pressure of the atmosphere during the earthquakes of the Ionian Islands, the observations I made were few : but they were sufficient to convince me that there was no constant relation between them. I have seen the mercury in the barometer fall considerably with a slight shock, and very little with a severe one.

Let us now consider briefly the movement and the effects of these earthquakes, with some of the phenomena accompanying them. As regards movement, they are commonly said to be of three kinds, subsultory, undulating, and vorticose. This division is founded partly on the sensations experienced, and partly on the manner in which heavy bodies have been shifted and displaced. The subsultory and the vorticose are held to be most dangerous. It is commonly stated that the earthquakes, generally, are accompanied by subterraneous sounds. I do not deny it; but I believe in many instances, the noises heard, have been more above ground than below, produced by the rattling of furniture set in motion, and the shaking of roofs, beams, and walls.*

In their effects they are very uncertain ; sometimes doing no injury to feeble buildings, and throwing

---

* By way of illustration, I shall transcribe from my note-books two instances, one which occurred at Zante, and the other in Cephalonia, the description of which was immediately written.

" Nov. 24, 1824.— This morning, between $5\frac{1}{2}$ A.M. and $8\frac{1}{2}$ A.M., there were four pretty smart shocks of earthquakes. Each shock was preceded a second or two by a rustling, or rather distant rattling noise ; it appeared to come from the southward, and was similar to that heard when the shock was felt, only less loud, more low and obtuse, as it were from a distance. The sensation from the shock was as if the house were seized by a gigantic being, and shaken forward and backward laterally. The noise accompanying the shock was produced by the furniture, &c., being set in motion.

" Besides the smart shocks, there were several very slight ones, as

down the strong,—the one in the immediate neighbourhood of the other; sometimes greatly injuring one side of a street, and sparing the opposite side; instances of which, in Zante, have been described to me by eye-witnesses. Their operation appears to be chiefly displayed on the works of man, which are resting only on the surface. Occasionally, indeed, the ground has been fissured, and portions of hills and cliffs thrown down; but these are rare occurrences.*

I am not aware of any instance in which any change of level, either by elevation of ground, or depression to any extent, has been produced; nor have I ever heard of any such throughout the Ionian Islands. The channels of water are sometimes affected, and the sources of springs, which is in accordance with the accidents of fissures alluded to.

When treating on the rocks of these islands and

it were tremors, which would not have been perceived, unless the attention had been directed to the subject. Such tremors are very common here."

"*Argostoli,* January 2, 1825.—This morning, when I was sitting with the Resident, an earthquake occurred. It lasted several seconds. It was preceded by no noise, and it was attended by no noise, excepting that made by the furniture in motion. The house was thrown into an undulatory motion, which was very sensible to the eye as well as to the feeling,—reminding one of the agitation of a ship in a cross sea, where the waves are only moderately high."

* The double-headed hill of clay, above the town of Zante, according to tradition, was divided by an earthquake in 1514; that which is now lowest, having separated and fallen. In the neighbourhood of Samos, in Cephalonia, on the way to Racli, are some fissured chasms in a horizontal bed of freestone, said to have been produced by an earthquake.

their springs, it was observed, that nowhere were there any traces of volcanic eruption or action, nor any vestiges even of trap-rocks, and no warm springs: I may add here, that during earthquakes, on no occasion, so far as I have been able to learn, has there been any appearance of the evolution of gas or vapour, or of the emission of flame or fire, or any elevation of temperature. The majority of earthquakes are slight, and do little harm. During the last half century, only four destructive earthquakes have occurred throughout the whole of the Ionian Islands, three of which were in Zante, and one in Santa Maura. In further illustration of the subject I shall briefly notice them.*

Of those in Zante, the first occurred on the 2d of November, 1791, at nine o'clock at night. A great part of the city was thrown down, or materially injured, as were also many of the adjoining villages below the mountainous district. Thirty persons only were killed; very many were wounded. The shock is described as having lasted about half-a-minute,—to have been preceded by a loud noise from the sea

---

* According to the researches of Count Paolo Mercati, the most remarkable earthquakes which have occurred in Zante in modern times, happened in 1514, 1593, 1664, 1710, 1742, 1743, 1767, 1791, 1809, and 1810. From a brief chronicle in the Royal Library at Paris, it appears that the earthquake of 1514, rent the Castle-hill from the top to the bottom, and threw down a part of it, which overwhelmed and buried a portion of the ancient city.—*Vide Saggio Storico Statistico della Città ed Isola di Zante compilato dal Co. Paolo Mercati nell' anno* 1811.

(*spaventoso muggito*) after a calm, in the morning following a storm. On this occasion, the buildings within the fortress, on the summit of the Castle-hill, suffered peculiarly, and especially the magazine, which was bomb-proof, and distinguished for solidity and strength of construction. The shock was sensibly felt at sea, and on the opposite shore of the Morea, where some houses were thrown down; and yet was very slightly felt in the mountainous part of Zante, and in some places there, not at all. These particulars I have extracted from a letter addressed by a nobleman residing at Zante to his friend in Corfu, written just after the catastrophe, with a trembling hand, and with a feeling of affright so powerful, that he was almost sceptical of his proper existence. " Io vivo, ma dubito ancora della mia esistenza, come egualmente vivono, e pur ne dubitano questi abitanti in generale, preservati dalla tomba per miracolo della Divina Providenza." He adds in the sequel, that it would be impossible to describe the terror produced at the time, and consequent on the calamity,—" the cries of women and children, the common lamentation, the misery expressed in every one's face, the implorings for help, the religious processions by day and by night, the severe fasts, the public prayers, the universal mourning."

The second occurred in 1821, on 29th December, the festa of the patron Saint of Zante, St Dionysius, at four o'clock in the morning.

A threatening state of atmosphere preceded it on

the 28th, when the barometer is stated to have been very little above 27 inches, the sky overcast, the wind southerly and gentle. A native writer, whose account of the catastrophe in manuscript I have consulted, opens his description with contrasting the melancholy aspect of the heavens on the eve of their saint's day, with the cheerful and serene countenances of the inhabitants, engaged in doing honour to his name.

The shock was succeeded, in the course of the same day, by many more, less severe, and by a violent storm of thunder and lightning, hail and rain. Some of the hailstones, it is said, weighed four ounces. This storm was followed at night by a deluge of rain (*un vero diluvio*), and for several successive days, by stormy weather, with heavy rains and frequent shocks of earthquakes. The loss of life was inconsiderable; only five persons were killed in the city by the falling of houses, and two drowned by the torrent which rushed through the streets. The damage to the buildings was great; the writer already referred to, says, the town had all the appearance of a dismantled and bombarded city; seventy-nine houses were entirely thrown down, and 100 considerably injured,— and he adds, that it would be difficult to find, out of the 4000 composing the town, a single one nowise damaged. The principal shock was felt over the greater part of the island, and in the villages situated low, it was more or less destructive; whilst the villages amongst the mountains escaped uninjured. It was felt at sea, as far as the Strophades, which are about fifty miles from Zante; a ship passing these islets felt it severely.

The third, of recent occurrence, took place on the 30th of October, 1840. It is well described by the then Lord High Commissioner, Sir Howard Douglas, in his despatches to her Majesty's government, relative to the event, parts of which have been printed by order of the House of Commons. I shall give some extracts, which, written in the midst of the catastrophe, portray, in a lively and forcible manner, both its ruinous effects, and the impression of alarm and terror produced on the minds of the inhabitants.

Writing from Zante, on the 6th of November, Sir Howard Douglas states, " I arrived on the morning of the 30th ultimo, half an hour after the occurrence of a dreadful calamity, which has irreparably injured the whole town and island. At half-past nine o'clock on that morning, when about three miles from the land, an extraordinary concussion was suddenly experienced, agitating violently the vessel and the machinery, and which it was quite evident was occasioned by an earthquake. The reality of this apprehension was immediately confirmed by the noises that were heard, and by several clouds of dust which were seen ascending from various points of the coast, and which were occasioned by the falling in of cliffs, and other effects of a violent shock. On approaching the port, the effects upon the buildings of the town were plainly visible. Several houses in the outskirts greatly injured; part of the prison unroofed, the body of the building cracked, and one of the outer walls thrown down. Onwards the ruins appeared more numerous; and, when we arrived in the port, so as to have a near view of the whole town, I perceived that a terrible and general calamity had fallen upon Zante.

" On proceeding through the streets, I found them filled or encumbered with ruins; the bulk of the population still out of doors; the tiles, and the shaken and disunited portions of houses fallen, or ready to fall; very few of the houses, not even those most solidly built, had escaped external and apparent injury; and, even where such was not visible, had suffered greatly internally in their furniture by the concussion.

" The consternation of the inhabitants was extreme; for I had scarcely entered the town when a considerable shock was felt, the dismay and confusion occasioned by which, it is impossible for me to describe; and, as I proceeded through the streets, constant successions of minor shocks were felt, which continued for many days ; and here I may add, in order to show your lordship how incessant has been the alarm and consternation, that, up to the 4th instant, ninety-five shocks of earthquakes, some very severe, were counted since the first great crash.

" I regret to acquaint your lordship that the devastation is still more general in the country than in the city, and that the distress is, and will be, infinitely greater; and the means of the inhabitants whose huts and houses have so generally been destroyed or injured, afford little or no resources for them to fall back upon."

Sir Howard Douglas mentions the villages which he visited, all of them on, or bordering on, the plain, and all of which he found had suffered more or less. They were the following :—Litakia, Pisimonda, Musaki, Romiri, Lagopado, Melinado, Bujato, Makirado, Pigadakia, and Catastari, which had suffered slightly; Sottiro, St Demetrio, Karkiesi, Draka, and Sculikado, which had suffered severely, the last named most of all. The state in which it was found is described in the following extract :—

" I then proceeded to Sculikado, and there I witnessed a scene of desolation and ruin, of consternation and misery, far exceeding any I had previously seen in the course of these visits, and I may well add in the whole course of my life. This village, containing a population of about 800 persons, is nothing but a heap of ruins; not a house untouched, and very few left standing. In all the other villages, even those most injured, there is covering left, which will enable the more fortunate to show their hospitality and feeling for their unfortunate neighbours, by giving them shelter; but here in Sculikado there is no shelter left. The site of the village is on a small hill, no part of the surface of which is free from ruins. The furniture, the beds, buried in the ruins of the houses; the devastation is so great that no parts of the fabric, in the shape of planks, are in a state to form fresh cover. I noted the cases of utter destitution; they are numerous. I intimated to those who had some resources of property, though at present none in ready money, that they might seek relief, in the shape of loan, out of the sum decreed by the senate ; and I acquainted the Capo that, if they would send to the town a sufficient number of horses to carry out seven or eight hundred planks for the use of the destitute, and to form covering for them, I would direct that these should be supplied gratuitously. This has been done ; and small sums of money have, by my directions, been dispensed to the most destitute for immediate necessities, and to enable them to get shelter put together, should their fellow-townsmen either refuse to labour for them gratuitously, or be too much involved in distress themselves to assist them."

Sir Howard Douglas, referring to the amount of injury occasioned, states,—" The material injury which the Island of Zante sustained is extensive, and cannot be rated at less than £300,000 sterling." No notice is taken of any damage occasioned in the mountain villages ; from whence it may be inferred that, as heretofore, they escaped the destructive effect of the shock.

The destructive earthquake in Santa Maura occurred on the 19th January, 1825, about noon. The greater part of the Fort and of the town of Amaxiki were reduced to ruins, as were also the majority of the villages throughout the island. Fifty-eight persons were killed by the falling of buildings, and ninety-two were wounded, seven of whom died of their wounds. The weather, both preceding the catastrophe and follow-ing it, was unsettled, and showery, and overcast, with a southerly wind. At Argostoli, where I was at the time, and where a severe shock, lasting near a minute, was felt about the same time,—the barometer fell a very little. At nine o'clock in the morning it was observed at 30.153; at twenty minutes after the earthquake, at 30.100. It was felt also about the same time in parts of Corfu, Ithaca, and Zante; its de-structive effects were confined to Santa Maura. About six weeks after the event, I visited Santa Maura, and made a tour of the island; and I can bear witness to the extent of its destructive operation. Referring to the notes which I made at the time, it appears, how-ever, that the different villages suffered in very dif-ferent degrees, and that two escaped injury entirely, the villages of Attani and Frini, both standing on limestone rock.*

Whilst the catastrophe was fresh in the recollec-tion of every one, I made minute inquiry relative to the circumstances attending it. I could not learn that any thing extraordinary either preceded, or accompanied, or followed it;—nothing indicative of the cause by which it was produced.

This part of the subject, the agency on which

---

* The village of Frini is about a mile from the town of Amaxiki. The ridge of secondary limestone on which it stands may rise about six hundred feet above the plain; it has very much the character of a mural precipice, formed of thick strata, perpendicular or approach-ing thereto, gradually tapering to the sea-shore.

earthquakes depend, is now almost universally admitted to be exceedingly obscure and difficult, especially in the instances, such as those of the Ionian Islands, which are not coincident with volcanic eruption, nor associated with phenomena indicative of suppressed volcanic action.

Electricity, by some inquirers, has been referred to as a cause of earthquakes. But the proofs of the operation of such a cause appear to be entirely wanting. What relation is there between the shock of an earthquake and an electrical shock? Who ever, during an earthquake, witnessed distinct electrical effects, excepting of the thunder-storm, which no one, I suppose, who reasons on the subject, will hold to be otherwise than accidental?

We are told by Aristotle that Anaximenes attributed earthquakes to excessive dryness and to excessive moisture, and that Democritus referred them to water penetrating into the earth.* If clay or marl is associated with these circumstances, are they not tolerably adequate to account for the phenomena, such as they present themselves in these regions; and especially if changes of temperature be called in as an auxiliary? The little compressibility of water; the relations of clay to water; the expansion of the earth from the excess of the fluid; its contraction from deficiency, as in drying,—are obvious qualities in favour of the views of the old Greek philosophers. Moist clay, which has been pressed between bibulous

* Meteorologicorum, cap. vii. viii., lib. ii.

paper, on being thoroughly dried, at a temperature below 212°, loses about thirty-three per cent., still, of course, retaining the proportion which constitutes it a hydrate. Now, may not the contraction connected with such a loss in a considerable mass or surface be adequate to the effect in question? And also, may not the absorption of so much water be likewise adequate to it?* And as moist clay is little permeable to water, and has the remarkable property of confining it, may not the admission of water between strata of clay have also an effect of the kind? In the hydraulic press its power is strongly exemplified. In the shrinking and cracking of wood from excessive dryness, we have a familiar instance of the operation of loss of water ; and in the cracking of glass from changes of temperature we have also an instance of an effect from this cause, analogous to that, which we are considering.

These conjectures I venture to throw out merely in relation to such earthquakes, as those of the Ionian

* It is universally known that when marl is thrown into water, this fluid is rapidly absorbed, and that the marl apparently expands and falls to powder. From the results of some experiments which I have made, I am disposed to believe that the expansion in this instance is not merely apparent, but is real. This appeared to be indicated by making the experiments in a vessel with a syphon-gauge attached to it, capable of showing very slight changes of pressure. After the admission of water by a stopcock to the marl, in the act of its falling to powder, a slight movement was perceived in the column of fluid in the gauge, indicative of a little increase of pressure ; and, from other trials, I had reason to infer that it was not owing to any change of temperature ; no heat appeared to be evolved.

Islands, of limited extent as regards the field of their operation, and of comparatively feeble effect, very different from those grand catastrophes which have desolated whole provinces, and have been felt over many thousand miles of the earth's surface, the causes of which are at present hid in complete darkness, as if to humble the pride of intellect and the reasoning powers of man.

CHAPTER VII.

ON THE TEMPERATURE OF THE MEDITERRANEAN SEA,
AND ON THE SPECIFIC GRAVITY OF ITS WATER.

Many Peculiarities of the Mediterranean, opening a wide field for Research. Results of Experiments on the Specific Gravity of its Water. Observations on its Temperature at different Seasons. Conjecture relative to the use of the Thermometer for determining its Currents. Observations on the Degree of Moisture of its Atmosphere. Reflections on the Proportional Saltness of this Sea. Conjectures on the same.

I KNOW no sea that presents so wide a field of research as the Mediterranean; that offers so many unsolved problems to the curious inquirer, and that has within it and around it so many circumstances of great and general interest. What a contrast between its shores, whether we consider them with a view to their physical or political condition; what a contrast between those of Africa and of Europe, between those of Europe and Asia. How remarkable and contrasted are the different islands; many of them, a large proportion, volcanic; many of them of an opposite nature, formed by deposition from water; all historically so ancient, that is, connected with the history of man; and yet the majority of them, in relation to the history of the globe, of most recent formation. Then,

the streams which flow into it, and supply its waste,—
they may well be mentioned as peculiar, and offering
further examples of contrast, as the comparatively
cold stream of the Hellespont, and the warm Nile;
the one a salt river, not differing very much in saltness from the almost perpetual current that pours in
from the Atlantic; the other differing very little in
quality from distilled water. Nor are its winds less
remarkable and contrasted, comparing the qualities
of the northerly with the southerly, the Sirocco with
the Etesian. Indeed, it is difficult to say where the
marvels of contrast cease; equally in the animal and
vegetable kingdom they are exhibited; the flying-
fish is seen in its waters; many of the birds of the far
north are its visitors; almost all its birds, and many
of its fishes, are migratory; the finest vegetable productions of its shores and islands, there is reason to
believe, were once exotics.

Of the problems which may be considered unsolved,
one, and not the least important, is the density of its
water at different depths; and connected with this,
its temperature at different seasons, the quantity of
water it loses by evaporation, and of salt water by
out-flowing currents,—the quantity of water which it
gains in the form of rains, and by rivers, and of salt
water by in-flowing currents. Could precise information be obtained on all these questions, there would
be little difficulty in solving the problem referred
to. Such information as I have been able to collect,
I shall give without hesitation, merely as an imper-

fect and very partial contribution, with the hope that it may have the effect of leading to further inquiry, and of promoting research; and I have an additional motive in making the offering, in consideration that some of the points of inquiry mentioned, are intimately connected with, and well adapted to throw light on, the climate of the Ionian Islands and of Malta (which will afterwards be treated of), as well as of the Mediterranean generally, and of its shores.

First, of the specific gravity of the water of the Mediterranean at its surface. On this subject I have made a considerable number of experiments. The specimens of water which I have examined, I have either collected myself, in passing from one part of the Mediterranean to another, in voyages undertaken at different seasons, or have been indebted for them to the kindness of individuals, on whose accuracy I could place reliance. The water has always been carefully preserved, in a manner to prevent evaporation; and on each different occasion, its weight has been compared with that of the same bulk of distilled water, by trial at the moment, both to ensure greater accuracy, and to obviate the necessity of correction for difference of temperature.

I shall give the results in a tabular form :—

I.—SPECIFIC GRAVITY OF SURFACE-WATER OF THE LOWER PARTS OF
THE MEDITERRANEAN, BETWEEN GIBRALTAR AND MALTA.

No.	Sp. Grav.	Situation.	Time.	
1	10273	About three miles off Tariffa, in the Strait of Gibraltar,	May 22,	1824.
2	10271	Lat. 37° 17′, off Carthagena,	25,	...
3	10281	37 22, Long. 9° E. .	June 3,	...
4	10271	37 22, 11 50, .	5,	...
5	10286	On the Sicilian coast, about a quarter of a mile off Augusta, . . .	September 6,	1826.
6	10309	Between Sicily and Malta, about ten miles from the latter,	8,	..
7	10309	Quarantine Harbour, Malta, in fourteen fathoms water,	8,	...
8	10287	About forty yards from Graham Island—the volcano in activity, .		
9	10287	About three miles from Graham Island, . . .		
10	10287	About three miles from Cape Bianco, in the neighbourhood of Girgenti, .	August,	1831.
11	10287	Between Girgenti and Gozo,		
12	10287	About a mile off Gozo, .		
13	10280	Off the Island of Galita, .	April 28,	1837.
14	10290	Off Cape Passero, . .	19,	...

II.—OF THE UPPER PART OF THE MEDITERRANEAN TO THE NORTHWARD AND EASTWARD OF MALTA.

No.	Sp. Grav.	Situation.	Time.
1	10286	Off Cape Spartevento, .	August 31, 1826.
2	10286	Between Cape Bianco, Corfu, and Paxo, . . .	29, ...
3	10288	Lat. 38° 20′; Long. 20° E. Off Cephalonia, . .	November 3, 1831.
4	10280	Between Paxo and Parga, .	April 7, 1826.
5	10280	Off Cape Ducato, Santa Maura,	7, ...
6	10280	Between Calamos and Castus,	6, ...
7	10292	Outside the mole of Zante, .	July 12, 1824
8	10289	Do. Do. Do.	March 14, 1826.
9	10289	About three miles off Point Skenari, Zante, . .	18, ...
10	10290	Entrance of Port Timone, Corfu,	August, 1825.
11	10487	Harbour of Asso, Cephalonia,	July, ...
12	10297	About three miles off Cape Scala, Cephalonia, . .	May 31, 1826.
13	10297	About three quarters of a mile off Asso, Cephalonia, .	7, ...
14	10289	About three quarters of a mile off Port Fiscardi, Cephalonia,	June 9, ...
15	10240	North of the Port of St Euphemia, Cephalonia, about a mile from land, . .	10, ...
16	10279	Close to the town of Argostoli, Cephalonia, .	January 11, ...
17	10303	About two miles off Cape Troy, out of the current of the Dardanelles, . .	16, ...
18	10300	About two miles to the southward of Mytelene, .	16, ...
19	10290	Between Negropont and Andros,	February 26, ...
20	10289	Lat. 39° 21′ Long. 25° 37′	July 26, 1833.
21	10292	39 54 26 8	... ...
22	10298	39 08 25 29	... ...
23	10297	38 45 25 04	... ...
24	10289	37 55 24 34	... ...
25	10294	37 35 24	... ...
26	10289	37 24 23 33	... ...
27	10294	36 03 30 20	... ...
28	10300	35 06 34 38	... ...
29	10300	33 43 34 16	... ...

III.—OF THE HELLESPONT AND THE SEA OF MARMORA.

No.	Sp. Grav.	Situation.	Time.	
1	10220	One quarter of a mile from the outer castle, on the European side of the Hellespont, where the current is strong, . . .	March,	1826.
2	10231	One half mile from the White Cliff, on the Asiatic side of the Hellespont, where there is little or no current, .	...	...
3	10193	Mid-channel between Galipoli and Lamsaki, . .	...	...
4	10201	Centre of basin, about two miles above the town of the Dardanelles, . . .	...	...
5	10190	About three miles from the north end of the Isle of Marmora, . . .	...	...
6	10190	About a mile southward of the Seraglio Point, . .	...	...

IV.—OF THE ADRIATIC GULF.

No.	Sp. Grav.	Situation.	Time.	
1	10242	About three miles off Ancona,	April 16,	1826.
2	10278	Off Genlia Nova, . .	...	...
3	10278	Off Manfredonia, . .	April 13,	...
4	10280	Off Lissa, . . .	...	...
5	10280	Off Brindizie, about 20 miles,	April 12,	...
6	10280	Between Cape Linguetta and Fano—Lat. 40° 6′, Long. 19° 20′, . . .	April 10,	...

These results show great variety in the specific gravity of the water of the Mediterranean at the surface, depending, no doubt, on local causes. The low specific gravity of the water of the Hellespont and of the upper part of the Adriatic is what might be expected, taking into account the large quantities of fresh water poured into the Black Sea and the Adriatic by rivers. The low specific gravity (No. 15) of the sea-water off the mouth of the port of St Euphemia, in Cephalonia, is probably owing to fountains of fresh water there bursting through the bed of the sea, similar to those which appear on the shore, already noticed, nearer Samos, on the same coast. And in favour of this conjecture it may be mentioned, that the extensive valley, at the mouth of which St Euphemia is situated, is without any perennial stream, and is, indeed, remarkably dry, as if the greater part of the rain which falls there were carried off by subterraneous chasms.* The high specific gravity of the water (No 11) off the harbour of Asso, in Cephalonia, taken up in the month of July, may be partly connected with the great aridity of the adjoining very lofty and precipitous shores, and partly to an unusual degree of evaporation of water in summer from the sea washing such a coast, well adapted to absorb and radiate heat, and to present an extensive surface in its rocks, on which the waves are perpetually breaking, for the formation of brine.

Considering the results generally, they seem to indicate a somewhat higher degree of density in the

---

* Occasionally, after very heavy rains, a destructive torrent descends through this valley, the traces of which, in water-worn stones, are very manifest along its course. When I passed through the valley in the latter part of the winter of 1825, the bed of the torrent was dry, though a good deal of rain had fallen about that time, and was then falling.

water of the Mediterranean at the surface than in that of the Atlantic. But the examination of the specific gravity of the water, both of the Atlantic and of the Mediterranean, has not yet been sufficiently extended to allow of arriving at a positive conclusion. I am disposed to think, that if there be a difference, it is small, much less than has been commonly supposed. For comparison, I shall insert here a Table, showing the specific gravity of sea-water, taken up during a voyage from Ceylon to England in 1820, ascertained by me with much care, and with an excellent balance, after the conclusion of the voyage.

No.	Sp. Grav.	Situation.			Time.
1	102667	Lat 30° 6' S.	Long. 11° 42' E.		April 21.
2	102671	26 55	7	3	24.
3	102667	6 N.	19	17 W.	May 17.
4	102671	9 1	25	8	21.
5	102671	12 6	28	28	23.
6	102762	15 56	32	38	25.
7	102762	18 15	34	6	26.
8	102762	20 55	35	49	27.
9	102823	23 27	37	8	28.
10	102823	28 1	37	57	30.
11	102762	31 8	38	27	June 1.
12	102823	34 8	37	57	4.
13	102762	42 10	30	36	8.
14	102721	44 51	26	37	10.
15	102721	47 5	14	12	17.
16	102721	49 3	8	1	19.
17	102648	Off Dover half-a mile,	.	.	22.

On the specific gravity of the water of the Mediterranean at different depths I have had very few opportunities of collecting additional information. The results of the small number of experiments I have made on water taken up from sixty to three hundred fathoms, have not shown any marked augmentation of density with the increasing depth. This accords with the results of Dr Wollaston's trials on two specimens of water of this sea, one from a depth of 450 fathoms, the other from 400 fathoms. Whether, at a very great depth, there is an augmentation of density remains to be ascertained. In one instance, water taken from a depth of 670 fathoms, in lat. 36°, long. 4° 40′ W., was found by the same inquirer to be of the high specific gravity, 1.1288.* As a solitary instance, however interesting, no general conclusion can be drawn from it with any confidence. As there are springs of fresh water in the sea, so there may also be brine springs; and the water in question, so strongly charged with saline matter, may have been obtained from such a source. It is to be hoped that so important a problem will not long remain unsolved; half-a-dozen specimens of water, brought up from such a depth, in different parts of the Mediterranean, well authenticated, would be amply sufficient, carefully examined, to set the question at rest. The great difficulty is in procuring water from so great a depth; even if provided with the proper apparatus, it is not practicable without the aid of a large number of men, and can hardly be accomplished, excepting in a man-of-war. In her Majesty's naval service, men of science now, happily, are not wanting, and to them we must look for the solution of this problem, whe-

* Phil. Trans., 1829, p. 31.

ther there is a stratum of brine in the depths of the Mediterranean; and whether it is probable that strata of rock-salt are now in the act of forming on its bed.

The temperature of the Mediterranean Sea is well deserving of attention, not only in connexion with the preceding subject, but also, and in a higher degree, in connexion with the Mediterranean climate. The observations I have been able to collect on it are not so numerous nor so continuous as I could wish, being chiefly confined to those which I have myself made when at sea, in passage from one port to another. I shall introduce them, not so much in the order of the time when they were made, as of the season, in relation to which they have a peculiar value. The temperature of the water was ascertained by placing a delicate thermometer, with an exposed bulb, into a bucket full of water, the instant it was drawn up from the sea. The temperature of the air was ascertained at the same time by a dry thermometer, exposed to the wind in the shade.

To prevent confusion, I shall place the broken series of observations under the different heads of the voyages in which they were made, and affix a slight notice of the weather and of the season.

VOYAGE FROM THE DARDANELLES TO ZANTE.—1826.

Situation.	Time.		Water.	Air.
In mid channel, off the White Cliffs,*	Feb. 24	2 P.M.	47.5	44
Entrance of the Hellespont, .	...	3	47	
Ægæan, about a mile from the entrance, ...	...	3½	49	
About five miles off the hummock, called the tomb of Antilochus,	...	3¾	52.5	
Midway between Cape Troy and Tenedos, ...	...	4	55	
Between Alexandria-Troas and the western extremity of Tenedos, ...	...	5½	55	
About ten miles northward of Ipsara, ...	25	8 A.M.	58	48
About fifteen miles northward of Andros, . . .	26	3 P.M.	57.5	56
Mid channel between Negropont and Andros, . . .		8	55	
Between Sirfo and Milo, .	27	8 A.M.	58	55
About twenty miles westward of Cape Matapan, . . .	March 1	10	60	54
About ten miles off Point Vasilico, (Zante), ...	2	8	60	52

The winter of 1826 in the Levant was unusually cold and tempestuous; northerly gales were prevalent. In February, at the town of the Dardanelles, the thermometer for several days was below the freezing point; on the 9th of that month, at 8 A.M., it was so low as 22°; and on the 16th, when I crossed the Mender, the ancient Scamander, near Coomcallè,

* These cliffs on the Asiatic shore of the Hellespont, have the appearance of chalk cliffs. The chalk-like material is a mixture of carbonate of lime and of magnesia. Silicious nodules in layers occur in them, of a quality intermediate between flint and chalcedony.

the greater part of that river, which was then of considerable size, was covered with ice.

FROM CORFU TO MALTA.—1828.

Situation.	Time.			Water.	Air.
Lat. 37° 11', Long. 17° 17', E.	March 3	12	M.	57	52
36 13 16 20,	9	12		57.5	52
About fifteen miles off Valetta,					
(Malta), ...	10	5	P.M.	57	57
About three miles from Valetta,	11	8	A.M.	57	57
In the Harbour of Valetta, .	...	12	M.	58	57

The weather during the voyage was boisterous; the winds chiefly northerly; the previous winter was cold, generally so in the Mediterranean, and especially in the Ionian Islands; at Corfu the temperature was several times below the freezing point. On the 9th of January a good deal of ice was collected in the neighbourhood of the town of Corfu, and brought in for use.

FROM MALTA TO MESSINA IN SICILY.—1829.

Situation.	Time.			Water.	Air.
Off Scalletta, ...	March 11	1	P.M.	57	60
Off Messina in mid channel, .	12	8	A.M.	56	57
Off the Faro, in shallower water,	...	10		55	54

The weather at the time was moderate; the preceding winter had been cold, especially the month of February in Malta; ice even had been seen there.

FROM ANCONA TO CORFU.—1827.

Situation.	Time.			Water.	Air.
At the mouth of the harbour of Ancona, ...	March 14	12	M.	52	60
About four miles off the Isle of Tremote, on the Apulian shore,	15	5	P.M.	54	54
At anchor in a little bay of the Isle of Curzola, . . .	16	3		55	47
Off Melita, about three miles,	17	5		56	45
At anchor in the channel of Curzola, ...	18	7	A.M.	56	45
Between Malada and Terra di Ragusa, ...	21	12	M.	55	51
Off Buda, about twenty miles,	22	12		57.5	56
A little to the eastward of Buda,	23	12		53	56
At the entrance of the Gulf of Ludrino, ...	24	12		57	57
About six miles off the headland of Durazzo, ...	25	12		57.5	59
At anchor in shallow water, close to the fortress of Durazzo, .	26	12		58	59
Between the Island of Fano and the Albanian shore, . .	27	12		56	40
In the channel of Corfu, .	...	4	P.M.	58	40

The weather during this voyage was boisterous; the wind was from different quarters, often violent, but without rain. The winter was unusually cold; the greater part of Italy, in the month of February, was covered with snow.

FROM MARSEILLES TO MALTA.—1830.

Situation.	Time.			Water.	Air.
In the harbour of Marseilles, about 100 yards from the Castle, at anchor, ...	April 22	12	M.	60	67
Lat. 41° 41 Long. 6° 35′ E.	23	10	A.M.	59	59
41 5 7 31 ...	24	12	M.	61	64
40 14 7 52 ...	25	12		63	62
38 9 20 ...	26	12		61	62
About fifteen miles to the westward of Pantalaria, . . .	27	12		62	61
Off Gozo about three miles, .	28	12		62	58

The weather during this voyage was moderate; the winds variable; the preceding winter had been severe, especially in the south of Europe.

FROM ENGLAND TO MALTA AND THE IONIAN ISLANDS.—1824.

Situation.	Time.		Water.	Air.
At the entrance of the Strait of Gibraltar, . . .	May 22,	6 A.M.	64	60
About two leagues within the Strait, ...	...	8	64	59
About three miles off Tariffa,	...	9	64	59
Off the Neutral ground, about six miles, . . .	...	12 M.	64	62
	...	2 P.M.	62	63
Course east, at the rate of about seven miles an hour, .	...	4	62	62
	...	6	63	62
	...	7	63	62
Lat. 36° 27′ Long. 2° W.	May 23,	12 M.	62	64
37 8 0 20′ W.	24,	2 P.M.	64	64
37 17	25,	12 M.	66	63
37 35 0 20 E.	26,	11 A.M.	65	66
37 46 0 20	27,	12 M.	65	66
38 10 0 40	28,	12	65	66
38 16 1 0	29,	12	65.5	66
38 24 1 40	30,	12	65.5	66
38 0 2 20	31,	12	66	67
38 14 4 10	June 1,	12	66	65
38 32 6 10	2,	12	65.5	65
38 25 9 0	3,	12	64.5	65
37 45 10 0	4,	12	65	63.5
37 23 11 20	5,	12	65	66
37 22 11 50	6,	12	65	66
36 30 13 10	7,	12	66.5	67
36 5 13 35	8,	12	67	69
About two leagues off Gozo, .	9,	12	66	66
About one mile off Gozo, .	...	4 P.M.	68	71
About one mile off Comino, .	...	6	68	70
In the great harbour of Valetta,	11,	4 A.M.	70	63
Lat. 35° 47′ Long. 16° 10′	20,	8	70	71
35 37 16 50	21,	8	69	73
36 57 18 40	22,	8	71	71
38 27 20 15	23,	8	70	69
About eight miles off Fano,	24,	5	70.5	69
Between Corfu and the Albanian shore, ...	...	4 P.M.	70	73
Between Cape Bianco, Corfu, and the Albanian shore, .	July 2,	6	75	75
Between Paxo and the mainland,	3,	8 A.M.	72	72.5
Off Santa Maura, . .	...	12 M.	72	72
Off the harbour of Argostoli (Cephalonia), . . .	...	7 P.M.	71	71
Off the western extremity of Zante,	4,	8 A.M.	72.5	74
At anchor in the bay of Zante, about a quarter of a mile from the town, in seven fathoms water, ...	...	7 P.M.	75	80

During this voyage the weather was moderate; the winds variable. The preceding winter had been mild.

FROM MARSEILLES TO MALTA.—1829.

Situation.	Time.			Water.	Air.
Lat. 42° 22′ Long. 6° 3′ E.*	June 20,	12	M.	63°	66°
41 40 7 30	21,	12		65	68
40 24 7 42	22,	12		68	71
39 43 7 50	23,	12		68	70
38 25 8 29	24,	12		69	70
37 40 9 10	25.	12		70	71
About 15 miles off Cape Farina, on the African coast, .	26,	12		72	71
Close to the island of Pantalerea,	27,	6	A.M.	71	70
About four miles to the southward of it, ...	...	12	M	76	75
About 15 miles to the S.E. of it,	...	7	P.M.	75	73
Off Gozo about one mile, .	28	7		74	74

The weather during the voyage was fine; the winds favourable.

FROM CORFU TO CERIGO.—1827.

Situation.	Time.			Water.	Air.
Between Corfu and the Albanian shore, ...	June 27,	7	P.M.	75°	74°
Between Antipaxo and the mainland, ...	28,	7	A.M.	72	69
About 10 miles off Santa Maura,	...	12	M.	73	72
Between Ithaca and Cephalonia,	...	6	P.M.	74	74
Between the Strophades and the Morea, ...	29,	8	A.M.	73	72
Off Coron, about 15 miles, .	...	6	P.M.	70	73
Off Cape Matapan, . .	30,	7	A.M.	69.5	72
Between Cape Matapan and Cerigo, . . .	...	12	M.	70	74
About a mile from Capsali (Cerigo),	...	6	P.M.	72	73

* By dead-reckoning.

During this voyage the weather was fine.

FROM CORFU TO CEPHALONIA.—1827.

Situation.	Time.	Water.	Air.
About five miles off Amaxiki, Santa Maura, ...	Aug. 21, 12 M.	80°	84°
About six miles off Asso (Cephalonia), ...	22, 10 A.M.	80.5	785.

FROM CORFU TO MALTA.—1826.

Situation.	Time.	Water.	Air.
Between Corfu and the Albanian shore, ...	Aug. 29, 12 M.	77°	78°
Between Cape Bianco and Paxo,	... 6 P.M.	76	75
About 100 miles from Corfu,*	31, 12 M.	78	77
About half-way between Corfu and Sicily, ...	Sept. 1, 12 M.	82	79
Off Cape Spartivento, . .	2, 6 P.M.	79	78.5
About 20 miles off Catania, .	5, 12 M.	79	80
About three miles off Augusta,	6, 12	77	80
About seven miles to the southward of Cape Porca, .	... 6 P.M.	80	78
About seven miles southward of Cape Passaro, . .	7, 10 A.M.	79	80
About one mile off Petsali, .	... 2 P.M.	74	7 7
About 35 miles from Malta, just visible, ...	... 6 P.M.	79.5	77
About ten miles from Malta,	8, 7 A.M.	79.5	78
About two miles from Valetta,	... 11	81	80
At anchor in the Quarantine Harbour, in about fourteen fathoms water, ...	... 2 P.M.	82	82

During this voyage the weather was fine; the winds light and variable.

* No regular reckoning was kept by the master of the little vessel in which this voyage was made;—he trusted to the compass and the headlands.

FROM MALTA TO GENOA.—1829.

Situation.	Time.	Water.	Air.
Off Tormino, about mid-channel,	Oct. 6, 11 A.M.	74°	73°
Off Reggio, ...	... 5½ P.M.	70	71
At anchor in the Harbour of Messina, ...	10, 12 M.	71	58
Just outside the harbour of Messina, in the current, . .	11, 8 A.M.	69	57
About mid-channel, in the narrowest part of the strait, .	... 11 A.M.	71	61
Close to the Faro, out of the current, ...	. ... 11¼ A.M.	69	
About four miles northward of the Faro, ...	... 1 P.M.	72	63
Off Stromboli, . . .	12, 12 M.	71	64
About 30 miles N.W. of Stromboli, ...	13, 12	70	63
About 60 miles N.N.W. of Stromboli, ...	14, 12	70	66
About 12 miles off the Isle of Ponza, ...	15, 12	68	67
About six miles off Civita Vecchia, the dome of St Peter's in sight,	16, 12	65	60
About eight miles from the little Isle of Monte Christi, .	17, 12	63	62
About six miles off the coast of Corsica ; its mountains covered with snow, . . .	18, 12	66	64
Between Elba and Capraia, .	19, 12	66	65
About 12 miles off Genoa, .	20, 12	64	64

The weather during the early part of the voyage
was tempestuous ; during the latter part, after leaving Messina, fine. Whilst in the port of Messina
there was a storm, accompanied with heavy rain and
a fall of snow, on the mountains of Calabria.

BETWEEN MYTELENE AND ALEXANDRIA.—1833.

Situation.		Time.	Water.	Air.
Lat. 39° 21'	Long. 25° 37' E.	July 26, 7 P.M.	74°	76°
39 54	26 8	Aug. 2, 2	71	74
39 08	25 29	6, 1	72½	73
37 55	24 34	8, 1½	74	79
37 24	23 33	9, 3½	77	80
36 03	30 20	{ Sept. 5, 12 M. } calm.	91	92
35 06	34 38	26, 3 P.M.	82	78
33 43	34 16	Oct. 3, 12 M.	77	75

These last observations were made by Mr John Maconochy when assistant-surgeon of H.M.S. Rainbow; and I am indebted for them to Captain Sir John Franklin, at that time commanding the Rainbow.

BETWEEN MALTA AND CAPE DE GAT.—1834.

		Water.			Air.
September 26, 7 A.M.	.	78°	.	.	76°
27,	.	77	.	.	75
28,	.	76	.	.	75
29,	.	76	.	.	75
30,	.	76	.	.	75
October 1,	.	76	.	.	75
2,	.	76	.	.	75½
3,	.	75½	.	.	76
4,	.	74	.	.	73

For these observations I am indebted to my friend Dr Nicholson, Deputy Inspector General of Hospitals.

FROM ENGLAND TO CONSTANTINOPLE.—NOVEMBER 1840.

Situation.	Time.			Water.	Air.
Entrance of the Strait of Gibraltar, Tariffa lighthouse in sight, ...	Nov. 8,	2	P.M.	68°	69°
About two miles off Tariffa, .	...	3		66	
Between Tariffa and Gibraltar,	...	3¼		68	
About fifteen miles off shore, the mountains of Grenada, their tops covered with snow, distinctly in view, Cape de Gat indistinctly, . . .	9	8	A.M.	64	68
The mountains of Grenada still in sight, ...	...	2	P.M.	65	66
Algiers about 30 miles distant to the eastward; the bold African coast distinctly in view, .	10,	8	A.M.	68	69
About two miles off the rocky islet of Galeta, . .	11,	3	P.M.	69	70

FROM ENGLAND TO CONSTANTINOPLE—NOVEMBER 1824.—(*continued.*)

Situation.	Time.		Water.	Air.
About 20 miles to the eastward of Pantelaria, . . .	Nov. 12,	8 A.M.	69°	
About 30 miles from Gozo, .	...	1 P.M.	70	71°
About eight miles to the northward of Gozo (almost calm),	...	3	72	75
Quarantine Harbour, Malta, nearly in its middle, . .	18,	4	72	70
Out of sight of land, about 100 miles to the eastward of Malta,	20,	8 A.M.	69	68
About 140 miles from that island,	...	1 P.M.	71	72
The Island of Falconera, about five miles distant to the northward,	21,	8 A.M.	68	68
Between the N.E. ends of Serpho and Serphanté, . .	...	2 P.M.	70	70
About a quarter of a mile from the shore of Syra, . . .	...	5	66	67
At anchor in the Harbour of Syra,	...	6	66	67
About a mile from the southern shore of Scio, . .	22,	8 A.M.	65	67
In the Gulf of Smyrna, about a mile from the south-west shore,	...	12 M.	65	70
About five miles from Smyrna, in shallow water of a light greenish hue, . . ,	...	1½ P.M.	67	70
At anchor about a quarter of a mile from the town of Smyrna, .	...	5	66	69
About mid-way between Tenedos and the Troad, . . .	23,	8½ A.M.	64	66
About a quarter of a mile from the hillock called the Tomb of Antilochus, . . .	...	9	64	66
At the entrance of the Strait of the Dardanelles, . . .	...	10	63	68
About three miles above the outer castle, ...	..	10½	63	68
About a quarter of a mile from the town of the Dardanelles, .	...	11¼	62	66
Nearly in mid-channel, opposite to the town of the Dardanelles,	...	11¾	61	66
Opposite the supposed sites of Sestos and Abydos, . .	...	12 M.	61	
Between Lampsacus and Gallipolis,	...	2 P.M.	62	71
In the Sea of Marmora, near the Island of Marmora, . .	...	7	59	62
At anchor in the port of Constantinople, ...	24,	7 A.M.	57	64

This voyage was made in steam-packets; from England to Malta, in the "Great Oriental" steam-vessel, at the rate, in the Mediterranean, of from ten to twelve miles an hour; from Malta to Constantinople, in the French government steam-packet "Tancrede," at the rate of about eight miles an hour. The weather was fine during the four days of passage between Gibraltar and Malta, and also during the four days and half that we were passing from Malta to Constantinople, excepting two or three hours of showery weather, with a strong wind, in the Gulf of Smyrna.

These observations on the temperature of the surface of the Mediterranean, few and limited as they are, are not without interest. They show, in part, the range of temperature of this sea throughout the year; how it varies with the different seasons, and what a great difference exists between the maximum summer heat of the surface-water, and its minimum in winter; and how, as a reservoir of heat, this sea, in common with all other great collections of water, must tend to equalize the temperature of the superincumbent atmosphere, and to affect the climate of its islands and shores. It is commonly believed that the temperature of the Mediterranean is generally higher than that of the ocean in corresponding latitudes. This, I am inclined to think, has been rather hypothetically assumed than proved by actual observation. From the results of my own observations, I am disposed to infer, on the contrary, that the temperature of the Mediterranean is rather lower than that of the ocean

The following observations made on approaching the Strait, in 1824 and 1840, are a few of the most decisive :—

Situation.	Time.	Water.	Air.
Lat. 38° 46', about thirty miles off the rock of Lisbon, .	May 18, 1824,12 m.	62.5°	63°
Lat. 38° 18', about thirty miles from land, . . .	19,	63.5	66
38°, about 28 miles from land,	20,	64	65
36° 28' Long. 8° west, .	21,	66	65
In the Strait of Gibraltar, off the neutral ground, about six miles,	20, 12 m.	64	62*
The rock of Lisbon in sight,	{ Nov. 7, 11 a. m.	64	68
	{ 8, 8½	69	69
Towards the entrance of the Strait, Tariffa Lighthouse in sight, †	2 p. m.	68	69

Probably an exaggerated idea of the high temperature of the Mediterranean has been acquired casually, from the remarks of travellers on the warmth of its waters in harbours and shallows, frequented in bathing in the hot season.

On the ocean, the thermometer has proved a useful instrument in navigation, for the purpose of detecting currents. Whether it admits of the same application in the Mediterranean, remains to be determined. It probably may be thus useful, especially in the Archipelago, through a considerable portion of which a cold current flows, derived from the Hellespont. It may be useful also in approaching the Straits of Gibraltar, from the Mediterranean, and perhaps in navigating the Straits of Messina, at night,

* *Vide* p. 208.   † *Vide* continuation of observations, p. 213.

and in other similar situations. The temperature of the current flowing into the Mediterranean, appears to be higher than that of the Mediterranean, at least in the cool season. The temperature of the current between Sicily and Calabria, too, is, it is probable, generally higher than that of the in-shore water out of its influence. These remarks are offered with much hesitation. Experience alone can determine the question,—experience consisting of extended series of observations carried on throughout the year, in many different parts, and especially in those parts where currents are known to prevail, and in their vicinity.

Of course, in connexion with the idea that the Mediterranean is warmer and salter than the ocean, the notion is entertained, that there is greater evaporation from its surface, and that the winds blowing over it are drier, so as to occasion evaporation in a greater degree. Of the correctness of this opinion, I am very doubtful. Looking over my sea-journals, the observations recorded with the hygrometer do not indicate generally a dry state of the atmosphere. The hygrometer used, was a delicate common thermometer, with a projecting bulb, covered with muslin, to be moistened when used, in which the cooling effects produced by evaporation, indicated comparatively the degree of dryness. The following are some of the results:—

FROM CORFU TO MALTA.—1828.

Situation.	Time.	Thermometer.		Diff.
		Dry.	Moist.	
Between Corfu and Vido, N.W. mod.; cloudy, after heavy rain, Lat. 37° 11' Long. 17° 17', N.W.	March 3, 8 A. M.	54°	52°	2°
gentle; clear, . . Lat. 36° 13' Long 16° 20' .	5, 12 M.	54	47	7
	9, 12	52	48	4
Off Malta, about 15 miles to the westward, N.W. fresh; clear,	10, 5 P.M.	57	52	5
About three miles off Valetta, N.E. moderate; clear, . .	11, 8 A.M.	57	51	6

FROM MARSEILLES TO MALTA.—1830.

Situation.	Time.	Thermometer.		Diff.
		Dry.	Moist.	
Lat. 38° 25' Long. 8° 29', E. by S. moderate; rather hazy, .	June 24, 7 P.M.	68°	66°	2°
Lat. 37° 40' Long. 9° 10' E. by S. moderate; slight haze, .	25, 9 A.M.	72	68	4
Weather and wind similar, .	12 M.	71	68	3
Ditto, Do. . . .	6 P.M.	70	68	2
About 15 miles off Cape Farina, on the African coast, .	26, 12 M.	1	67	4
About 15 miles S.E. of Pantaleria, S.S.W. moderate; cloudy, .	27, 7 P.M.	73	68	5

FROM CORFU TO CERIGO.—1827.

Situation.	Time.	Thermometer.		Diff.
		Dry.	Moist.	
Between Corfu and the Albanian, shore, S.E. moderate; overcast,	June 27, 7 P.M.	74°	69°	5°
Off Antipaxo, N. moderate; clear,	28, 7 A.M.	69	60	9
Off Santa Maura, about 15 miles, N. moderate; cloudy, .	12 M.	72	64	9
Between Ithaca and Cephalonia, N. moderate; cloudy,	4 P.M.	74	65	9

FROM CORFU TO CERIGO, 1827.—*(continued.)*

Situation.	Time.	Thermometer.		Diff.
		Dry.	Moist.	
Off Coron, about 15 miles, N.W. moderate; cloudy, . .	June 29, 6 P.M.	73°	68°	5°
Off Cape Matapan, calm; clear,	30, 7 A.M.	72	65	7
Between Cape Matapan and Cerigo, S.E. by E., moderate ; cloudy,	12 M.	74	69	5
About a mile from the shore of Cerigo, N.W., gentle; cloudy,	6 P.M.	73	69	4
At anchor in the harbour of Capsali, N., strong; blowing off land; clear, ...	July 1, 7 A.M.	79	62	17

FROM CORFU TO MALTA, SICILY, AND NAPLES.—1826.

Situation.	Time.	Thermometer.		Diff.
		Dry.	Moist.	
Between Corfu and the Albanian shore, S E. moderate; clear,	Aug. 29, 12 M.	78°	70°	8°
Out of sight of land ; squally, S.E. after heavy rain, . .	30, 8 A.M.	75	74	1
N.N.W. gentle; fine, . .	31, 12 M.	77	72	5
About half way between Corfu and Sicily ; calm, . . .	Sept. 1, 12	79	74	5
W.S.W. gentle ; pretty clear,	6 P.M.	77	71	6
S.S.W. ditto, ditto, . .	2, 10 A.M.	79	75	4
Ditto, ditto, ditto, . .	12 M.	80	74	6
S. by W. moderate; hazy, .	3, 12	79.5	76	3.5
S. by W. gentle; slightly hazy,	4, 12	82	77	5
Off the Sicilian shore; weather and wind similar, . . .	6 P.M.	80	75.5	4.5
Off Mount Etna, wind from land ; S. moderate; clear, . .	5, 8 A.M.	78	70	8
About 20 miles off Catania, weather and wind similar, . .	12 M.	80	76	4
About 10 miles from Malta, W. by S. gentle; clear, . .	8, 7 A.M.	78	74	4
At anchor in the quarantine harbour, N.W.; weather the same,	2 P.M.	82	75	7

FROM MALTA TO GENOA.—1829.

Situation.	Time.	Thermometer. Dry.	Thermometer. Moist.	Diff.
In the harbour of Messina ; N.W., strong ; after heavy rain, .	Oct. 10, 12 M.	58°	54°	4°
Just outside the harbour of Messina ; calm ; clear, .	11, 3 A.M.	57	50	7
In the narrowest part of the strait; N.W.; moderate ; cloudy,	11 A.M.	61	54	7
About four miles north of the Faro, N.W. ; moderate, . .	1 P.M.	63	54	9
Off Stromboli, N.W. ; moderate, clear, ...	12, 12 M.	64	53	11
About 30 miles N.W. of Stromboli, N. W. gentle, . .	13, 12 M.	63	54	9
About 60 miles N.N.W. of Stromboli, N.W. gentle, . .	14, 12 M.	66	57	9
About 12 miles off the isle of Ponza, N.W. gentle, . .	15, 12 M	67	61	6
Off Civita Vecchia, about six miles, N.W. nearly calm ; overcast,	16, 12 M.	60	56	4
Between Corsica and the mainland, about eight miles from the isle of Monte Christi, N.W. moderate ; clear. . . .	17, 12 M.	62	56	6
About six miles off the coast of Corsica ; calm, clear, .	18, 12 M.	64	59	5
Between the Islands of Elba and Capraia, S.E. ; gentle, .	19, 12 M.	65	60	5
Off Genoa, about 12 miles, N.W. moderate ; pretty clear, .	20, 12 M.	64	57	7

Comparing these results with some which I obtained during a voyage from Ceylon to England, in 1820, on the ocean, at a very great distance from land,* it would appear that the atmosphere of the

* *Vide* the Edinburgh Philosophical Journal, vol. x. for 1824, 1st series, edited by Professor Jameson and Sir David Brewster; and the journal of the same name, in continuation, edited by Sir David Brewster, for the latter results.

Mediterranean generally more abounds in moisture or aqueous vapour, than the atmosphere over the Atlantic, excepting near shore, or where the wind blows off shore.

Dew, I believe, never forms on the ocean; at least I have never witnessed it there; but I have witnessed it occasionally in the Mediterranean, thereby indicating a greater degree of dampness of atmosphere. I shall mention an instance, extracting it from my sea journal, kept on first going into the Mediterranean, in 1824:—" *May* 30.—The air has been the whole day exceedingly damp; the atmosphere hazy; the sun, towards its setting, seen through the haze, of a light silver hue, rather resembling the full moon. Soon after sunset, every thing on deck became moist, and some things wet, as if from the deposition of copious dew; a wine-glass, carefully washed with fresh-water, and well dried, after ten minutes exposure on deck, had become damp; its surface was just obscured, as if from the deposition of a very slight dew." This was in Latitude about 38° 24', and Longitude 1° 40' east, just within sight of the Spanish coast; the wind was easterly, and gentle; the thermometer 65°.

I am inclined to think that the degree of dryness of the atmosphere over the Mediterranean, may have been rated too high, from observations with the hygrometer, made on land, than which nothing can be more deceptive, especially in the summer season, when the ground is parched, and its drying effect on the air is great. I shall introduce an instance, showing the remarkable difference which may exist in the air over the sea and land, in the season alluded to. In the middle of August 1827, I went in a steamer from Corfu to Cephalonia; at sea, on the 22d of that month, the thermometer was about 80°, and the moist thermometer about 77°; at Argostoli, the former was about 90°, and the latter about 70°; the wind at sea and on land the same, south-west.

The facts which I have brought forward relative to the specific gravity and the temperature of the surface-water of the Mediterranean, and relative to the quantity of vapour in the superincumbent atmosphere, if they do not prove that the commonly received opinions referred to, are not correct, at least show that these opinions are not sufficiently founded on precise observations, and that at present, therefore, they ought not to be received as demonstrated.

Further, on certain general considerations, I think we may arrive at the same conclusion. No sea is so well, and has been so long known, as the Mediterranean. During the last 2000 years, it appears to have undergone no material change. It is inhabited by the same fishes now as in the time of Aristotle,—a circumstance strongly in favour of its degree of saltness being the same. * If there be a tendency to an aug-

* As many of the fishes of the Mediterranean are migratory, and at different seasons of the year pass to and from the Black Sea, a fresher body of water, it may perhaps be said, that the argument adduced above does not hold good : be this as it may, the objection, I apprehend, cannot be urged, in the instance of one fish, the torpedo. In the

mentation of salt, as there is in the ocean generally, and in all close seas, probably it is very slight, not greater than may be, and is, counteracted by the necessities of man, requiring a constant supply of this indispensable necessary of life. The salt extracted from the Mediterranean for use annually, must amount to many millions of pounds, probably to four times, or even ten times as many millions as there are human beings dependent on it. The adaptations in the economy of nature are generally admirable ; and it would be extraordinary indeed, and contrary to the analogies of that general economy, were it true, as it is supposed, that the saltness of this sea is constantly increasing, and is so far tending ultimately to become a dead sea.

The principal argument employed by those who have adopted the view of the greater and increasing saltness of the Mediterranean, is the circumstance of the current flowing into it from the Atlantic. That there are counter-currents along shore is certain, and that there is a deep current flowing from the Mediterranean is probable.* Should the latter be proved

time of Aristotle, as now, this fish was found in the Archipelago : had that sea, then, been fresher than at present, it is not probable it could have existed there ; for it is not met with, that I can learn, either in the sea of Marmora, or in the Black Sea, both, independent of being less salt, not differing materially from the Mediterranean and parts of the ocean in which this fish is common. The young torpedo dies more rapidly in fresh water than in the air.—*Vide Researches, Anat. and Physiol.* vol. i. chap. i.

* The following passage is from Mr Montgomery Martin's History

to exist, and be constant, it may, with the superficial along-shore currents, be equivalent, or nearly so, to the inflowing ocean current; and if there be at any time an increase of density of water, it may thus, in part, be carried off: the increase of density may give rise to the currents.

If the current flowing from the Atlantic into the Mediterranean were chiefly owing to greater evaporation from the surface of the Mediterranean than of the ocean, it might be expected that the flow of the current would be strongest in summer and autumn, —that it would be very feeble in winter, and cease towards the beginning of spring, after the heavy rains and cool and moist weather. But what is the fact? Not in accordance with the supposition. In Appendix C. to Mr M. Montgomery Martin's "History of the British Colonies," designated "Sailing Directions for the Straits of Gibraltar, written by Mr Ignatius Reiner, from his own experience," the concluding remark is as "*N.B.* In the middle of the Straits, the current generally runs towards the east, without

of the British Colonies, vol. v. p. 47. "Through these straits the current on the *surface* of the ocean sets constantly from the Atlantic into the Mediterranean. Beneath the surface there is doubtless an under current *from* the Mediterranean into the Atlantic. This idea is confirmed from the circumstance of a Dutch merchant ship being sunk by one broadside of a French privateer in the middle of the gut (as the straits are termed), between Tarifa and Tangier, and a few days after, the sunken ship, with her cargo of brandy and oil, was cast ashore near to Tangier, twelve miles to the westward of the place where she went down."

being influenced by the moon." No difference is mentioned in connexion with season.*

* Since the above was written, looking into Dr Birch's History of the Royal Society, vol. ii., I find in p. 213 a statement—founded on the observations of a Mr Sheres, who had resided for a considerable time at Tangier—to the following effect :—

" 1. That the ocean runs into the Mediterranean, at the Straits' mouth, about nine months in the year, viz. from February to November.

" 2. That the water of the Mediterranean runs backward into the ocean for one month in the year, viz. December, or about the winter solstice : that in November and January it ebbs and flows at the Straits' mouth about six feet.

" 3. That, about the summer solstice, the current inward is so strong, as that a boat of ten oars can but well stem it.

" 4. That the Levant wind blows there most part of the summer, and that when the wind blows a storm outwards, there is a torrent inwards of counter-moving water."

Though this statement does not appear to be probable, it may deserve to be inquired into ; if true, it might be supposed it would have been long ago confirmed ; it was made in 1675.

CHAPTER VIII.

ON THE CLIMATE OF THE IONIAN ISLANDS.

General Character of Climate, as regards the Seasons. Yearly Range
and Mean Annual Temperature. Temperature of Springs.
Monthly Temperature. Observations on Rain. Thunder Storms.
Range of Barometer. Dryness and Humidity of Atmosphere.
Variable Condition in relation to Atmospheric Transparency,
and Production of Dew. Observations on prevailing Winds.
Peculiarities of Climate in connexion with Elevation. Observations on the Temperature of particular spots in mountainous
and hilly situations, suitable for Summer Residence. Points of
difference in the Climate of the different Islands. Special observations on the Climate of Cerigo. Incidental notice of the fall
of Rain at Gibraltar, illustrated by Tables.

IN the climate of these islands there is a general
resemblance, depending on the little difference in
their geographical position. There are also certain
peculiarities of character belonging to each of them,
arising out of local circumstances.

The seasons generally are tolerably well marked
and characteristic. The summer months are hot and
dry; the autumn showery and mild; the winter rainy
and tempestuous; the spring mild and showery.
The month of August may be considered most cha-

racteristic of summer; October of autumn; January of winter, and April of spring. The summer season is the most constant in character; next, perhaps, the winter; the autumn and spring (at least, the early spring) are more uncertain. Occasionally, the summer is protracted into the autumn, and occasionally the winter into the spring. The transition of the seasons, excepting from spring to summer, is generally abrupt. The hot and dry weather of summer is commonly brought to an end by thunder-storms, attended with copious showers. The mild and agreeable weather of autumn, following the first rains (known by the name of the Little Summer), is also generally terminated by storms,—the influx of a vast volume of cold air from the north, and a fall of snow on the mountains. Northerly winds maintain the winter season, and often prevail in March; the southerly bring in the spring, and, when they predominate, as they generally do in the beginning of April, then spring is truly established—the foliage may almost be seen to expand, there is such a sudden burst of vegetation. The transition from spring to summer is almost insensible, and yet rapid. May, the most delicious of months in these islands, deserving of all the praise bestowed on it by poets (truly the poet's May), belongs rather to summer than spring.

The variations of temperature, whether annual or diurnal, are not very considerable. The extreme range of the thermometer throughout the year, at the level of the sea, may be stated at about 50° or 60°, in the hottest weather seldom rising above 90°, and in the depth of winter rarely falling below 46°, and very rarely, indeed, descending so low as the freezing point. The mean annual temperature of the atmosphere is highly favourable to excellence and agreeableness of climate. At and near the sea, I believe, it varies between 61° and 64° of Fahrenheit. This I infer from observations which I have made on the temperature of perennial springs. Few as they are, I shall give the results in detail in the subjoined note,* as a

* At Ipsa in Corfu, there is a large stream which bursts out from beneath a mass of gypsum, close to the sea ; on the 1st of April, 1825, its temperature was 62° 5'.

In the same island, close to the sea, near the lake Carissia is a copious spring : the locality of which is tolerably well marked on that little frequented shore, by a conspicuous layer of lignite ; on the 29th August, 1825, its temperature was 62° 5'. Dr Hennen, in his valuable work, the Medical Topography of the Ionian Islands, states that this is a salt-water lake, and that it discharges its waters by a narrow outlet into the Mediterranean. The two circumstances are hardly compatible : the latter is correct, the former erroneous. When I visited the lake in the spring of 1825, I tasted the water and found it fresh, and was assured by the natives that it is always fresh.

The copious fountain of Crissida, in the vicinity of the town of Corfu, only a very few feet above the level of the sea, on the 9th April, 1825, was 62°.

The springs of saline water which break out on the shore near Samos in Cephalonia, have already been noticed ; their temperature in February 1825, was 62°.

In the lagoon of Cutavo, at the foot of the ancient Cranii, in the same island, are several large springs of fresh water ; on the 15th of February, 1825, the temperature of the most considerable was 64°,

contribution to the subject, with the hope that such observations will be multiplied and made at different seasons.

To show the monthly range of temperature, the following Tables are given, kept in Corfu, Cephalonia, and Zante. For the first I am indebted to Dr Roe, who for several years was stationed in Corfu, when surgeon of the 28th regiment. The thermometer was kept in a room without a fire, well ventilated; and it was observed twice a-day, viz. at eight A.M., and at three P.M., during the first four years, and thrice a-day during the three last, viz. at eight, twelve, and three; and from these daily observations, the following monthly averages were taken.

that of the smallest 62°, and that of the brackish water of the lagoon, through which they rose, 51°.

In the town of Lixuri, in the same island, only a few feet above the level of the sea, is a very abundant spring, already noticed; in January 1825, its temperature was 63°; and it was the same on the 17th of February.

In Santa Maura, the very fine fountain called the Bassa's Fountain, breaks out near to the sea-shore, and a few feet (perhaps twenty) above it; on the 13th March, 1825, its temperature was 61°.

In Ithaca, at Perivoli, the supposed garden of Laertes, there is a spring near, and a very few feet above the sea; its temperature in January 1825, was 64°.

In Zante, the temperature of a well, in August 1824, in the village of Catastari, a few feet above the level of the sea, was 63°; that of another in the plain of Zante, not more elevated, was of the same degree of temperature; and that of an abundant spring, close to the sea-shore, near the " Grease-Spring," on the 27th of August of the same year, was 65°.

MONTHLY AVERAGE HEIGHT OF THE THERMOMETER IN CORFU FOR
SEVEN YEARS.

Months.	1821.	1822.	1823.	1824.	1825.	1826.	1827.
January, . .	52°	53°	52°	52°	52°	53°	54°
February, . .	53	49	53	54	51	50	53
March, . . .	56	53	56	56	51	55	55
April, . . .	63	59	59	56	57	57	57
May, ...	74	66	68	65	66	61	67
June, . . .	74	76	75	71	69	70	71
July, ...	79	80	79	$77\frac{1}{2}$	76	73	$79\frac{1}{2}$
August, . . .	84	84	80	$81\frac{1}{2}$	77	80	$82\frac{1}{2}$
September, . .	78	82	79	$80\frac{1}{2}$	74	79	$75\frac{1}{2}$
October, . . .	67	75	73	73	65	72	71
November, . .	63	65	63	62	$62\frac{1}{2}$	$66\frac{1}{4}$	$64\frac{1}{2}$
December, . .	59	58	54	58	61	59	60
Mean annual,	66	67	64	$65\frac{1}{2}$	$63\frac{1}{2}$	$64\frac{3}{4}$	66

The second Table is formed from observations
made by the late Major Temple, who for many years
was Commandant and Resident of Santa Maura,—
one of the many British officers who have fallen
victims to the pestilential climate of Western
Africa. The thermometer was kept in an open
verandah of the Resident's house in the Fort of
Santa Maura, and was observed twice a-day, viz. at
eight A.M. and three P M., with occasional interrup-
tions.

MONTHLY AVERAGE HEIGHT OF THE THERMOMETER AT SANTA MAURA, AT EIGHT A.M. AND THREE P.M., FOR A PERIOD OF FOUR YEARS.

Months.	1820.		1821.		1822.		1823.	
	8 A.M.	3 P.M.	8 A.M.	3 P.M.	8 A.M.	3 P.M.	8 A.M.	3 P.M.
January, .	55°	60°	57°	57°	53°	55°	50°	53°
February, .	54	57	52	52	52	55	53	57
March, . .	57	61	55	57	59	62	55	60
April, . .	63	70	63	64	65	69	60	64
May, . .	66	73	69	71	67	70	69	72
June, . . .	76	80	73	75	77	80	75	79
July . .	78	84	77	81	77	84	77	81
August, .	82	85	77	83	80	83	78	82
September,	78	80	77	77	77	81	72	76
October, .	71	72	65	70	67	72	67	73
November, .	61	62	59	61	57	63	52	...
December, .	55	58	56	58	51	54	52	...
Mean, .	66	70	65	65.5	65.4	67	63.4	...

The third Table is framed from observations made in the town of Zante by Captain Cranfield, late of the 90th regiment, whilst stationed in that island. The meteorological journal, from which the averages of temperature are derived, he was so obliging as to send to me before he quitted the Mediterranean, with permission to use it.

MONTHLY AVERAGE HEIGHT OF THE THERMOMETER IN ZANTE, AT
8 A.M. AND 3 P.M., FROM APRIL 1822 TO JANUARY 1826.

Months.	1822.		1823.		1824.		1825.	
	8 A. M.	3 P. M.	8 A. M.	3 P. M.	3 A. M.	3 P. M.	8 A. M.	3 P. M.
January, .	...°	...°	54°	57°	53°	56°	52°	54°
February, .	...	...	58	61	54	55	53	54
March, . .	...	...	58	61	55	57	54	56
April, . .	64	65	63	65	57	61	60	62
May, .	71	71	71	73	68	71	69	72
June, . .	77	81	76	78	73	76	72	75
July, . .	80	85	78	81	77	82	77	81
August, . .	81	86	80	82	82	86	79	83
September,	78	83	74	77	76	78	76	77
October, .	71	75	69	71	71	73	68	69
November, .	63	68	59	61	62	64	62	65
December, .	58	60	56	60	57	60	59	61
Mean,	...	...	66	69	65	68	65	66

As the observations in these Tables were made
under cover, they necessarily indicate a steadier temperature than belongs to the atmosphere.

The mean annual temperature deducible from them
is higher than that of the springs, even confining the
deduction to the results of the morning's observations, which is also what might be expected.

I shall now notice some of the other general qualities or circumstances of atmosphere intimately connected with the character of the climate.

No observations having yet been made with a pluviometer in these islands, the exact quantity of rain
which falls has not been ascertained. That it is considerable is certain; it probably occasionally exceeds
forty inches per annum, and on an average is not less

than thirty inches. It varies much in different years, and also in the different islands in the same year. This, however, is common to all of them, that the greater quantity falls in showers of shorter duration, and that continued rain beyond a few hours is nowise frequent.

The following Table is constructed with the intention of showing the frequency of rain, the number of days in which rain fell, in the Islands of Corfu, Santa Maura, and Zante, formed from the meteorological journals already referred to.

NUMBER OF DAYS IN WHICH THERE WAS RAIN DURING A PERIOD OF THREE YEARS IN THE TOWNS OF CORFU AND ZANTE AND THE FORT OF SANTA MAURA.

Months.	1823.			1824.			1825.		
	Corfu.	Santa Maura.	Zante.	Corfu.	Santa Maura.	Zante.	Corfu.	Santa Maura.	Zante.
Jan.	14	13	11	15	24	18	6	10	11
Feb.	16	6	5	10	8	8	8	5	6
Mar.	14	11	11	14	16	14	11	5	10
April,	10	6	3	24	12	7	7	3	2
May,	3	...	...	4	1	...	5	5	2
June,	3	5	3	4	1	...	8	3	2
July,	1	...	...	2	1	1	4	1	2
Aug.	...	...	...	1	1	1	1	1	1
Sept.	3	9	10	7	4	3	10	7	4
Oct.	12	3	7	7	5	5	12	9	4
Nov.	10	8	13	6	7	3	16	6	13
Dec.	13	13	12	11	7	5	16	...	7
Total,	99	74	75	105	87	65	104	...	64

According to these results (and observations in the Mediterranean generally, I believe, accord with them), the greatest and principal quantity of rain falls in the six months when the sun is south of the equator; the least when it is north: when, in one instance, the temperature is low and the clouds are low, and there is much moisture in the air; and in the other, when the temperature is high, clouds unfrequent, floating chiefly in the upper regions of the atmosphere, and when the air is rarely, if ever, nearly saturated with moisture. At the end of this chapter will be found the results of observations made with the pluviometer at Gibraltar, during nearly half a century, and which are in accordance with the remarks just offered.

In variable and rainy weather, especially in the beginning of autumn and in winter, electrical phenomena are common in the atmosphere; thunder storms are not unfrequent, and they are often severe; hail is an occasional, and rain is an almost constant accompaniment, with a great reduction of temperature; and the latter has been known to fall in destructive torrents.

The following Table, made from the registers already referred to, shows the frequency of thunderstorms in Zante and Santa Maura, during the different months of the year:—

NUMBER OF DAYS IN EACH MONTH, DURING A PERIOD OF TWO YEARS
IN WHICH THERE WERE THUNDER-STORMS IN ZANTE AND SANTA
MAURA.

Months.	1823.		1824.	
	Zante.	Santa Maura.	Zante.	Santa Maura.
January, .	4	3	2	...
February,	1	...	1	...
March, .	3	1	...	1
April, . .	1	1	...	...
May, . .	...	...	...	...
June, . .	...	1	...	...
July, : .	...	...	...	...
August, .	...	...	...	1
September,	6	3	2	3
October, .	2	...	3	1
November,	1	1	3	...
December,	1	...	1	...
Total,	19	10	12	6

Little attention has yet been paid to the state of
the barometer in these islands, and I regret that I
have no series of barometrical observations to be depended on, to offer to supply the deficiency. It may
be remarked generally, that during the settled fine
weather of summer, the range of the mercurial column
is exceedingly small; its height is about thirty inches;
and further, that, during this season, as within the
tropics, it is subject to a well marked diurnal variation.   In the winter, on the contrary, the fluctuations
of the mercury are great and sudden, hardly less so
than in our own climate.   In spring and autumn,
the variations are less; they are most remarkable
when the weather is unsettled.

In relation to dryness and humidity, the atmosphere of the Ionian Islands is exceedingly variable. In winter, spring, and autumn, the dryness is never remarkable; the moist thermometer used as an hygrometer may fall from 10° to 2° lower than the dry thermometer. In the height of summer the dryness of the air is occasionally extreme : in Zante, in 1824, on the 8th August, at one o'clock in the afternoon, the difference of temperature between a moist and dry thermometer, exposed to the wind, was the very remarkable one of 32°, the greatest I ever witnessed in any country; the dry thermometer stood at 99° ; the wind was about W.N.W. For several days previously, the weather had been hot and parching. During this season, there is a strongly marked difference of degree of moisture with the direction of the winds; the northerly land-winds are commonly very dry as well as hot, whilst the southerly, especially the south-east or Sirocco wind, is invariably damp. Fortunately this latter wind is never in these islands of high temperature ; it rarely exceeds 84° or 85° of Fahrenheit, and its degree of moisture is such, that it seldom reduces the moist thermometer more than 5°. The contrast between the hot dry northerly winds and the warm moist southerly, in relation to sensation, is very remarkable. The former are infinitely less oppressive than the latter, when the moist thermometer falls from 25° to 30°, though the temperature is above 90°,—though every thing metallic feels hot, and the furniture and wooden work of one's room may be cracking with explosive violence,—yet the sensation of heat is not disagreeable, the skin is dry, and exercise may be taken in the open air with pleasure and alacrity, and with little feeling of fatigue. With a Sirocco wind at 85°, one is bathed in perspiration,—one feels as in a vapour bath,—and life is almost a burden. When I come to treat of the climate of Malta, I shall make some further remarks on the character of this wind.

In relation to transparency, the atmosphere is exceedingly variable. When the weather is fine, and the winds northerly or westerly, the air is generally admirably clear, and its hues are exquisitely beautiful. On the contrary, when the winds are southerly, the atmosphere is always more or less hazy. In some situations, a change of wind, from the S.E. to the N.E. or N.W., has a remarkable effect;—the atmosphere of a sudden becomes clear,—a new landscape opens before one,—as if a curtain were withdrawn from a picture;—at first one can hardly credit the senses; it looks like illusion. In all the Ionian Islands, looking towards the continent, these effects may be witnessed, but nowhere in a more remarkable manner than in Zante. A stranger may be there several weeks with a southerly wind, without seeing the Morea, and with a change of wind and consequent sudden clearing of the atmosphere of the obscuring vapour, he will witness before him a most extensive and varied view of a great part of this classical and picturesque region.

Connected with clearness of sky, is the cooling effect from radiation of heat, and the consequent production of dew. The cooling effect from radiation is often very considerable, especially in autumn and in winter; and, as in Bengal, is occasionally sufficient to produce ice, when the temperature of the air is three or four degrees above the freezing point. A series of observations with the aetheriscope, throughout the year, in these islands, is a desideratum. I suspect it would show that, during the summer, there is little radiation of heat,—that there is a great deal during the autumn, and that it is very variable in winter and spring. I am induced to draw these inferences from the partial observations which I made with a thermometer applied as an aetheriscope, and from remarks on the appearance of dew, which is rare in summer, common and abundant in autumn, and uncertain and not common in winter and in spring.

The direction of the winds is exceedingly uncertain. The natives pay great attention to them, and have assigned them different names, according to the points from whence they blow. Baron Theotoky, in his work on Corfu,* has given the character of the winds, according to their effects, in thirty different directions. His description of them is too general to be useful. On such a subject the nicest discrimination is necessary, and a variety of associated circum-

* " Details sur Corfou."

stances require to be taken into account and noticed. The same wind, at different seasons, may have in these islands a very different character. The northerly winds, during a considerable part of the year, when the adjoining mountains over which they pass are covered with snow, are necessarily cold ; but in summer, when there is no longer any snow on the mountains,* and their arid surface is warmed by the sun, they may be the reverse of cold and unusually hot. The same remark applies to the southerly winds, with a uniform character for humidity throughout the year; yet, their temperature differing so much in summer and in winter (the difference being from twenty to twenty-five degrees), their sensible character and their effects on the system may be totally dissimilar,—in winter mild and not unpleasant, in summer distressingly hot and relaxing.

Although the winds generally are very irregular in their occurrence, an exception, in the instance of breezes, may be mentioned. It is most distinctly marked during the summer season, and in that inland sea bounded outward by Santa Maura, Cephalonia, and Ithaca, terminating in the Gulf of Corinth. Here the movement of the air observes a certain regularity, analogous to the land and sea breeze on tropical shores. During part of the twenty-four hours

* None of the mountains of the adjoining continent are within the range of perpetual snow ;—before the great heats of summer commence, snow has disappeared even on the highest of them.

the breeze blows down the Gulf of Corinth, extending to or beyond Santa Maura; and during another part of the same period, it flows in a contrary course from the west or north-west, over the same track. The easterly breeze commences a little after midnight, and continues nearly till mid-day; the westerly sets in soon after noon, and lasts till nearly midnight. The constancy of these breezes is such, that the natives, with perfect reliance, avail themselves of them in their little trading voyages along the coast. Coming from the Gulf of Corinth, proceeding westward, they start before the earliest dawn; in returning, no early exertion is made; they patiently wait for the afternoon breeze.

The preceding remarks on the climate of the Ionian Islands chiefly refer to their shores, and to those parts of them which are very little raised above the level of the sea. Their hilly and mountainous districts have a climate in some respects peculiar, varying in degrees of coolness or of coldness with their elevation.

The highest mountain in the Ionian Islands, is Mount Ænos of antiquity, the Black Mountain, as it is now commonly called, occupying the central parts of Cephalonia. According to the admeasurement of it by Commander Slater, R.N., its perpendicular height above the level of the sea is 5306 feet; owing to this considerable elevation, a large portion of it is every winter covered with snow. When I ascended it on the 19th February, 1825, nearly one-

third of it was so covered,—the cold was severe,—
the thermometer fell to 24°. It was then a most
dreary and wintry scene. In summer, the climate of
this mountain is most delightful; it has been described to me by a native as a spot of peculiar enjoyment,—the air fresh, light, and invigorating,—the
nights invariably cool.

The following Table, extracted from the Appendix
to Sir Charles Napier's work on the Ionian Islands,
in which a comparison is made between the height
of a thermometer on the mountain and at Argostoli, is
well adapted to show the fitness of the former, as
regards temperature, for a summer residence.*

* Sir Charles Napier, in his "Memoir on the Roads of Cephalonia," says:—"On the Black Mountain a gentleman might build a
villa, and pass the heats of summer in the midst of woods and the
most beautiful scenery, and from his windows would have one of
the most extensive and interesting views in the world; would see
the whole of Cephalonia, Ithaca, and Santa Maura, with the small
islands, spread like a map beneath him; and beyond them, all Acar-
nania, Mount Pindus, the Gulph of Corinth, Patras, Clarence, and
the Arcadian Mountains. His ice-house might be filled as late as
the end of May, his table furnished with the finest fruits and vegetables; and the height of the situation would give him an atmosphere many degrees cooler than Argostoli, to which place he might
drive in two hours, and return in three."

1830.	\multicolumn{4}{c}{Copy of the Register of a Thermometer, kept in Captain Kennedy's hut, situated at about two-thirds of the height of the Black Mountain, in Cephalonia.}				\multicolumn{3}{c}{Copy of the Register of a Thermometer, kept in the Hospital of Argostoli.}		
	8 o'clock A.M.	3 o'clock P.M.	8 o'clock P.M.	WINDS.	8 o'clock P.M.	3 o'clock P.M.	8 o'clock P.M.
July 22,	74°	78°	:	E. E. E.,	85°	91°	:°
26,	65	71	:	N.E., E., N.W.,	84	86	:
27,	64	72	:	E.,	84	87	:
28,	64	:	:	E.,	84	:	:
29,	70	72	:	E.,	84	88	:
30,	66	72	:	N.E.,	84	88	:
August 5,	74	78	69	N.E.,	84	87	84
6,	74	77	70	E. N.E.,	85	88	84
7,	71	72	70	S.W., N.E., with fog,	83	87	84
8,	70	73	66	S.W., N.E.,	83	88	84
9,	65	79	70	E.,	84	87	84
10,	66	74	:	N.W.,	84	86	84
11,	68	:	63		84	86	:
19,	:	67	60	N.W.,	:	88	82
20,	63	66	64		82	86	81
21,	62	68	70	N.E.,	81	86	82
22,	70	77	64	N.W.,	83	85	84
23,	68	72	65	N.W.,	84	85	84
24,	68	71	:		83	86	85
25,	62	:	71	S.W., heavy fog all day,	81	88	:
September 2,	71	75	64		86	87	86
3,	66	66	68	W. fog and rain at night,	83	91	83
4,	66	74	64	N.W.,	82	85	82
5,	68	66	:	W., fog and rain,	82	85	81
6,	60	:	:		80	84	:
7,	62	61	:		79	78	:

From the above it appears that, during summer,

The mean temperature in Argostoli would be about . . . . 84°
The mean temperature of the mountain would be about . . . 68
—————
The mean difference of temperature, ... 16

The other larger islands have mountains, varying in height from 1000 to about 3000 feet above the level of the sea. Vrachiona, in Zante, was measured by Captain Slater, and found to be 2274 feet; Mount Scopo, in the same island, 1509; Mount Neritos, in Ithaca, 2476. The higher mountains of Santa Maura are probably very little under, or rather above, 3000 feet; and the highest mountain in Corfu, Mount St Salvadore, is probably nearly as high; and each of these islands has mountainous inhabited districts, varying in elevation from 1000 to 2000 feet in perpendicular height. The more elevated of these are delightful retreats in summer, and are deserving of being better known to the English inhabitants, especially the village of Perithra and Seignes, on the side of St Salvadore, in Corfu; those of Vathkirri and Englavi, in Santa Maura; and that of Maries, in the mountainous district of Zante. All of them are easily accessible, and may be reached in a few hours from the principal stations of the respective islands. The air in all of them is salubrious as well as cool, and what is hardly less important in relation to comfort, the water also is cool. Moreover, the scenery in their neighbourhood, without exception, is of an interesting character, the views,—especially the distant ones, magnificent; and, in consequence, there is much inducement to take exercise (an important circumstance in relation to health), and in doing so great and varied enjoyment. When I visited Vathkirri and Englavi, in the middle of March 1825, the temperature of a spring in the latter village was 54°, and of a very copious one, sufficiently large to turn a mill, in the vicinity of the former, 54.5. Then the adjoining mountains were covered with snow, in which, in some places, we sank knee-deep; and the wild and Alpine character of the scenery was heightened by tracks of wolves in the snow. These villages are so cool that the oak flourishes there, not the olive. In the beginning of April, when I was at Perithra and Seignes, the temperature of the springs in both was only 50°. The inhabitants are familiar with frost and snow,—a winter does not pass without them;—indeed, their complexions were indicative of the climate; they had more of the fresh colour of a northern than the olive hue of the southern races.

The climate of the hilly districts, those elevated between 300 and 1000 feet above the level of the sea, in relation to temperature, is intermediate between the low country and the mountainous regions. They are commonly cooler in summer than might be expected, and especially at night, particularly in certain favoured situations, probably owing to the effect of free radiation of heat into the upper ethereal space. Such a situation is the Castle of Zante, the elevation of which, according to the admeasurement of Commander Slater, is 719 feet. No near height commands it; no object radiates heat to it; it is so much cooler than the town below, that it is a favourite summer residence; and many of the wealthy inhabitants have houses within its precincts.

On the climate of the islands individually, I shall here limit myself to a very few general remarks. More rain, I believe, falls in Corfu than in any other of the Ionian Islands, or, at least, showers are more frequent there.

It is commonly supposed that Santa Maura differs very little from Corfu in its quantity of rain, or the number of its rainy days. The Tables given are not in favour of this popular notion; they rather show that in this respect it approximates more to Zante.

It is also commonly supposed that the southern groupe of islands, Zante, Cephalonia, and Ithaca, are exceedingly alike in their summer season; that the summer season in them is hotter than in Corfu and drier; and that therefore they are better fitted for the cultivation of the currant-vine,—an opinion, I believe, founded on truth; although of questionable accuracy when extended to Santa Maura.

In relation to temperature, limiting remark to the principal towns or stations, I believe it may be stated that the climate of Corfu is most equable; that it is cooler in summer than either Zante, Argostoli, or Santa Maura, and less cold than the two latter in winter; and that Zante, I mean the city, is hottest in summer, and mildest in winter. Their peculiarities in these respects are perfectly in accordance with their situations and relative positions.

I shall conclude this chapter with a few observations on the climate of Cerigo, respecting which less is known, and still less has been published, than on any other of the Ionian Islands. The information I have to offer was collected in the summer of 1827, during a visit to this island, when I had the advantage of consulting a meteorological journal kept by Mr Huthwaite, then assistant-surgeon of the 90th regiment, for a period of twelve months.

As might be expected from its situation, the climate of Cerigo is mild, perhaps milder and more equable than that of any other of the Ionian Islands, or of any part of continental Greece. Fires are very seldom required in winter, and the heat is not often oppressive in summer. Ice is rarely seen, and snow still seldomer, excepting in the distance, on the mountains of the Morea, or on Mount Ida, in Candia.

The following Table, framed from Mr Huthwaite's Journal, shows the maximum and minimum temperature at noon for twelve consecutive months. His observations were confined to that time of the day, and they were made in the Castle, the principal military station, which stands on the summit of a hill, close to the sea, and about 300 feet above it, on the south-west shore, commanding the town and bay of Capsali.

February,	1826,	maximum	53°	minimum	46°
March, .	...	...	59	...	50
April, .	...	...	68	...	58
May, . .	...	...	72	...	60
June, . .	...	...	76	...	69
July, . .	...	...	83	...	75.5
August, .	...	...	82	...	77
September,	...	...	83	...	72
October, .	...	...	74	...	68
November,	...	...	70	...	62
December,	...	...	65	...	52
January,	1827,	...	60	...	52

The climate of Cerigo is comparatively dry; rain is neither very frequent there, nor heavy, and it falls rather in showers of short duration, than uninterruptedly for many hours; indeed, a day of continued rain is considered by the natives as an uncommon occurrence. During a period of twelve months, the number of days in each month in which there was rain, was the following :—

In March,	1826,	.	.	.	5 days.
April, . .	...	.	.	.	2 ...
May, . .	...	.	.	.	2 ...
June, . .	...	.	.	.	2 ..
July, . .	...	.	.	.	1 ...
August, .	...	.	.	.	2 ...
September,	...	.	.	.	...
October, .	...	.	.	.	2 ...

(N.B.—No observations from the 6th to 27th)

November,	...	.	.	.	3 ...
January,	1827,	.	.	.	1 ...
February,	...	.	.	.	5 ...

In November there was one entire day of rain : with this exception, on all the other days, in accordance with the preceding remark, there were only showers, or a shower.

Cerigo is almost proverbial for gales, which is not surprising, considering its exposed and peculiar position, open on one side to the Archipelago, and on the other to the Mediterranean. Notwithstanding, the number of fine days is large in comparison with the stormy. In the period last referred to, they were the following :—

In March,	1826,	fine days	20,	stormy	5	days.
April, .	...	...	21,	...	3	...
May, .	...	...	23,	...	5	...
June, .	...	...	27,	...	2	...
July, .	...	...	28,	...	1	...
August, .	. .	...	25,	...	1	...
September,	...	...	22,	...	1	...
October,	...	(Only a few days' observation.)				
November,	...	...	20,	...	1	...
December,	...	...	10,	...	3	...
January,	1827	...	9,	...	4	...
February,	...	...	12,	...	5	...

The days in Mr Huthwaite's Journal, which were not marked " fine," were marked " cloudy," or " moist," or " overcast."

The direction of the winds, is, I believe, less variable than in any other of the islands. The spring and autumn are principally the seasons of variable winds ; in summer the Etesian winds, blowing down the Hellespont, mostly from the north-east, are prevalent ; in winter the southerly winds ; the one in summer cooling the atmosphere, the other in winter bringing warmth.

As in the other islands generally (excepting on the mountains), in common with the whole surface of the Mediterranean, mist and fog are of exceedingly rare occurrence in Cerigo. I have heard the master of a Mediterranean trader, of many years' experience, assert, that the breath, at no season of the year, is ever visible after passing the Straits of Gibraltar. This assertion is not perfectly accurate; it would be more correct to say, that the breath is commonly invisible, with occasional exceptions, chiefly in winter, the air being seldom saturated with moisture, or seldom of sufficiently low temperature to condense the vapour contained in the warm air expelled from the lungs. The same circumstances will serve to account for the rareness of fog or mist. And, in confirmation, it may be remarked, that where these circumstances do not exist, as in hilly regions, where

" The south wind wraps the mountain top in mist," *

and as in the sea of Marmora and the Hellespont, there fogs are not unfrequent. In the instance of the latter, they occur on the gentle setting in of the moist warm southerly wind, which, mixing with the cold air incumbent on the cold surface of these waters, has a portion of its aqueous vapour precipitated. In consequence, fog is a common indication of a southerly wind, and is considered by the Turks,

* Iliad, translated by Cowper, p. 67.

who see the effect before they feel the wind, as a certain herald of this welcome event.*

In Cerigo, during the summer months, as in the other Ionian Islands, there is great dryness of the atmosphere, and that by night as well as by day. At this season dew is rarely seen, excepting in low and moist situations. Whilst I was there, in July, there was commonly a difference of 20° between a moist and dry thermometer exposed to the wind by day, and at night the difference generally exceeded 15°. On the 2d of the month, at five o'clock in the morning, when the air was 75°, a thermometer, the bulb of which was moistened, fell 17°. The wind was then northerly—the prevailing summer wind. These observations were made at the Castle, or on the high grounds adjoining. In lower situations, and close to the sea, the air at night was generally damper; and it was often remarkably so just after sunset, and at the same time the air was cooler. I may mention a particular instance as an example :—On the 7th of July, being in a boat in the harbour of Capsali, I noticed the temperature of the air and of the water;

* During about two-thirds of the year, northerly winds prevail at the Dardanelles, and ships bound for Constantinople cannot make head against the current; this they can only effect with a leading southerly wind ;—the setting in, therefore, of this wind, is a welcome event. The fog attending it on the sea of Marmora, I have been informed, is sometimes so dense and so low, that whilst the hulls of adjoining ships are completely hid, the stars at night may be seen from the top-masts, and that, for security, it is necessary to keep the ships' bells constantly ringing.

the former was 76°, the latter 73°, the moist thermo-meter 74°; the evening was calm and serene. At the Castle, to which I ascended almost immediately, the temperature of the air was 80°, and the moist thermometer was reduced by evaporation 14°. Elsewhere in the Ionian Islands, I have made similar observations, especially in Corfu. There, very often, I have found the hollows amongst the hills, just after sunset, many degrees cooler than the decli-vities and summits, and even of the western declivi-ties, which had been shaded equally long. The difference was often so striking as to be obvious to sensation. This greater coolness of the hollows and low situations is probably owing to the effect of radiation of heat; and the higher temperature of the sides and summits of the adjoining hills to ascending currents of warm air. And the greater dampness of the air in the lower situations, is most likely con-nected in part with greater coolness, and in part with greater humidity of surface. The fact, I believe, is very general. It may help to account for the greater apparent magnitude of the harvest-moon, especially as it appears immediately after sunset. From the observations which I have made, there has appeared to be more moisture in the atmosphere at that time, in its lower region, than in any other part of the twenty-four hours.

In a preceding note, I have alluded to the obser-vations which have been made with the pluviometer at Gibraltar for a period of nearly half a century. I am indebted for an account of the results to a friend, now no more, who, in compliance with my request, procured them, through the aid of Mr Barron Field, late Chief Justice of Gibraltar, from the office of the commanding engineer. For the sake of facility of reference, the observations will be given in three Tables, in which an arrangement will be followed different from that adopted in the construction of the original register.*

* The pluviometer was kept in the garden of the commanding engineer, about 100 feet above the level of the sea.

I.—NUMBER OF DAYS IN EACH MONTH IN WHICH RAIN FELL AT GIBRALTAR, FROM SEPTEMBER 1811, TO DECEMBER 1836.

Months.	1811.	1812.	1813.	1814.	1815.	1816.	1817.	1818.	1819.	1820.	1821.	1822.	1823.	1824.	1825.	1826.	1827.	1828.	1829.	1830.	1831.	1832.	1833.	1834.	1835.	1836.	Mean number of days in each month, in which rain fell in twenty-five years.
January,	:	11	12	16	•12	10	6	7	7	15	14	3	17	11	8	15	8	2	15	20	18	15	14	6	12	16	10.6
February,	:	8	3	6	3	11	:	10	2	9	10	6	9	10	4	5	23	11	9	7	7	12	7	10	3	9	7.7
March,	:	10	7	12	:	4	:	1	11	11	8	1	9	4	8	8	3	:	21	3	6	6	13	9	8	13	7.0
April,	:	10	9	9	10	16	11	11	9	13	9	9	12	2	12	5	7	6	12	3	20	7	9	6	11	6	9.4
May,	:	3	3	3	5	8	10	8	2	1	1	13	4	1	:	4	3	9	9	8	11	1	5	8	5	4	5.2
June,	:	:	2	:	5	2	3	:	1	1	:	:	4	:	2	1	:	:	2	4	1	1	:	1	6	:	1.4
July,	:	:	:	:	?	:	:	:	:	:	:	:	:	:	:	:	:	:	:	:	:	:	:	:	:	:	:
August,	:	:	:	:	:	:	1	:	1	1	:	1	2	4	4	:	:	1	:	:	5	:	:	:	1	:	0.8
September,	1	3	6	4	8	2	5	4	2	2	:	1	4	1	5	2	7	:	3	:	4	3	2	:	5	4	3.0
October,	9	7	10	11	4	9	13	4	8	5	4	6	8	8	2	8	13	1	5	4	7	5	9	8	5	3	6.9
November,	6	5	1	9	16	13	5	14	14	11	3	10	14	4	8	8	8	12	13	8	4	9	11	23	13	3	9.5
December,	10	20	13	6	8	4	8	14	10	11	9	10	5	2	18	7	9	8	18	14	6	:	:	13	17	2	9.3
Total,	:	77	66	76	71	79	62	73	67	80	58	60	88	47	71	55	81	50	107	71	79	59	69	84	86	60	71

11.—QUANTITY OF RAIN WHICH FELL AT GIBRALTAR DURING EACH
SEASON, FROM 1790 TO 1812.

Date.		Inches.	Total per annum.
From 2d October to 31st December	1790,	18.65	
... 1st January to 20th June .	1791,	6.44	} 22.13
... 21st September to 31st December	...	15.69	
... 1st January to 7th June .	1792,	28.36	} 39.85
... 13th August to 31st December	...	11.49	
... 1st January to 29th May .	1793,	7.59	} 19.27
... 23d September to 31st January	...	11.70	
... 1st January to 16th June .	1794,	10.66	} 18.66
... 8th September to 31st December	...	8.00	
... 1st January to 19th June .	1795,	13.56	} 23.63
... 3d September to 31st December	...	10.07	
... 1st January to 28th May .	1796,	15.57	} 62.87
... 19th August to 31st December	...	47.30	
... 1st January to 11th May .	1797,	17.30	} 33.05
... 10th August to 31st December	...	15.75	
... 1st January to 16th June .	1798,	14.80	} 31.28
... 5th October to 31st December	...	16.48	
... 1st January to 3d July .	1799,	14.71	} 37.17
... 3d September to 31st December	...	22.46	
... 1st January to 11th June .	1800,	19.75	} 26.54
... 5th August to 31st December	...	6.79	
... 1st January to 19th May .	1801,	8.33	} 16.45
... 14th September to 31st December	...	8.12	
... 1st January to 8th July .	1802,	21.37	} 39.91
... 9th September to 31st December	...	18.54	
... 1st January to 8th July .	1803,	24.10	} 47.71
... 9th September to 31st December	...	23.61	
... 1st January to 4th May .	1804,	27.30	} 39.30
... 25th August to 31st December	...	12.00	
... 1st January to 27th March .	1805,	18.61	} 47.50
... 1st October to 31st December	...	28.89	
... 1st January to 5th June .	1806,	10.56	} 14.76
... 1st October to 31st December	...	4.20	
... 1st January to 18th June .	1807,	25.49	} 39.81
... 24th September to 31st December	...	14.32	
... 1st January to 7th May, .	1808,	18.69	} 32.13
... 3d September to 31st December	...	13.44	
... 1st January to 18th May, .	1809,	17.78	} 36.57
... 10th October to 31st December	...	18.79	
... 1st January to 16th June .	1810,	18.57	} 28.33
... 21st August to 31st December	...	9.76	
... 1st January to 18th June .	1811,	17.92	} 30.94
... 12th September to 31st December	...	13.02	
... 1st January to 7th May .	1812,	24.77	} 43.31
... 1st September to 31st December	...	18.54	
Mean of 22 years,		......	33.23

III.—QUANTITY OF RAIN WHICH FELL IN EACH MONTH, FROM SEPTEMBER 1811, TO DECEMBER 1836.

Months.	1811.	1812.	1813.	1814.	1815.	1816.	1817.	1818.	1819.	1820.	1821.	1822.	1823.	1824.
Jan.,	..	7.545	5.025	11.320	7.420	2.330	3.070	2.530	3.700	10.420	15.890	0.300	3.830	7.180
Feb.,	..	5.195	0.430	0.975	0.430	3.580	..	3.850	0.480	5.290	3.140	1.900	3.550	3.540
March,	..	4.740	0.910	3.860	..	1.550	..	0.090	4.940	4.990	1.760	0.050	2.200	0.610
April,	..	5.050	5.450	2.460	6.830	3.525	8.400	3.210	2.180	3.660	2.460	2.940	3.290	0.240
May,	..	2.240	1.310	0.600	3.010	1.400	2.190	1.560	0.370	0.060	0.030	2.580	1.770	0.080
June,	..	..	1.360	..	2.530	0.160	0.350	..	0.100	0.050	..	..	1.770	..
July,	..	..	..	..	..	..	..	..	..	..	..	..	..	..
August,	..	..	..	..	..	..	0.060	..	0.180	0.020	..	0.280	0.800	0.990
Sept.,	0.030	0.440	3.740	0.860	2.455	0.310	1.730	1.970	0.750	0.560	..	0.200	0.380	0.070
Oct.,	2.615	1.280	7.790	3.760	4.230	5.320	6.460	0.200	3.220	4.370	0.650	1.740	1.910	4.240
Nov.,	6.665	2 840	0.150	2.250	4.620	5.340	1.250	10.800	2.640	3.630	0.290	6.320	5.210	1.050
Dec.,	3.710	13.985	5.465	0.960	4.730	1.720	3.180	6.760	5.020	3.640	8.570	1.700	0.780	0.060
Yearly Quant.	..	43.315	31.630	17.045	36.255	25.235	26.690	30.970	23.580	36.690	22.790	18.110	25.490	18.060

TABLE *continued.*

Months.	1825.	1826.	1827.	1828.	1829.	1830.	1831.	1832.	1833.	1834.	1835.	1836.	Mean Monthly.
Jan.,	6.960	94.40	3.090	0.550	5.650	13.110	17.080	6.590	4.090	0.540	3.230	2.760	6.15 Jan.
Feb.,	1.330	2.450	7.350	4.520	2.280	1.370	1.210	4.240	1.740	8.310	0.240	3.940	2.85 Feb.
March,	3.930	2.890	0.190	..	7.320	0.300	2.310	1.270	5.520	5.200	4.290	3.370	2.41 March.
April,	2.990	1.320	1.890	4.250	3.830	0.530	7.080	1.670	3.270	2.200	2.310	0.510	3.26 April.
May,	..	1.380	0.880	3.910	4.820	0.510	2.310	0.020	2.210	2.550	0.590	0-920	1.49 May.
June,	0.230	0.370	..	..	0.100	0.280	0.010	0.050	..	0.210	1.080	..	0.33 June.
July,	..	..	..	..	..	..	..	..	..	..	..	..	.. July.
August,	0.800	..	..	0.070	..	..	2.610	..	..	..	0.020	..	0.23 Aug.
Sept.,	0.990	..	3·390	..	0.680	..	0.520	0.270	0.080	..	0.630	0.250	0.78 Sept.
Oct.,	0.470	0.250	4.770	0.180	0.440	2.270	7.930	1.850	4.370	2.280	0.630	1.010	2.85 Oct.
Nov.,	3.950	8.070	2.940	6.710	25.770	2.290	0.400	2.980	5.450	12.550	9.490	1.160	5.18 Nov.
Dec.,	7.720	2.010	1.490	1.310	10.260	2.830	1.440	..	..	8.280	9.550	0.240	4.00 Dec.
Yearly Quant.	29.370	28.180	25.990	21.500	61.150	23.490	42.900	18.940	26.730	42.120	32.060	14.160	Mean yearly, 29.29.

From the results contained in the first Table, it appears that the average number of days in which rain fell at Gibraltar, between 1811 and 1836, were 71 per annum, that the greatest number in any year was 88, and the smallest 50 ; that of the months the greatest number was in January, and the least in July ; and, lastly, during the half-year the sun is south of the Line, the mean number was 51, and when north 19.8.

From the second Table it appears that the average quantity of rain which fell per annum, during a period of 22 years, was 33.23 inches; the greatest quantity in any year 62.87 inches ; the least quantity 14.76 inches.

From the third Table it appears that the average quantity which fell per annum during the second period, extending to 25 years, was 29.29 inches ; the greatest quantity in any one year 61.15 inches ; the least 14.16 inches ; that of the months the greatest quantity of rain fell in January (averaging 6.15 inches), and the least (none) in July ; that the greatest quantity in any one month was 25.77 inches ; and, lastly, that the average quantity which fell when the sun was south of the Line was 23.44, and when north 6.20 inches.

Many particulars in these Tables are deserving of note, and illustrative, not only of the climate of Gibraltar, but of that also of the Mediterranean generally, especially the variableness of the quantity of rain annually, and its comparative constancy in relation to seasons, and even particular months, and the immense quantity which has fallén at particular times. Thus, in the winter of 1829-30, in the three months of November, December, and January, there were 51 days of rain, in which the very large quantity of 49.14 inches fell, and of these 25.77 inches in 13 days in November. Knowing these facts, we are not surprised to hear of the floods produced, and of their disastrous consequences. Mr Barron Field, in the letter which accompanied the register of the pluviometer, addressed to my friend, alludes to some of the more remarkable. He states that, in 1755, the rain caused a flood, which rose to the second storey of the houses in Irish Town ; that, in 1766, on the 30th of January, there was a storm of lightning hail, and rain, which drowned sixty persons, and did L.20,000 worth of damage; and that, on the 17th November 1834, there was a storm of rain, which drowned ten persons, and carried away the Castle ramp.

CHAPTER IX.

ON THE CLIMATE OF MALTA.

Points of Difference in the Climate of Malta and of the Ionian Islands. Marked Difference of Temperature between the town of Valetta and Malta generally, illustrated by Tables. Prevailing Winds and their character. Sirocco Wind. Opinions and Remarks on its Peculiarities. Conjectures on its Origin, in connexion with its Qualities. Gales. Proportion of Cloudless and Cloudy Days. Observation on the Radiation of Heat. Suggestions for making Cool Sleeping Apartments. Observations on Freezing at a temperature of Atmosphere above 32°. Remarks on Dew. Question of its Influence in Bleaching considered. Notice of Experiments on the Light of the Moon. Observations on Rain. Description of a Shower of Dust of remarkable extent. Barometrical Observations. Notice of Thunder and Hail-Storms. Brief mention of the Climate of Gozo.

MANY of the remarks which have been made on the Ionian Islands, in relation to climate and seasons, are necessarily applicable to Malta. Situated farther south, its mean annual temperature is higher; its surface being less elevated, its highest hills not exceeding 600 feet, and being farther removed from lofty mountains, and surrounded by a greater expanse of sea, its temperature during the greater part of the year is more equable; and, lastly, being nearer the coast of Africa, it is more liable to be invaded by hot winds,—and in summer to experience excessive degrees of heat.

As regards temperature, in considering the climate of Malta, it is necessary to distinguish between the town and the country, the circumstances of the two being in many respects peculiar, and occasioning a marked difference in the results of thermometrical observations. The town of Valetta, by its massive buildings, and comparatively narrow streets, is well fitted to equalize temperature; the country, on the contrary, being almost entirely destitute of wood, its surface rocky, its soil scanty, is better adapted to radiate heat. This distinction is commonly neglected, and in consequence, the observations which have been made in the city, have been applied to the whole island, and an exaggerated idea has been formed of the equability of the temperature of Malta, and especially during the heats of summer.*

To avoid the error in question, I shall first give

---

* Mountains and vallies, the former considerably below the region of perpetual snow, the latter moderately open and exposed to sunshine, appear to have an effect in equalizing temperature, somewhat similar to that of massive buildings in towns and narrow streets. In travelling on the Continent, late in autumn, and in the depth of winter, in passing from a low plain country, as from France into Savoy, or from Lower into Upper Austria, I have been struck with surprise at the mildness of air of the mountain vallies, compared with the cold experienced in the lower and open country. But, on reflection, is not the difference such as might be expected, considering the causes in operation which have an effect on atmospheric temperature, and especially those connected with the radiation of heat? The damp mountain forests, in absorbing and giving out heat, may act like moun-

some Tables illustrating the temperature of the town, framed from a register of weather, for the use of which I am indebted to the kindness of Major-General Sir Howard Elphinstone, of the royal engineers, by whom it was kept. The thermometer used was of Sixe's construction; it was suspended from a window having a northern aspect, and where the sun never shone, in the house of the commanding engineer in Strada Britannica, standing about 100 feet above the level of the sea, and altogether in a situation favourable to the equalizing effect already referred to.

I. MEAN MONTHLY MAXIMUM AND MINIMUM TEMPERATURE, FROM MAY 1832 TO AUGUST 1834, IN VALETTA.

Months.	1832.		1833.		1834.	
	Max.	Min.	Max.	Min.	Max.	Min.
January, ...	...°	...°	546°	50.7°	58°	53.8°
February, ...	...	...	57	52	55.6	50.3
March, ...	...	...	58	53	57	49.4
April, ...	...	...	61	56	60	54
May, ...	68	63.5	68	62.7	70	65
June, ...	73	67.6	73	73	74.5	70
July, ...	78	72	76	74.6	80	77
August, ...	79	72	77	76	80	78
September, . . .	76	69	73	71	...	...
October, ...	68.6	64	70	66	...	...
November, ...	65	60	63	59	...	...
December, ...	56	51.6	60	55	...	...

tain lakes and streams. The rocks on the mountain sides, besides absorbing and giving out heat, must throw back heat which they receive from the vallies. In the economy of nature, the circumstances alluded to seem to be a beautiful provision for softening the severity of winter, and rendering habitable, regions which the imagination is disposed to conceive the seat of storms and inclemency during the winter season.

II.—THE MAXIMUM AND MINIMUM TEMPERATURE OF EACH MONTH,
DURING THE SAME PERIOD.

Months.	1832.		1833.		1834.	
	Max.	Min.	Max.	Min.	Max.	Min.
January, . . .	...°	...°	60°	42°	60°	44°
February, . . .	...	...	60	46	59	46
March, . . .	...	...	62	49	61	45
April, . . .	...	...	65	52	62	47
May, . . .	72	59	73	52	74	59
June, . . .	78	63	79	68	80	66
July, . . .	84	66	79	63	88	74
August, . . .	83	68	82	74	84	76
September, . .	83	61	78	69	...	...
October, . . .	73	59	73	61	...	...
November, . .	69	56	68	55	...	...
December, . .	63	45	63	43	...	...

II.—THE GREATEST VARIATION OF TEMPERATURE IN TWENTY-FOUR
HOURS, DURING THE SAME PERIOD.

Months.	1832.	1833.	1834.
January, . .	...	9°	7°
February, . .	...	10	9
March, . .	...	10	14
April, . .	...	9	9
May, . .	8	8	7
June, . .	8	7	9
July, . .	8	4	7
August, . .	9	4	5
September, .	12	4	...
October, . .	8	7	...
November, .	7	8	...
December, . .	8	8	...

According to these observations, the greatest diurnal variation of temperature observed in Valetta,

during a period of nearly three years, was 14°; the greatest range of the thermometer in any month was 25°; the greatest range of the instrument in the whole period was 46°; its highest elevation 88°, its lowest depression 42°, and the mean annual temperature, deduced from the observations of 1833, 64°.

I regret that no perfectly corresponding series of observations were made in the country during the same period; the difference, I am satisfied, in some particulars, would be great; the range of the thermometer would be found to be much more consider able; its occasional elevation in summer very much greater, and its depression in winter greater, though in a less degree. I shall give some observations in illustration, confined to the summer season, and first at the Inquisitor's Palace, which stands on a rocky platform, at the head of a valley, elevated about 550 feet above the level of the sea, and about a mile distant from the nearest sea-cliff on the western coast of the island,—a situation of remarkable coolness and freshness, and strongly contrasted with Valetta.

The following are the results of the observations made with the thermometer during three of the hottest months of the year in 1834:—

Months.	Mean.		Extreme.		Greatest Variations in 24 hours.
	Maximum temperature.	Minimum temperature.	Highest temperature.	Lowest temperature.	
June, ·	74.5	65.5	85	61	15
July, .	81.6	72.6	86	66	14
August,	82.3	73	90	66	13

The thermometer used was a delicate one, with a projecting bulb, which was exposed to the open air. The observations were commonly made at three P.M., the hottest part of the day; about ten o'clock at night, and between five and seven in the morning. Had a register thermometer been used, the difference of temperature indicated between the town and the country, would doubtless have been greater; and it would also have been greater, of course, had the early observations been made just before sunrise.

As the difference of temperature, in connexion with health and enjoyment between the town and country, is important in the hot summer climate of Malta, for the sake of closer comparison, I shall place side by side the daily observations for one month, of Sir Howard Elphinstone, taken with a register thermometer, in Valetta, and those which I made at the Inquisitor's Palace, selecting July, when the climate approaches nearest to a tropical climate, and when the high temperature is most equable :—

TOWN.				COUNTRY.						
No.	Max.	Min.	Wind.	No.	Time	Min.	Wind.	Time.	Min.	Wind.
1	79*	74°	E.	1	3 P.M.	78°	W. by S., mod.	6 A.M.	66°	Calm.
2	79	74	E.	2	3	82	S.W. ..	6	73	
3	79	76	S.	3	3	81	S.by W., strong.	6	74	
4	80	77	E.	4	3	86	E. moderate.	10 P.M.	74	E., moderate.
5	79	77	E.	5	3	80	E.S.E., strong.	10	75	E.S.E., strong.
6	79	77	S.E.	6	3	77	W., moderate.	10½	71	W., moderate.
7	81	75	N.W.	7	3	81	N.W., ..	6 A.M.	70	N.E., gentle.
8	78	75	N.	8	3	82	N.W., ..	6½	72	Calm.
9	79	76	N.W.	9	3	82	E., gentle.	11 P.M.	71	N.W., gentle.
10	80	76	W.S.W.	10	3	82	N.W., gentle.	11	71	N.W., moder.
11	78	75	N.N.W.	11	3	77	E. by N., strong.	11	68	E., gentle.
12	80	76	N.N.E.	12	3	80	S., moderate.	11	73	Calm.
13	81	76	N.E.	13	3	84	N.W., ..	10	73	W., gentle.
14	82	76	N.N.W.	14	3	84	N.W., ..	6 A.M.	73	N.W., mod.
15	84	78	N.	15	3	86	N.W., ..	7	76	Calm.
16	81	78	N.N.W.	16	3	83	N., .	6	73	N., moderate.
17	81	79	N.	17	3	81	S.E., gentle.	10 P.M.	73	S.E., gentle.
18	80	77	N.	18	3	83	N.E. ..	10	74	N., ..
19	82	77	N.	19	3	83	N.W., mod.	10	73	N.W., mod.
20	83	77	N.N.W.	20	3	82	N.W., ..	10	71	Calm.
21	80	77	N.N.E.	21	3	82	W., ..	6 A.M.	73	
22	83	78	W.N.W.	22	3	83	W., strong.	8	75	W., moderate.
23	84	79	N.W.	23	3	82	W., moderate.	10 P.M.	73	W.N.W., mod.
24	82	77	N.W.	24	3½	82	W.N.W., mod.	10	73	W.N.W. gentle.
25	81	77	S.E.	25	3	80	S., moderate.	6 A.M.	74	W.N.W., ..
26	82	79	S.S.W.	26	3½	83	E., gentle.	11 P.M.	77	E., in gusts.
27	80	78	N.N.W.	27	3	83	N., ..	10	73	N.W., mod.
28	81	79	E.	28	3	81	E., moderate.	6 A.M.	73	N., gentle.
29	81	79	E.	29	3	80	S.E., strong.	10 P.M.	74	S.E., strong.
30	81	79	S.E.	30	3	80	S.S.E. ..	10	73	S. by E , gentle.
31	88	81	S.S.E.	31	3	79	S., moderate.	6 A.M.	74	Calm.

Further, in illustration of the difference in regard to temperature between the town and the country, I shall give a few detailed observations, made at the Pietà during the summer season, at a house only a few feet above the level of the sea, and not above 100 yards from the water's edge. I shall confine myself to the summer of 1833, for the sake of comparison with Sir Howard Elphinstone's observations made in the town.

August 17,	3	P.M.	98°	S.W., strong.
...	6		90	S.W., moderate.
...	7		83	S.W., gentle.
...	9		82	S.W., very gentle.
...	11		78	almost calm.
18,	8	A.M.	84	S.W., gentle.
.	9		89	N.W., gentle.
...	3	P.M.	102	W. by S., moderate—unsteady
...	5		96	
...	6		88	
22,	10½		67	calm; very clear: during the day a gentle N.W. breeze.
Sept. 1,	1		89	S.W., strong; violent gusts.
...	6½		78	W. by N.
2.	8	A.M.	72	N.W., moderate.
3,	8		67	N.W., strong.
4,	6		63	calm,
5,	7		78	S.E., strong.
...	3	P.M.	84	S.E., tempestuous.
6,	8	A.M.	77	calm.
...	2		89	S., strong.
...	11		78	S.E., gentle.
16,	7½	A.M.	63	calm.

How great is the contrast between these observations and those made in the town; in the town, in August and September, the greatest diurnal variation of temperature was 4°; in the country 20°: in the town the greatest variation, in the course of the two months, was 13°; in the country, in less than one month, 39°, almost equal to the greatest range of the thermometer observed in Valetta during the whole year.

In considering the climate generally, other illustrations of this difference will offer, and the causes will be developed on which it depends.

The mean annual temperature, 64°, deduced from Sir Howard Elphinstone's observations during the year 1833, is probably near the true one. The temperature of a few fountains that I tried was tolerably in accordance.*

The winds which prevail in Malta, and which influence chiefly its climate, are the south-east, or Sirocco, and the south-west, the north-east, and north-west.

The latter winds generally are cool; the degree of coolness depending very much on their strength, especially in winter. At this season I have known the thermometer, with a northerly wind, fall so low as 41°; during seven years I never saw it lower. The north-east and north-west winds (especially the latter, in summer), are usually cool, dry, and invigorating, excepting when gentle and partial, then they are commonly hot. The difference between a moist thermometer and a dry one, exposed to them in the hot season, varies from 12° to 20°. In winter they are more moist, and their character is more variable.

The north-east wind is occasionally of great violence, and is sometimes the cause of much damage, especially in the harbour of Valetta, into which it

* The temperature of a copious fountain at the Inquisitor's Palace, called Fontana Grande, on the 10th June 1834, four days after a heavy shower, was 64.5; on the 27th July, no rain having fallen intermediately, it was 63; on the 15th September, after heavy rain, by which the water was slightly discoloured, it was 65.5. The temperature of another spring, in the adjoining valley of the Boschetto, which probably has a deeper source, was, during the whole summer, whenever I tried it, the same, 64.5.

blows directly: it is called "Gregale" by the natives.

The character of the southerly winds, excepting when they are very gentle, is different from that of the northerly, as might be expected, considering the regions over which they come; and is in many respects peculiar. Warmth is their general characteristic; in other qualities they vary, according to their easterly or westerly inclination. Their peculiarities are most strongly marked in summer. I shall notice only the south-west and the south-east; the wind blowing from the intermediate points approaches in qualities one or other of these very much according to its degree of proximity.

The south-west winds (including the variations between south and west) in summer are the hottest and driest that blow, which a reference to the map will help to explain. I have witnessed with these winds a temperature so high as 105°, and a degree of dryness so great, that a moist thermometer, exposed to the wind, fell from 105° to 73°, and on another occasion from 101° to 69°,—a difference of 32°. In both instances the wind was south by west. More frequently, the temperature of these winds varies between 88° and 98°. They are commonly of short duration, seldom blowing more than a few hours, and are always, as far as my experience allows me to speak, marked by great dryness. When they prevail, they are best guarded against by shutting closely the windows, so as to exclude the heated air. By such precaution, taken in time, the unpleasant effects within doors may be avoided, and the house be kept comparatively cool. If the windows are left open, either through ignorance or the carelessness of servants, the ordinary dwelling apartments soon become almost uninhabitable, and refuge is gladly sought in cellars and stables, as I have more than once witnessed.*

* On the 16th August 1833, when the thermometer in the country, exposed to the south-west wind, rose in the open air to 98°, the temperature of the house, by closing the windows, was kept down to about 86° ; and the temperature of a small room, carefully kept cool during the hot season, was preserved so low as 79°. This room was well adapted for the exclusion of heat: it was beneath another, its walls very thick, always shaded, and it had only one small window, which was always closed during the heat of the day ; indeed it was rarely opened, excepting for a short time in the cool of the early morning.

Further, in illustration of the difference of temperature connected with situation, I may introduce the following observations, made on the 18th July 1831, in Valetta. The thermometer exposed to the open air in the yard of the General Hospital, was 84°; taken into a vaulted room, perfectly dry, hewn out of the rock, under the Pharmacy, it was 74° ; and plunged into a cistern under the yard of the same building, supplied with rain-water, and from which the atmosphere was as much as possible excluded, it fell to 64°.

The luxurious ancients had their subterranean palaces and baths, in which they avoided the extreme summer heats, much in the same manner as some of the Oriental nations do at the present time. At Syracuse, in the hottest weather, I visited an ancient bath, about fifty feet under ground; it was about 20° cooler than the atmosphere. How delightful, in the south of Europe, during the extreme heats, would under-ground houses be, such as the natives of Cabul enjoy themselves in, as described by Mr Elphinstone ; and to which the summer palaces of the Romans appear to have been analogous, at least in design.

The south-east wind is well known, and of evil report, under the name of Sirocco. Respecting this wind much variety of opinion exists, and very contradictory accounts are to be found in authors. By some it is described as excessively damp; by some as extremely dry; it has even been described as both damp and dry, and one writer denies that it is possessed of any peculiar qualities. This discordancy has probably arisen from partial and superficial observation on the part of travellers, who may have drawn their inferences from exceptions in particular situations, and have generalized from them.

The Sirocco wind in Malta, and, it may be added, in the Mediterannean generally, as well as in the Ionian Islands, is invariably charged with moisture, and even more so in summer than in winter. When it blows with any strength, the difference between a moist thermometer and a dry one, exposed to it, seldom exceeds 4° or 5°. Its temperature is never very high, even in the height of the hot season. I have never seen it raise the thermometer above 86° The atmosphere, when this wind prevails, is always hazy, as if palpable vapour were suspended in it. Dust is raised by it in a remarkable manner, and carried along with it.* The sensations which it produces at different seasons are far from being the same. In winter, when its temperature may be about 60°, it

* Perhaps in consequence of the specific gravity of the dust being diminished by the absorption of moisture.

feels mild and agreeable. In spring and early summer, when its temperature may be about 70°, it is not generally unpleasant. It is chiefly in summer and autumn that it is disagreeably felt and complained of, when its temperature ranges between 75° and 85°. The higher its temperature, so much the more distressing are its effects, owing to the little evaporation which it produces. This is connected with its comparative humidity ; and this, its humidity, is, I believe, the principal cause of all its peculiarities,— of the oppressive sensation of heat—of the perspiration in which the skin is bathed,—of its relaxing and debilitating effects on the body, and its lowering and dispiriting effects on the mind. Other effects, too, which are unquestionable, may be referred to the same quality,—as its retarding the drying of paint,* —the promoting the decomposition of animal and vegetable matter,—the rusting of metals,—the fermentation of wines, and the acetous fermentation,— to which may be added the propagation of odours.†

Some effects attributed to it are, I believe, imagi-

* Its bad effects, in connexion with the operation of house-painting, appear to be of two kinds—retarding the drying, and preventing the due adhering of the paint. The former may be from the little evaporation going on; the latter from the humidity of the surface to which the paint is applied, and to the incorporation probably of moisture with the substance of the paint.

† Dr Hennen, in his Medical Topography of the Mediterranean, in p. 32, noticing a similar effect of the easterly winds at Gibraltar, in connexion with the sewers, which, with easterly winds, are peculiarly offensive, asks, " Is this the result of the humid atmosphere

nary and false. I shall mention only a few of them. It has been said to interfere with the operation of vaccination and of inoculation for small-pox, and to render it inert.*   This is not the case, as I have

softening the soil of the sewers, and occasioning an increased exhalation ?" As moisture appears to be almost essential to the propagation or dispersion of odours, probably the effect in question is chiefly owing to the increased power of the air, as a carrier of odorous particles, in consequence of increase of humidity.

     * Dr Hennen has too readily adopted the above opinion; in page 157, of the work already quoted. speaking of the effects of the Sirocco wind, he says, " It is a remarkable fact that wounds and ulcers, and the discharge from mucous surfaces, generally deteriorate during the prevalence of a Sirocco ; and it is equally certain that if vaccination or small-pox inoculation, are performed at this period, they are extremely liable to fail ; and if they succeed, the progress of the pustule is often suspended, and it is frequently ten or twelve days in reaching the state usually attained in six or eight." He refers to the seventy-first volume of the Philosophical Transactions. In that volume there is an account, not of the Sirocco, but of the Harmattan, a wind of a character totally different, cool, and excessively dry, which frequently prevails on the African coast, between Cape Verd and Cape Lopez (an extent of coast upwards of 2100 miles), during the months of December, January, and February. It is an easterly wind, and blows from the interior towards the Atlantic. Amongst the effects attributed to it by Dr Dobson (the author of the account drawn up from the observations of Mr Norris) is its stopping the progress of epidemics, as small-pox, &c., and preventing inoculation for small-pox from taking effect. It is remarkable that this wind, though extremely dry, is accompanied with a hazy state of atmosphere, a dry mistiness from subtile dust suspended in it. Although most salubrious to animals, it is described as very injurious to vegetables ; by its drying power, it exhausts their moisture and withers them, " the grass withers, and becomes dry like hay."

     Many mistakes respecting the Sirocco of the Mediterranean have arisen, probably from confounding it with the Harmattan of the Gold Coast.

been assured by a very experienced vaccinator. Wine, it is said, bottled during a Sirocco, will not keep. I have made the trial, and the result has not confirmed the saying. Sound wines may, I believe, be bottled at any time with safety. Light wines, those not thoroughly fermented, will be in more danger, especially immediately after the vintage, when the Sirocco is commonly very warm as well as moist, the vinous fermentation being exceedingly prone to pass into the acetous.

The beneficial effects of this wind, which have generally been less dwelt on, and are less commonly known than its disagreeable ones, are dependent, I believe, chiefly on the same quality of humidity,—as its promoting vegetation, by preventing the parching of the soil,—its favouring the corn-harvest, by preventing the sudden drying of the ear, and the falling out and loss of the grain,—and its favouring the olive crop in ripening, by preventing the olives from becoming shrivelled on the trees. In the month of May, the period of corn-harvest in Malta, a hot parching south-west wind is as much dreaded by the natives as a cold and parching north-east wind is feared in Corfu, in February, the time of the olive crop. A good word, too, is sometimes spoken of this wind by sportsmen, on account of the flights of quail which it brings in ; and occasionally, also, by invalids, such as happen to like a warm moist atmosphere, and muzzy weather ; and occasionally, too, by young ladies, performers on the guitar, the sounds of which it softens and improves, by its relaxing effect on the chords. It is, perhaps, partly on this account as well as on account of the warmth of the Sirocco, that it is peculiarly influential in the Ionian Islands on the musical natives; when it blows, especially in winter and spring, serenading parties perambulate the streets, and the guitar, in accompaniment with the voice, is to be heard very commonly. Besides humidity, other causes have been supposed to exist, in connexion with the Sirocco, to which its peculiarities have been attributed. Some have considered them owing to a peculiar electric state, and some to deficiency of oxygen. The experiments which I have made on it with much care, have not been favourable to either of these conclusions.

In a series of experiments which I made on atmospheric electricity, for several months in Valetta, in 1835, the results of which have been given in a paper published in the thirteenth volume of the Transactions of the Royal Society of Edinburgh, no well marked difference was perceptible in the electrical condition of the atmosphere, from whatever quarter the wind blew, under ordinary circumstances,—whether the clear north-east or north-west wind prevailed, or the hazy Sirocco, the electrical state of the atmosphere was found to be opposite to that of the earth, —the former negative, the latter positive. And this condition was less frequently reversed with a Sirocco wind than with other winds; when the change did occur, there were commonly indications of a disturbed electrical equilibrium, the accompaniments of the thunder or hail-storm.

In another series of experiments which occupied me more than a year, viz. from September 1830 to December 1831, I carefully weighed a certain portion of atmospheric air, to endeavour to ascertain, if, with different winds and at different seasons, there is any change in its specific gravity. I engaged in the inquiry at the suggestion of my friend Dr Prout, with a delicate apparatus specially procured for the purpose. The results were negative. There was no appreciable difference of specific gravity between the air of the moist Sirocco and of the sultry and excessively dry south-west wind, or of the very clear north-east or north-west wind; nor was there any difference of specific gravity appreciable during the different seasons.* The necessary deduction from these negative results is, that the ponderable elements of the Sirocco are nowise different from common atmospheric air, and, *à fortiori*, that the proportion of oxygen is not less.

Whether the Sirocco is impregnated with any subtle substance analogous to the matter of malaria, or that which produces intermittent and remittent fever, —a matter so subtle that it escapes our senses, eludes every chemical test, and is known only by its effects on the animal economy,—it is difficult to determine. I am more disposed to infer that it does not bear with it such a substance than that it does, principally

---

* In these trials, the air, previous to weighing, was kept over water, and saturated with moisture.

because I am not aware that any of its effects are similar to those of malaria : I am not aware that it exercises any *specific* effect injurious to the constitution,—that it occasions any specific morbid action or disease. If a known cause is sufficient, it is not philosophical to have recourse to an imaginary one; it appears to me that all the ordinary effects of the Sirocco may be referred to its humidity and comparatively high temperature combined. Those who have doubts on the subject, will do well to submit them to the test of experiment, and endeavour to collect and demonstrate the existence of foreign matter. In such an inquiry, it will be necessary carefully to discriminate between what is constantly present in the Sirocco, and that which may be accidentally wafted, as the occasional matter of blight, affecting vegetation,* and the earthy and saline matter, in the form of impalpable dust, of which it is occasionally the vehicle.

Another interesting subject of inquiry is, the origin of this wind, or the circumstances to which it owes its peculiar qualities, especially its high degree of humidity.

The hypothesis which appears to me most accordant with facts (I do not know whether it has been proposed before) is, that the humidity of the Sirocco, its most characteristic quality, is owing to the admix-

---

* It has been said that the Sirocco, though moist, scorches vegetation; when any such apparent effect is produced by it, it is probably owing to an accompanying blight, or peculiar matter injurious to vegetation, of which the wind is merely the vehicle.

ture of warm with cool strata of air in the atmosphere of the Mediterranean,—of warm air, already abounding in moisture, though in less degree than the Sirocco.

On this hypothesis, the different degrees of dryness of the south-east wind, in different situations, do not appear difficult of explanation, and some apparently contradictory statements as to the nature of the Sirocco admit of being accounted for.

In Upper Egypt, at Tripoli, on the African coast of the Mediterranean generally,* also at Palermo, the south-east wind is described as excessively dry and hot in the summer season. In the former instances, it blows over a parched and heated desert; and in the last, that of Palermo, it crosses a considerable portion of Sicily, also heated and dry, and well fitted to deprive it of its moisture, abounding as that part of the country does in clay and limestone formations, and naturally arid.

In Lower Egypt, especially towards the coast, and at Alexandria, the south-east wind (there not common),† is described as moist and hazy; qualities which it may derive in its passage over a considerable tract of country, either under water, or nearly satu-

* Pliny says:—"Humidus aut æstuosus (auster) Italiæ, Africæ quidem incendia cum serenitate affert."

† Some of the ancients supposed that this wind is unknown in Egypt: Pliny says " in Ægyptum penetrare (austrum) negat Fabianus." And Aristotle in his Problemata asks, why does this wind prevail above Memphis, and not blow within a day and night's journey from the coast?

rated with water, according to the season of the year and the state of the Nile.

At Tripoli, the east wind is the most humid, and approaches nearest to the character of the Sirocco of Malta; and that wind also passes over a comparatively moist surface, along-shore, and over the Great Syrtis, an extent of nearly 400 miles, low, sandy, and marshy.*

At Gibraltar, too, this wind has the same character; whilst at Aleppo it is the reverse : at the former it is exceedingly moist; in the latter, excessively hot and dry.† The circumstances are perfectly in accordance with these qualities. In the former instance, passing over a great tract of the Mediterranean, it is necessarily damp and warm ; in the latter passing over a dry heated country, it becomes parched and hot ; and moreover, at Gibraltar, the elevated cold rock, against which the current of air strikes, acts the part of a refrigeratory, and precipitates, in the form of mist, a portion of the aqueous vapour, producing a singular and very striking appearance, as if the rock were smoking and on fire.

Whether the Sirocco comes from Africa, or is air set in motion over the Mediterranean, towards the African shore, is a problem of no easy solu-

* I have been informed by Dr Dickson, many years resident at Tripoli, that a moist thermometer exposed to the east wind, falls 8° or 9° in summer, and that with a south-east wind, he has seen it fall 30°. There is commonly there, in the hot season, a land and sea-breeze.

† *Vide* " A General Description of the Seasons at Aleppo," in the Appendix to Dr Russel's work on the Plague.

tion. The circumstance that this wind does not prevail in Africa, in the countries bordering on the Mediterranean, is in favour of the latter supposition. So also is its apparent lowness; it is called " *basso vento*" now; Pliny speaks of it even as if it rose from the sea, "infernus ex imo maris spirat."* The manner too in which it blows, alluded to by Aristotle in his problems (if a fact), is in favour of the same notion. " Cur auster parvus oritur, magnus desistat ?"

On this hypothesis, its humidity would be perfectly explained as a " basso vento"—considering it, as a stratum of air immediately incumbent on the sea, set in motion, and from its situation, nearly saturated with moisture. And it would account equally well, for the greater prevalency and heightened character of the Sirocco wind in autumn, than at any other season, the Mediterranean then being of highest temperature, and the atmosphere comparatively cool above it.

* The circumstance that this wind is occasionally saline, may have led to the above idea respecting its origin. By saline, I mean impregnated with, or holding suspended, saline matter, of which I had proof on the night of the 2d of August 1834, and it was the only time I witnessed what I had frequently heard asserted. On that night, the wind in question was blowing moderately. I perceived a slight saline moisture, like dew, on the naked bulb of a thermometer exposed to it ; and I farther satisfied myself of the fact, by exposing glass vessels to the wind. The saline matter was in exceedingly minute quantity ; it appeared to be principally sea-salt. The thermometer at the time was 76°, the air saturated with moisture. The observation was made at the Inquisitor's Palace, between three and four miles from the south-east shore.

The following Table shows the frequency of gales
in the different months, during a period of nearly
three years, extracted from Sir Howard Elphinstone's
Register.

Months.	1832.	1833.	1834.
January, .		7	4
February,		5	6
March, .		7	3
April, . .		8	3
May, . .	...	...	...
June, . .	...	1	...
July, . .	...	1	...
August, .	...	...	...
September,	...	...	1
October, .	5	...	2
November,	...	1	1
December,	5	6	...

Few regions are less liable to calms than Malta, especially by day. A calm of twenty-four hours' duration,
has perhaps never been experienced there in the
memory of man. During the hot season, this perfect
ventilation of the island is on the whole a fortunate
circumstance. But whether it is to be considered so
in winter and early spring, when the winds are particularly rude and boisterous, is doubtful. The strong
winds then prevalent, render the climate far from
agreeable, and more trying to invalids than might be
expected, from its comparatively high and equable
temperature. I shall recur to this subject in considering the climate of Malta, in connexion with
health.

The atmosphere of this island, as of the Mediterranean generally, is distinguished for its clearness. During a considerable portion of the year, it is cloudless to excess; the incessant brightness is almost as wearisome to the mind as it is trying to the eyes; when clouds do appear, they are welcomed much in the same manner as sunshine is in England in the winter season, and their effect is very grateful.

The following Table, formed from the Meteorological Register, kept by Sir Howard Elphinstone, shows the number of cloudless days in each month, of days in which there was partial sunshine, and of those in which the sun through the day was entirely hid.

Months.	1832.			1833.			1834.		
	Constant sunshine.	Partial.	Absent.	Constant.	Partial.	Absent.	Constant.	Partial.	Absent.
January, ...				6	13	12	20	8	3
February, ...				14	6	8	9	11	8
March, ...				17	7	7	16	10	5
April, ...				21	6	4	16	8	6
May, ...	14	5	2	19	7	5	23	6	2
June, ...	25	3	2	16	6	8	24	4	2
July, ...	29	2	...	26	5	...	31	...	...
August, ...	31	...	...	30	1	...	29	1	1
September, . . .	26	3	1	14	15	1	18	10	2
October, . . .	13	8	10	14	15	2	16	12	3
November, . .	8	10	12	19	6	5	11	5	5
December, . . .	13	11	7	19	9	3			6

During the dry season, the sky generally at night is even clearer than by day; whilst during the rainy season, it is commonly the reverse. These are happy circumstances, both of them conducive to the equalization of the temperature;—the former favouring this effect by radiation from the earth into ætherial space, and consequent loss of heat, so preventing excessive accumulation in summer; the latter having a contrary tendency in winter.

In illustration of the cooling effect of radiation, which acts so important and beneficial a part in the economy of nature in warm climates, I shall give here the results of a series of observations made on the subject, in the summer, autumn, and early winter of 1830, and continued during part of the following summer. I hope they will not be considered without interest to the meteorologist. That they may not be valueless, I shall give them in detail, and as they were noted down at the time. The place of observation was the terrace-roof, either of the house at the Pietà, already referred to, well adapted to the purpose, or of a house in the town of Valetta, not commanded by any near building, and about thirty feet above the level of the street. Delicate thermometers, with projecting bulbs were used, both for trying the temperature of the air, the effect of evaporation (the bulb being moistened), and the effect of radiation. For this last mentioned object, the instrument was placed on a surface of cotton-wool, either loosely attached to a flat piece of cork, or collected in an open wicker basket. In this way the thermometer was effectually defended from heat rising from below, and the effect of radiation was, I believe, as great as possible, or very nearly so. In a comparative trial with an aetheriscope of the best construction, the reduction of temperature was greatest on the cotton, greater than in the concave mirror by 2°.*

1838.	Hour.	Therm. in Air.		Therm. on Cotton.		Dew.	Weather, &c.
		Dry.	Moist.	Dry.			
July 13,	4½ A.M.	67°	64°	58°		Slight dew.	Calm—clear.
14,	4¾	73	63	57	...	Very slight.	Ditt o
15,	4¾	74	70	63	...	Dew.	Ditto.
16,	4¼	74	73	67	...	Ditto.	{ N.W., gentle—low gray clouds.
	3 P.M.	84	73	112	In sun.	...	N.W., strong.
	6 30	83	78	72	In shade.	..	N.W., gentle.
	7 30	78	...	72	{ ½ hour af. sunset.	..	} Ditto.
	10 45	78	72	68	...	Much dew.	Calm—clear.
17,	4 47 A.M.	73	71	67	...	Ditto.	{ Nearly calm—horizon hazy.
	11 P.M.	74	70	64	...	Ditto.	Calm—clear.
18,	4 45 A.M.	69	67	63	...	Ditto.	Nearly calm—clear.
	6 45 P.M.	80	...	70	In shade.	Very slight.	{ Nearly calm—clear.—N.B. Just before sunset.
	9	78	73	67	...	Copious.	N.W., gentle—clear.
	11 10	76	...	64	...	Much dew.	Calm—clear.
19,	4 40 A.M.	70	67	60	...	Ditto.	Almost calm—clear.
	7 P.M.	80	74	70	...	Slight.	N.W., gentle—clear.
	9	...	...	66	...	Much dew.	Nearly calm—clear.
20,	4 35 A.M.	70	68	63	..	Ditto.	
22,	3 P.M.	86	75	...	...	...	N.W., strong—clear.
	11	77	72	66	...	Dew.	Calm—clear.
23,	5 A.M.	73	70	66	...	Much dew.	} W., very gentle—clear.
24,	4 40	70	67	61	...	Ditto.	
25,	5	74	68	68	...	Slight.	{ W., gentle—a few clouds—in clear sky.
26,	3 P.M.	83	72	...	...	...	{ Variable—thunder from 5 to 7 P.M. heavy rain & hail.

* The aetheriscope belonged to the late Dr Turnbull Christie, whose premature death in India science has to deplore. When I recollect the ardour, the ability which he displayed in making observations, and how well he was provided with instruments, I cannot but express regret that the results of his even unfinished inquiries have not been given to the world, especially on the climate of Egypt, and of those parts of India which he visited.

TABLE (*continued.*)

1830.	Hour.	Therm. in Air. Dry.	Moist.	Therm. on Cotton. Dry.	Dew.	Winds, &c.
July 26,	10 P.M.	68	64	63	No dew.	W., gentle—zenith clear — violent thunderstorm and hail.
30,	4 40 A.M.	68	68	65	Much dew.	Calm—clear.
Aug. 3,	5	76	71	70	No dew.	S.E., gentle — hazy—cloudy.
	6 30 P.M.	75	69	70	Ditto.	S.E., very gentle—pretty clear, after rain.
	12 M.	75	71	70	Ditto.	S.E., very gentle—light clouds.
4,	11 P.M.	77	74	70	Much dew.	S E., gentle — pretty clear—light clouds.
5,	5 A.M.	75	73	68	Ditto.	S.E., very gentle—pretty clear—light clouds.
6,	5	71	71	65	Ditto.	Calm—hazy—smoke descending.
7,	5 20	77	74	73	Very slight.	W. by N.—moderate—cloudy.
	11 P. M	78	67	72	No dew.	W., moderate—clear.
8,	5 25 A.M.	74	74	69	Slight dew.	W., gentle—clear.
	10 45 P.M.	74	71	66	Dew.	Calm—clear.
9,	5 15 A.M.	71	70	64	Much dew.	Ditto
	3 P.M	81	73	...	...	N.W., fresh.
	6 30	79	72	71	...	Ditto.
	11 30	78	72	66	No dew.	Calm—very clear.
10,	5 A.M.	70	67	64	Much dew.	Calm—clear.
	7	77	72	70	...	Ditto.
	6 30 P.M.	80	70	75	...	N.E., gentle—clear—the cotton in shade.
	7	79	72	70	...	N.E., gentle—clear just after sunset.
	9 30	74	70	65	Slight dew.	Calm—very clear.
11,	5 A.M.	68	67	64	Much dew.	W., very gentle—clear.
	7 25	79	72	69	...	Ditto.
	10 11 P.M.	75	73	68	Ditto.	W., gentle—clear.
12,	5 10 A.M.	72	70	66	Ditto.	Ditto.
	11 P.M.	79	74	72	Slight.	Ditto.
13,	5 10 A.M.	73	68	64	Pret. much.	Calm—clear.
	1 P.M.	84	79	...	...	S.E., moderate—light low clouds.
	10	80	76	74	Dew.	E. by S., gentle—clear.
14,	5 25 A.M.	72	72	66	Much dew.	Calm—Zenith clear.
	11 P.M.	76	72	66	Ditto.	W., very gentle—clear.
15,	5 15 A.M.	72	70	64	Ditto.	Calm.
	3 P.M.	84	75	...	...	S. W., pretty strong—low gray clouds.

TABLE (*continued.*)

1830.	Hour.	Therm. in Air. Dry.	Moist.	Therm. in Cotton. Dry.	Dew.	Winds, &c.
Aug. 15,	6 40 P.M.	81	74	72	Much dew.	W., nearly calm—clear —sun just gone down.
	10 30	76	74	64	Pret. much.	Calm—clear.
16,	4 55 A.M.	71	70	65	Much dew.	Ditto.
	10 30 P.M.	77	73	63	Ditto.	Ditto.
17,	4 55 A.M.	72	70	61	Ditto.	Ditto.
	10 P.M.	79	75	69	Some dew.	S.W., very gentle.
18,	5 A.M.	77	74	70	Ditto.	N.W.,fresh—gray clouds in clear sky.
	11 F.M.	74	67	73	No dew.	N.W., strong—clear.
19,	5 15 A.M.	73	67	73	Ditto.	Ditto.
	5 26	73	67	67	...	N.W., a sudden lull— sun rising.
20,	5 30	71	64	66	No dew.	W.N.W., mild—clear.
	9 P.M.	71	69	58	Dew.	S.E., very gentle—clear.
21,	5 15 A.M.	68	63	57	Much dew.	Calm—Zenith clear.
22,	5 25	79	77	76	Ditto.	S.E., mild — cloudy— hazy.
	3 P.M.	81	77	...	...	S.S.E., strong—hazy— overcast.
	8	79	76	75	...	W.N.W., strong—hazy.
	10 30	79	76	73	Very slight.	W., gentle—pretty clear.
23,	5 A.M.	79	72	72	No dew.	NW.,moderate—hazy— cloudy.
	11 15	72	67	61	Dew.	Calm—clear.
24,	5 30 A.M.	72	69	65	Much dew.	Nearly calm — light fleecy clouds.
	4 P.M.	75	68			
	11	...	...	62	Slight dew.	
25,	5 A.M.	68	64	56	Much dew.	Clear, N.W.—very gentle.
	3 P.M.	79	68	...		
	11	72	68	63	Ditto.	Clear—W., very gentle.
26,	5 20 A.M.	67	66	59	Ditto.	Clear—calm.
	3 P.M.	81	75	...	...	S.E., moderate — light clouds.
	10 ½ P.M.	73	68	65	Ditto.	Clear—W., very gentle.
27,	5 30 A.M.	67	67	59	Ditto.	Clear—calm.
	9 20 P.M.	74	68	64	Ditto.	Ditto.
28,	5 24 A.M.	67	64	57	Ditto.	Ditto.
	1 P.M.	80	...	78	...	Clear—N.W., gentle.
29,	5 15 A.M.	65	64	56	Ditto.	Calm—very clear.
	10 P.M.	73	...	65	...	Clear—W., very gentle.
30,	5 15	67	...	60	Ditto.	Clear—almost calm.
31,	5 25	67	63	54	Little dew.	Calm—clear.
	3 P.M.	84	70	...	...	E., gentle.
	6 30 P.M.	81	71	64	Very slight.	Clear—calm.

TABLE (*continued.*)

1830.	Hour.	Therm. in Air.		Therm. on Cotton.	Dew.	Winds, &c.
		Dry.	Moist.	Dry.		
Aug. 31.	7 25 P.M.	80	...	60	Slight dew.	Clear—calm.
	8 40	77	69	62	...	Clear—S.W., very gentle.
	10 30	71	67	59	Dew incrsg.	Clear—nearly calm.
Sept. 1,	5 35 A.M.	69	69	53	Much dew.	Calm—clear.
	3 P.M.	90	68	115	...	Clear—W.N.W., mod.
	10 30	77	65	64	No dew.	Clear—W., gentle.
2,	6 A.M.	70	68	60	Slight dew.	Calm —hazy—low clouds.
	3 P.M.	87	70	...	...	
	11 A.M.	77	74	64	Much dew.	Calm—clear.
3,	6 A.M.	71	71	65	Much dew.	{ Calm—hazy—masses of vapour on the higher ground.
	4 P.M.	84	76	...	...	Clear—S. by E., moderate.
5,	5 45 A.M.	78	73	72	No dew.	{ Hazy—S.E., strong, in gusts.
	3 P.M.	85	76	...	...	{ S.W., strong — stormy —hazy and cloudy— obscured by dust.
	6 30	79	71	77	...	{ W. by N., tempestuous —hazy.
6,	6 A.M.	72	65	70	Ditto.	N.W., moderate—clear.
	3 P.M.	77	68	...	...	N.W., moderate —cloudy.
	10	75	64	65	Ditto.	N.W.,gentle—pretty clear.
7,	5 40 A.M.	67	66	63	Slight dew.	W., very gentle—clear.
	3 P.M.	80	70	...	...	N.W., mod.—light clouds.
	6 25	77	69	76	...	W., strong—overcast.
8,	5 45 A.M.	69	66	63	Ditto.	{ Calm — gray clouds—a little blue sky.
	3 P.M.	78	71	...	...	{ S.E., variable — cloudy —overcast — after a little rain.
9,	5 50 A.M.	73	66	70	No dew.	W., mod.—horizon cloudy.
	3 P.M.	77	62	...	...	{ N.W., blowing strong in gusts—light low clds.
	10	72	62	66	Ditto.	W., rather strong—clear.
10,	5 50 A.M.	67	62	55	Slight dew.	{ Calm—clear—the night windy.
	3 P.M.	78	68	...	...	N.W., moderate—clear.
	11	68	62	59	Dew.	Calm—clear.
12,	5 45 A.M.	69	66	62	Slight dew.	{ W., very gentle—zenith clear.
	10 P.M.	72	64	58	Ditto.	Calm—very clear.
13,	6 A.M.	72	65	65	No dew.	Calm—cloudy.
	10 P.M.	72	65	58	Dew.	Calm—clear.
14,	5 50 A.M.	73	67	66	No dew.	N.W., moderate—clear.
	3 P.M.	79	69	...		N.W., strong—clear.
15,	5 50 A.M.	67	63	57	{ Pretty much dew. }	Calm—clear.

TABLE (*continued.*)

1830.	Hour.	Therm. in Air. Dry.	Moist.	Therm. on Cotton. Dry.	Dew.	Winds, &c.
Sept. 15,	10 P.M.	71	65	57	Much dew.	Calm—clear.
16,	6 A.M.	65	64	55	Ditto	Ditto.
	3 30 P.M.	79	72	...	...	N.W., moderate.
17,	5 55 A.M.	64	64	58	Ditto.	Calm—clear.
	9 P.M.	72	68	62	Ditto.	Ditto.
18,	6 A.M.	66	64	58	Ditto.	Ditto.
	3 P.M.	81	72	...	...	S.W., moderate—low clds.
20,	6 A.M.	67	87	63	Slight dew.	S.E., gentle—hor. cloudy.
	3 P.M.	78	72	...	...	S.E., moderate—cloudy.
	10	72	67	62	Much dew.	Calm—clear.
21,	6 A.M.	65	65	58	Ditto.	Calm—pretty clear.
	3 P.M.	81	73	...	...	S.W., strong—cloudy.
24,	6 A.M	69	59	65	No Dew.	N.W., strong—clear.
	9 45 P.M.	70	63	64	Ditto.	W.by N., moderate—clear.
25,	6 30 A.M.	63	58	56	Very slight.	N.W., gentle—very clear.
	10 P.M.	70	66	65	Ditto.	N.W., mod.—scatt. clouds.
28,	6 30 A.M.	61	57	57		W., gentle — dark low clouds — rain during night.
	3 P.M.	67	60			W., cloudy—showery.
	10	60	56	52	Much dew.	W., very gentle—hazy—stars of 1st and 2d magnitude only visible
29,	6 40 A.M.	57	57	53		Nearly calm — zenith clear—night squally, with heavy rain.
	11 P.M.	62	59	55	Ditto.	W., very gentle—clear—heavy rain about noon.
Oct. 1,	1 A.M.	63	60	50	Ditto.	Calm—clear.
	6 10	60	59	50	Ditto.	Ditto.
	3 P.M.	73	66	...	...	N.W., gentle—clear.
	9 30	66	63	57	A little dew.	Calm—clear.
2,	6 A.M.	62	62	55	Much dew.	Ditto.
	11 P.M.	63	63	57	Ditto.	Ditto.
4,	6 A.M.	72	70	68	A very little dew.	S.W., gentle—sky overcast with gray clouds.
6,	7	66	65	65		N.E., strong — dark clouds — after heavy rain.
	11 P.M.	65	62	58	Slight dew.	W., very gentle—clear—scattered white clds.
7,	6 20 A.M.	60	60	52	Much dew.	N.W., very gentle—zenith clear.
	3 P.M.	72	65			E., moderate—light clouds.
8,	6 30 A.M.	68	62	62	No dew.	E., fresh—scattered silvery clouds.
	9 30 P.M.	61	58	49	Much dew.	Calm—clear.

TABLE (*continued.*)

1830.	Hour.	Therm. in Air.		Thermometer on Cotton.		Dew.	Winds, &c.
		Dry.	Moist.	Dry.	Moist.		
Oct. 9,	6 15 A.M.	61	58	55	...	Dew drying.	E., mod.—zen. clear.
	2 P.M.	70	60				E., moderate—clear.
	10	61	55	50	...	No dew.	Calm—clear.
	10 45	61	55	46	...	Slight dew.	Ditto.
10,	6 20 A.M	61	58	55	...	...	{ E. by S., gent.—gray —clds in clear sky rain during night.
12,	6	54	54	46	...	Much dew.	Calm—zenith clear.
	2 P.M.	67	63	...	...	Raining.	S.E., moderate.
19,	6 25 A.M.	61	54	54	...	No dew.	{ E., moderate—dark clouds in'clear sky.
22,	6 15	61	55	53	...	Ditto.	{ E., moderate—clear —some clouds.
29,	10 P.M.	60	55	52	...	Ditto.	{ N.W., moderate— clear—light clds.
30,	6 35 A.M.	55	55	52	...	Dew.	{ W. by N., very gentle—clear.
Nov. 2,	10 30 P.M.	56	53	46	...	Dew.	{ W., almost calm— very clear.
3,	7 A.M.	52	52	46	...	Much dew.	{ W. by N., very gentle—very clear.
	3 P.M.	67	60	...	...	...	N.W., very gent.—clr.
	6	63	59	48	...	Slight dew.	Calm—clear.
	10 30	55	55	45	...	Much dew.	Calm—very clear.
4,	6 40 A.M.	52	52	40	...	Very much.	Ditto.
5,	6 40	62	60	59	...	Dew.	{ E., very gentle— grey clouds—part of night sky clear.
10,	6 40	53	53	43	...	Much dew.	Calm—zenith clear.
20,*	7		65	63	58	...	Much dew.	{ S.E., moderate — zenith clear.
21,	7		58	53	50	...	No dew.	{ N.W., moderate— zenith clear.
22,	7		57	53	48	...	Slight dew.	Ditto.
23,	7		57	50	48	...	Ditto.	N.W., mod.—clear.
27,	7		55	51	48	...	No dew.	N.W., gentle-zen. clr.
28,	7		59	56	50	...	Much dew.	W., very gent.—clear.
Dec. 9,	11 30 P.M.	60	56	53	...	Slight dew.	W., gentle—clear.
10,	7 A.M.	62	59	55	...	Dew.	{ S.W., very moderate—pretty clear.
1831.							
July 10,†	5	71	...	66	...	Much dew.	Calm—clear.
15,	8 P.M.	82	72	65	64	No dew.	Calm—clear.
	9	80	70	67	64	Ditto.	N.W., gentle—clear.
	10	78	63	64	59	Ditto.	Ditto.
16,	5 A.M.	72	64	60		Ditto.	{ N.W. nearly calm— zenith clear.

* In Valetta, on a terrace-roof.   † Pieta.

TABLE (*continued.*)

1831.	Hour.	Therm. in Air.		Therm. on Cotton.		Dew.	Winds, &c.
		Dry	Moist.	Dry.	Moist.		
	3 P.M.	90°	70°	...	...	No dew.	N.W., gentle.
July 24,	10 30	76	74	64	64°	Much dew.	Calm—clear.
25,	5 A.M.	67	65	60	60	Ditto.	Calm—zenith clear.
Aug. 21,	6	83	...	...	...	...	{ W. by S. stormy-- hazy—cloudless.
	10 30 A.M.	101	73	...	...	...	W. by S., in str. gusts.
	1 P.M.	105	73	...	...	...	{ N. mod.—gray clds. forming.
	3	99	75	...	...	...	N. gentle—light clds.
	5	92	76	...	...	...	S.W., gentle—clear.
	7	89	76	77	74	No dew.	SW.,nrly calm—z. cl.
	11	85	76	72	...	Ditto.	W., str.—partial cl.
22,	6 A.M.	90	75	...	...	...	{ W. by S. strong— cloudy hazy.
	2 P.M.	97	78	...	...	...	
	10 0	79	74	69	69	Much dew.	{ N.W., nearly calm very clear.

I have already pointed out the great difference of temperature at night between the town and the country in Malta. These observations on the radiation of heat, and reduction of temperature in consequence, may help to explain the rationale of the difference; and, further, they may lead to some practical results, and perhaps useful applications.

Were I asked an opinion respecting the most effectual way of obtaining coolness, combined with safety to health, at night, so desirable in the hot nights of Malta, I would suggest an apartment, made as much as possible of glass,—in fact, an apartment all window,—provided with thick wooden shutters, lined on the inside with cotton-wool, and painted white on the outside. Were the shutters closed by day, the sun's heat would be very much excluded, and the apartment

would be kept cool. And were they opened after
sunset (glass interfering very little with the radiation
of heat), the apartment would have the advantage of
the cooling produced by radiation. The windows
even might be thrown open till protection from the
open air became advisable; or musquito blinds might
be partially substituted for glass frames. They would
allow of a circulation of air, exclude insects, and
permit of a certain degree of cooling effect from
radiation.

I may mention a few results in illustration. At
five o'clock in the morning, on the 14th August 1830,
when the thermometer in the open air was 72°, one
placed on cotton naked was found to be 67°, and
another on cotton covered with glass 68°; and again,
at eleven o'clock at night, when the thermometer in
the air was 76°, that on the cotton exposed was 66°,
and that on the cotton under glass was 68°. On another occasion, when the temperature of the air was
78°, a thermometer on cotton naked was 66°, one on
cotton covered with thin muslin, at the height of two
feet, was 71°. This was at eleven P.M. on the 14th
of August. On the following morning at five A.M.,
the thermometer exposed to the air was 72°, that
under muslin on cotton 69°, and that on cotton
naked 66°.

Were an apartment such as I have imagined constructed, with all due attention to comfort, and in a
proper situation,—as on an elevated terrace, or any
other more convenient site not exposed to reflected

heat,—I cannot but infer that it would prove of incalculable use, both as regards comfort of sensation
and health, and especially through the means of refreshing sleep, which it would greatly help to procure.
Even against warm winds the glass would serve as
a protection;—not only by excluding the current of
heated air, but also by allowing of the radiation of
heat from within through the heated air. Thus, on
the 20th August 1830, at half-past five A.M., when the
wind was of moderate strength, and a thermometer
exposed to it stood at 71°, and a moist thermometer
at 64°, a thermometer on cotton exposed was 66°,
whilst another covered with thin glass was 63°.

It is to be regretted that, in modern times, science
has been so little applied to the regulation of temperature and ventilation, especially in the south of
Europe. We cool wines for the table ; we cool water;
but no precautions are taken to cool our sitting-
rooms, or even ventilate them. The company is at
the mercy of chance ; and the chances are that an-
noyance from heat and close air will be great, and
spoil all enjoyment. At Malta, indeed, at the height
of the hot season, social intercourse, at least in the
form of dinner parties, is almost entirely interrupted.

To return to radiation of heat :—Some of the
observations contained in the preceding Tables may
deserve to be particularly pointed out ; first, as
showing the very rapid manner in which the temperature falls immediately after sunset ; and, secondly,
how the effect of radiation may be combined with

that of evaporation in lowering temperature. The observations made on the evenings of the 16th, 18th, and 19th of July 1830 ; on the 10th, 15th, 20th, and 31st of August; and on the 2d of November of the same year, particularly bear on the first point; and those made on the 15th of July and the 21st of August 1831, on the second.

The very rapid cooling from radiation, as soon as the sun has sunk below the horizon in a clear sky, has often surprised me. I have seen it strikingly displayed in a very simple manner, by exposing a wine-bottle of green glass, filled with water and corked, to the open sky on a terrace-roof, resting on cotton. On the 20th August, at three P.M., when the temperature of the air was 79°, the moist thermometer 66°, and the wind blowing briskly from the N.W., the temperature of the water in the bottle, which had been exposed several hours, was 126° ; at nine P.M. it had fallen to 74°; at half-past ten, to 71° ; and at five A.M. the following morning to 62°, and then the temperature of the air was 68°. To this happy and beautiful provision, no doubt, we owe the delightful evenings, which in the south of Europe, to those who go forth into the open air, compensate for the hot days, and afford so much enjoyment to the natives, who at this season almost live in the open air.

Relative to the conjoint effect of radiation and evaporation in cooling, above noticed, it probably is not inoperative in the economy of nature ; it may equally serve to explain the production of ice artificially procured in Bengal, when the temperature of the atmosphere is above the freezing point; and the fact of snow not thawing, as is often witnessed in northern regions, when it might be expected from the higher temperature of the air. Sir Robert Baker's account of the " Process of making Ice in the East Indies" appears to me to accord with this idea. According to his statement, the greatest quantity of ice was produced " when the atmosphere was perfectly serene, sharp and thin, with very little dew after midnight."* I need not point out how all the precautions taken in conducting this curious process are almost equally favourable for promoting evaporation and radiation. At home we sometimes witness this joint effect, not only in preventing the thawing of snow, but also in producing the freezing of water. In the spring of 1837 I observed it, on the 24th of March, when the thermometer in the shade was 33°, just after sunset; water then trickling on the ground from a pump was freezing; a thermometer placed on cotton fell to 30°, and a moist thermometer to 26°: and again, on the 16th of the same month, at ten P.M., when the thermometer in the air was 34°, one on cotton was 31°; and when the moist thermometer in the air was 31°, on the grass it was 29°; and water exposed in a shallow earthen pan, resting on cotton, was covered with ice.

Dews are not so frequent in Malta nor so copious

* Phil. Trans. abridged, vol. xiii., p. 643.

as might be expected from the general clearness of the atmosphere and its calmness after sunset, so common during the hot season, probably owing chiefly to the parched state of the surface of the island at this season. An erroneous idea relative to the frequency of the occurrence of dew would be formed from the preceding observations, were not allowance made for the circumstances under which it appeared. Very frequently dew formed on the cotton, exposed on the elevated terrace, when the shrubs in the adjoining garden remained perfectly dry. The period of dew is considered by the Maltese as commencing about the time of the Festa of St Lorenzo, which is on the 10th of August, when the heat is supposed to be at its maximum ; the duration, however, of the period, I believe they have not attempted to assign ; this is necessarily uncertain, as well as its commencement. The popular opinion on such a subject should perhaps be received only as indicative of a general fact—a rule to which there are many exceptions ; in the same manner as the notion that the greatest heat of the season is about the time of the festa just mentioned ; and the greatest cold about the time of another festa, that of S. Antonio, in the month of January (the 17th), and the heat and cold each of short duration, according to the saying,—

> Festa di St Lorenzo gran caldura,
> Festa di St Antonio gran freddura
> E l'uno e l'altro poco dura.*

* The period of disagreeable cold is not expected to last more than fifteen days.

When making observations on the effects of radiation of heat, and the production of dew, I paid some attention to the composition of dew. I made some trials with different specimens, collected with care, on the quality of the air which it contains. The results proved that it contained very little air, and that common air. I could detect no saline matter of any kind in it, and only a very slight trace of foreign matter ;* it was detected by means of solution of nitrate of silver, a most delicate test of organized matter, and was probably vegetable.

I was induced to make these trials in connexion with bleaching, a process for which Malta is very favourable. Dew is commonly supposed to have a bleaching effect ; and this supposed effect has been explained by another supposition, that dew is oxygenated water, or that it abounds in oxygen, by means of which it operates in the process in question.

Finding no excess of oxygen in dew, I was led to question the correctness of the common opinion ; and the few experiments I made confirmed me in my disbelief, and have led me to the conclusion that dew, by itself, has no active power in bleaching, and that if it at all contributes to the effect, it is merely as moisture after sunrise, when (if there be dew) the atmosphere is commonly very clear, and the sun's rays conse-

* The dew was collected in glass vessels ; the nitrate of silver had no effect at first, but, after exposure to sunshine, the dew acquired a faint purplish tint, probably owing to a very minute quantity of subtile vegetable matter precipitated from the atmosphere.

quently powerful. The operation of bleaching is a subject requiring further investigation. It is generally supposed that light, moisture, and oxygen, are all concerned in it. From some experiments which I have made I am inclined to think that sunshine is the principal agent, and moisture merely auxiliary; and that by the sun's rays alone, without moisture being present or oxygen, colouring matter may be destroyed. I shall insert, in the form of a note, the experiments alluded to, with the hope that the inquiry will be prosecuted further.*

---

* On the 17th August 1830, exposed two portions of brown cotton, one on water, the other dry, both day and night to the atmosphere, on an open space; and two other portions by night alone. On the 23d of September, the results were as follow:—The portions of cotton exposed only by night retained the colour undiminished, both that on water and that not; almost every night dew formed on the cotton. Of the portions exposed both by day and night, that which was placed on water, was bleached white; that without water was faded a little. In the instance of the bleached cotton, there was no appearance of any air being disengaged,—no appearance of the colouring matter having been dissolved by the water.

On the 17th of September of the same year, exposed lavender-coloured silk to sunshine, in hydrogen, azote, and common air, confined in glass tubes over mercury.

On the 24th September, the silk in hydrogen was almost deprived of colour. (A little moisture was present. The hydrogen was tried after the experiment by nitrous gas; no fume was produced).

That in azote showed no sensible change of colour.

That in common air showed very slight change.

On the 24th September, exposed green, yellow, and lavender-coloured silks to sunshine, in common air, in azote (the oxygen of common air having been removed by phosphorus), and in hydrogen. On the 9th of October the results were the following:—

In consequence of the clearness of the atmosphere, especially at night, during the summer season, the moonlight in Malta is extremely bright; but I am not aware that any particular effects are attributed to it by the natives. They sleep exposed to it without dread; and there being little malaria in Malta, they have not followed the example of the inhabitants of countries in which malaria is active, in attributing to the moon's rays effects on the constitution, strictly owing to the latter cause. The brightness of

1. Common air, with a little moisture;—the lavender-coloured silk had become almost white; the green had faded a little, and the yellow a little. The same apparently dry,—the lavender had faded considerably, but less than the moist; the green and yellow very slightly.

2. Azote, slightly moist;—the lavender had faded very much, it had acquired a slight tingr of red; the green and yellow were slightly faded. The same apparently dry,—the lavender was slightly faded, the green and yellow hardly perceptibly.

3. Hydrogen gas, slightly moist;—the lavender was very much faded, and had acquired a very slight tinge of red; the yellow and green were very slightly faded. Apparently dry,—the lavender was less faded than in azote; the yellow and green were not distinctly faded.

August 15, 1830. Exposed some olive oil, of a bright yellow colour, in two wine glasses, one floating in water, the other without water. In rather less than twenty-four hours both portions of oil had become colourless like water. The bleaching was effected by day; no disengagement of air could be detected.

This bleaching effect of the sun's rays on olive oil may admit of useful application, especially in preparing the finest and colourless kinds; and it is the more deserving of attention, as the discoloration appears to take place without any unpleasant smell being acquired; rancidity is the effect of the absorption of oxygen.

the moonlight in Malta induced me to make some trials with it, in connexion with the questions—Has it any heating power—has it any chemical power—or any magnetizing power? The results were all negative. I shall mention particularly only one, relative to the question of chemical power. Moist chloride of silver, freshly precipitated, was exposed several hours to the brightest light of the full moon, and not the slightest discolouration appeared.

The quantity of rain which falls annually in Malta has not been measured by the pluviometer. It is considerable; probably as great as in either of the Ionian Islands. As in these islands, it is liable to much variation, and that both as regards quantity and the time when it falls.* The following Table, shewing

* During the last three years so small has been the quantity of rain which has fallen that much distress has been experienced, especially in the country and by the agricultural population. The wretched state of the island, the consequence of this drought, is strongly and well expressed in the following passage from a letter of a friend, written in Malta, in the last week of May 1841. " I fear I am within bounds when I say that about a third of the country people, women and children particularly, are living, day after day, upon a pennyworth of dry beans or carrubi. The country is quite ruined. The great drought of last and two preceding winters has quite dried up the ground. All the crops have failed. Even the cotton, which was their last hope, has withered away; and they are all obliged to sell their cattle to support themselves and to keep from starving. In some casals they have no water to drink; it has to be brought from a great distance, and they pay one shilling for a small barrel. In town most of the houses are without water in the wells, and many families have to pay from four to five taris a day for water. Considerable emigration is taking place from the country, and it would, no doubt, be more extensive could the necessary funds be raised to pay the first expenses.

the frequency of rain, during the best part of three years, is formed from Sir Howard Elphinstone's Meteorological Journal.   The observations commenced on the 12th May 1831, and ended on the 21st November 1834 :—

NUMBER OF DAYS IN EACH MONTH IN WHICH THERE WAS RAIN IN VALETTA.

Months.	1832.	1833.	1834.
January, .		23	8
February,		10	14
March, .		8	7
April, .		6	10
May, . .	5	3	5
June, . .	4	5	2
July, . .	1	...	...
August, .	1	...	2
September,	3	9	9
October, .	12	11	5
November,	12	9	4
December,	13	6	

The summer has already set in with severity, and it is sad to look forward to the privations which must be undergone." These winters of drought were accompanied by unusually mild and fine weather, very favourable for invalids, with whom Valetta was crowded.   The prosperous state of the town, in consequence of an unusual influx of opulent strangers, crowding the inns and lodging-houses, was singularly contrasted with the suffering and wretched state of the country. The scarcity of water mentioned has produced much exertion on the part of the local government, to prevent a recurrence of the evil to the same extent.   Neglected cisterns have been repaired ; additional springs have been brought into communication with the aqueduct; and an attempt, it is said, is in progress, to obtain water at St Elmo, by boring, on the plan of the artesian well, with the bold idea of finding a spring fed from Sicily.   As the rains, this last winter, are reported to have been abundant, it is to be hoped that the period of distress is past, and that, with increased means of supply, the agriculture of Malta will again flourish.

A day of incessant rain in Malta is not common; the rain falls principally in showers, and they are more frequent by night than by day. The autumnal showers are occasionally very heavy and destructive. Fortunately, they are of very limited extent. One of the heaviest falls of rain experienced for many years occurred on the 26th October 1830. Its violence was confined chiefly to the least cultivated part of the island—the north-west part. The havoc it made was great; the damage to public property alone (chiefly the Government farms) was estimated as equivalent to L.2500. The removing of stones washed from the surrounding high grounds into the salines, or salt-works, it is said, cost L.500. The rain appeared to fall as a body of water. A person who witnessed the phenomenon where it was most remarkable, compared it to the fall of water in mass from a cistern, on a terrace-roof, supposing the roof suddenly broken down. There was little wind at the time, and no appearance of a water-spout. So very partial, occasionally, are the heavy autumnal showers, that I have known an instance of a road being flooded and rendered impassable by a torrent, the consequence of a shower at the head of a valley, not more than three or four miles distant, though no rain, excepting a few drops, fell where the road crossed the outlet of the valley.

From the nature of the medium through which rain falls, it might be expected that its water would never be perfectly free from impurities. In the

Ionian Islands, I never chemically examined rain; in Malta, I repeatedly subjected it to this examination, and always found it slightly impregnated with foreign matters. In October 1833, and in April 1834, I had rain water carefully collected in vessels of glass or porcelain, previously washed with distilled water. Every specimen that I tried (and I tried several, collected at different times) was similar, yielding a very minute quantity of saline matter, and a trace of vegetable matter. In the saline matter were detected the muriatic and sulphuric acids, and lime and magnesia. The principal ingredient appeared to be muriate of lime; in consequence of which the minute residue obtained by the evaporation of the water was always deliquescent. Even without concentration by evaporation, the presence of the muriatic acid or chlorine could always be detected. On the addition of solution of nitrate of silver, the rain water invariably became faintly, just perceptibly, clouded. Trial was made of rain water, in October and in April, shortly after the first rains, and just before the commencement of the dry season, with an expectation that some difference might be detected, which was not realized. The April rain did not appear to contain less foreign matter than the October. Trial, too, was made of rain which fell in different places, as in Valetta, close to the sea-shore, and at Citta Vecchia, several miles inland, and standing about four or five hundred feet above the level of the sea, but without any difference of results.

Common salt was sought for, but could not be detected in the saline matter; from whence it may be inferred, that this matter was not derived from the sea, mechanically suspended in the form of spray. Perhaps the acids were exhaled from volcanoes; and the earth with which they were combined, and also the very little vegetable matter, were raised in the form of impalpable dust.* It has been asserted that nitric acid has been found in rain water, supposed to be formed from its elements in the aerial elaboratory by the action of lightning. I carefully sought after this acid in the rain water of Malta, but without being able to discover any traces of it, not even in the rain of the thunder-storm.

Showers of dust are recorded to have fallen at different times in various parts of the globe. A striking example of the kind occurred in Malta and in some of the adjoining and even distant parts of the Mediterranean, on the 15th of May 1830. In the morning of that day, a strong Sirocco wind prevailed; the atmosphere was hazy; the sky overcast, of a sooty hue; at eight A.M. the dry thermometer was 69°, the moist 63°. Towards noon, the wind moderated, and at the same time the obscurity of the atmosphere increased; so that the natives became alarmed

---

* These specimens of rain water were not tested for ammonia, which, from the results of recent inquiry, it would appear is commonly present in such water in a very minute quantity; and by Liebig has been considered as one of the causes of the fertilizing influence of rain.

and apprehensive of some impending calamity, such as an earthquake or something extraordinary. Between one and two o'clock it became almost calm, with the same state of atmosphere. About that time, I believe the falling of dust was first perceived. I happened then to be riding into the country, and was surprised to perceive that the rain-drops, of which there were but few, left a reddish stain on my linen; and on going into a garden, I found the leaves of the plants generally covered with a reddish dust of extreme fineness. The exact time the dust was falling was not ascertained; it probably did not exceed two or three hours. It ceased soon after four P.M., about which time the wind changed to westerly, and the haze diminished. When the dust was falling fastest, and the obscurity was greatest, there was sufficient light to see objects distinctly. The quantity, too, of dust which fell was inconsiderable; what was swept from the deck of the Windsor Castle, a ship of the line of seventy-four guns, then lying at anchor in the great harbour of Valetta, was supposed sufficient to fill two buckets. This I was told by an officer who was present; it may help to give some idea of the quantity.

The extent of surface over which the dust fell was the most remarkable circumstance. There are authentic accounts of its having fallen in many distant parts of Sicily; indeed there is reason to suppose that no part of that island escaped it. There are also authentic accounts of its having fallen at Naples, Rome, and Lucca, at Palma Bay in Sardinia, and at Cagliari in the same island. In Sicily and Sardinia, the fall of dust was on the same day, and about the same time of the day as in Malta; in Italy, it was a 'day or two later. I could not learn that it was observed either in the Ionian Islands or in Greece, or on the coast of Asia Minor.

The quality of dust, wherever it fell, appears to have been very similar. It was invariably described as very fine, and of a reddish or brownish hue. I examined three specimens of it collected in Malta, and one collected in Palma Bay in Sardinia. Of the three Malta specimens, one was gathered from a terrace-roof of a house in Valetta, one from the floor of a balcony in Vittoriosa, and one from the leaves of a vine in a garden at the Pietà. That from the terrace consisted of 43.4 per cent. of carbonate of lime, and of 56.6 per cent. of matter insoluble in dilute muriatic acid; that from the floor of the balcony consisted of 51.6 carbonate of lime, and of 48.4 of insoluble matter; and that from Palma Bay of 38.7 carbonate of lime, and of 61.3 of insoluble matter. The insoluble matter was chiefly very fine silicious sand, with which were mixed some particles of clay. The dust which fell in Malta was slightly saline, from the admixture of a very minute quantity of common salt; that which fell in Palma Bay was destitute of saline matter. All the specimens I examined had slight traces of vegetable matter, in the form of fine fibres.

For the sake of comparison, I examined shortly after, some of the common dust of Malta, which, when the wind is high, especially the Sirocco, is very troublesome and penetrating, drifting in clouds, and even obscuring the atmosphere. One specimen of it, collected from the terrace-roof of a house, was composed of 97.4 per cent. of carbonate of lime, and of 2.6 per cent. insoluble matter : another specimen, collected from a table in an unoccupied room in Valetta, the windows of which were open, was composed of 89.7 per cent. of carbonate of lime, and of 10.3 of matter insoluble in nitric acid. The insoluble matter in each instance consisted of very fine silicious sand, a little clay coloured red by oxide of iron, with a trace of vegetable matter. A trace of common salt, too, was detected in each. Thus, the Malta dust, and that which which fell on the 15th of May, chiefly differed in the proportion of insoluble silicious matter.

I shall give some extracts from notices of the phenomenon, as it appeared in some other places, especially in Sardinia, where, perhaps, it was most remarkable.

For the first extract which I shall introduce, I was indebted to the late Sir Robert Spenser, then commanding H. M. frigate, Madagascar, from whom also I received the specimen of dust ; it was collected on the deck of the Madagascar.

" On arriving off the coast of Sardinia, the wind, which had previously been about south-west, became variable both in strength and direction, until the evening of the 12th, when a fresh south-easterly breeze commenced, with the usual dull sky attending it; there was some lightning to the southward, a little rain fell, and some thunder was heard in the night. Thermometer, 68° at noon; barometer fell from 29.92 in the morning, to 29.80; the hygrometer, contrary to its usual practice with south-easterly winds, indicated less moisture in the atmosphere; it stood at 3.500.

" The next morning the weather was beautifully serene, until about four P.M., when the wind freshened; it became overcast, and a few drops of rain fell occasionally during the night; thermometer, 66°; barometer, from 29.71 at eight A.M., to 29.74 at night; hygrometer, in the morning, 4.25; wind, south-east.

" On the 14th, the breeze freshened, and brought with it an additional portion of the heavy lead coloured nimbus looking clouds; these in the course of the day, as the wind increased to a strong gale, gradually approached the horizon, and formed a heavy fog. Thermometer, 68° and 70°; barometer at eight A.M., 29.68, fell to 29.61 at two o'clock, and rose between that and eight P.M., to 29.64; hygrometer, 3.90, six P.M., 3.55; wind, south-east by east.

" On the morning of the 15th, the wind still blowing hard, as the sun arose, the fog took a reddish appearance, which increased to a horrid looking glare; about noon the light was very obscure, out of the sun it was barely possible to see without candles. In the afternoon a very slight shower of dirty rain fell; it soon dried in a uniform coat of dark brown dust, on every part of the rigging and decks exposed to the wind. It was so very fine, that every attempt to sweep it carefully together was baffled, as the wind carried it away as soon as disturbed, and only some portions which had drifted into corners could be collected. The wind moderated soon after it fell, and a drizzling rain continued, until we ran off the coast on the 17th.

" The direction of the breeze never varied more than from south-east to east-south-east. Barometer, at eight P.M., 29.59, rose after four P.M. to 29.65 ; hygrometer at eight, 2.98, at noon, 3.40, at four P.M., 3.75."

The following extract is from the *Malta Gazette*, of the 4th August 1830, taken from a French journal. " On the 15th May, a phenomenon, similar to that which appeared in Italy, occurred at Cagliari, in Sardinia. The Sirocco came on with unusual force, and about mid-day the sky became so completely overcast, that lights were required. The darkness broke off about three o'clock, after the fall of a great quantity of red ashes or dust, which covered the foliage of the trees. The sea was violently agitated, and several vessels were wrecked. On the 8th (18th?) the same kind of ashes covered the whole of Lucca. It was on the 16th and 17th of May that the first of these extraordinary effects was felt in Calabria, Rome, and Lucca."

The next extract is also from the *Malta Gazette*, taken from the *Gazette* of the Two Sicilies ; the notice is dated Palermo, June the 7th.

" While the hurricane of the 15th ultimo filled the minds of the inhabitants of this city with terror, cinders were falling in the island of Ustica. Professor Ferrara having analyzed them, has made the following statement. ' On account of the small quantity that was sent me, I have been obliged to have recourse to re-agents, and obtained the following results:—1. carbonate of lime; 2, alumine; 3, oxide of iron; 4, silex. I should mention that similar cinders fell almost throughout the whole of Sicily, but more abundantly towards the southern part of the island. A smaller quantity fell on Etna than on the towns of Licata, Peazza, or Aidone; and as these cinders were brought by the Sirocco, we have every reason to believe, they did not proceed from Mount Etna. Secondly, according to the result of the analysis, they should not be called cinders, but from the nature of the component parts, might not improperly be called marble dust. Similar dust fell in Sicily in 1807 and 1813. It is very probable that a powerful Sirocco, after raising the dust from the barren sands of the African coast, to the higher regions of the atmosphere, drove it in the direction of Sicily. The cinders which Mount Etna ejects at the time of its eruptions, have been carried by north winds, as far as Malta, a distance of 180 miles. It is, therefore, probable, that a Sirocco of extraordinary force, may transport dust to a still greater distance."

Relative to the source of this dust, the opinion of Professor Ferrara, just quoted, appears to be highly probable, much more than that it was of volcanic origin. Its composition accords with its being dust of the desert, and militates against its being thrown up by a volcano. But the manner in which it was raised, and how it was so widely spread, is not a little mysterious ; nor is it less uncertain from what part of the desert exactly it came. I was not able to learn that any dust had fallen on the African shore. A vessel, which was nearly lost in the gale of the 15th of May, off Cape Bon, arrived soon after, at Malta. The master was particularly questioned on the subject. He replied that he perceived no dust, and was of opinion that none had fallen where he was. This, too, is in accordance with Professor Ferrara's opinion, that it was raised from the desert to a great height, and from thence carried away by the wind.

I shall give one extract more, with a different intention from the preceding, to show the great disposition there is to exaggerate on the occurrence of a remarkable phenomenon such as the preceding, and to state what is merely imagined as if it were fact,— and so to falsify.

" PARIS, June 8th.

" Private letters from Palermo, of the 20th ultimo, speak of a violent eruption of Etna. Seven different openings were made in the sides of the mountain, and several villages have been completely destroyed. The atmosphere at Palermo was so completely overcharged during two days, that objects at five and twelve paces distance could scarcely be discerned. The cloud of ashes borne away by the hurricane which at the time prevailed throughout the Mediterranean, and destroyed several vessels, reached as far as Rome. It carried desolation into Calabria, where the olive trees have suffered severely."

I need not observe that this circumstantially described eruption of Etna, and the seven openings in the side of the mountain, were entirely imaginary. There was no eruption at that time—nothing that occurred to justify the report—which seems to have arisen entirely out of its being probable, and was so circumstantially detailed to make it plausible.

The remarks made respecting the barometer in the Ionian Islands, are applicable to this instrument in Malta, as will appear in part from the following Table, in which the maximum and minimum height of the mercurial column is given for each month,— extracted from Sir Howard Elphinstone's register.

Months.	1832.		1833.		1834.	
	Max.	Min.	Max.	Min.	Max.	Min.
January, . .			30.40	29.62	30.35	29.51
February, . .			30.24	29.50	30.62	29.50
March, . .			30.02	29.10	30.30	29.38
April, . .			30.10	29.54	30.09	29.55
May, . . .	30.10	29.70	30.12	29.60	30.15	29.58
June, . .	30.15	27.77	30.05	29.69	30.20	29.86
July, . .	30.10	29.92	30.14	29.74	30.05	29.80
August, . .	30.15	29.87	30.01	29.81	30.04	29.73
September, .	30.32	29.84	30.05	29.55	30.15	29.76
October, . .	30.17	29.62	30.05	29.75	30.30	29.65
November, .	30.08	29.63	30.25	29.45	30.35	29.52
December, .	30.20	29.44	30.25	29.70		

The height of the barometer was noted by Sir Howard Elphinstone three times a-day, viz. at eight A.M., four P.M., and at ten P.M. The two Tables annexed show the daily range of the mercury in August and March 1834 (one in which the fluctuation is least

March 1834.

	1	2	3	4	5	6	7	8	9	10	11	12	13	14	15	16	17	18	19	20	21	22	23	24	25	26	27	28	29	30	31
BAR.																															
RAIN														Hail Storm													Gale	Thunder Storm–Hail			
WIND	WNW	N	NE	NE	W	ESE	WSW	W	NNE	NW	NW	N	E	NE	NNW	ENE	E	NNW	SSW	NE	N	N	NW	S	SSE	W	WNW	NW	NW	N	N
TEMP.	57 50	56 60	57 54	38 50	50 49	59 49	37 50	58 56	38 57	60 52	60 53	59 54	53 57	53½ 49	47 49	54 46	56 49	37 47	60 50	50 47	53 45	56 48	59 47	60 46	61 53	61 56	53 48	55 46	56 47	58 48	60 50

August 1834.

	BAR.	RAIN	WIND	TEMP.
1			ESE	82 / 80
2			E	89 / 80
3			NNW	82 / 80
4			NW	83 / 79
5			NW	81 / 78
6			N	80 / 76
7			WNW	79 / 77
8			ENE	86 / 77
9			NNE	81 / 77
10			W	81 / 78
11			NNE	80 / 77
12			S	80 / 76
13			ESE	80 / 77
14		Thunder	ENE	79 / 77
15		Thunder	WNW	78 / 77
16			E	79 / 76
17			ENE	78 / 77
18			SW	79 / 76
19			N	80 / 78
20			E	81 / 80
21			SSE	81 / 80
22			Variable	81½ / 81
23			ESE	83 / 81
24			E	83 / 80
25			Variable	82 / 80
26			E	82 / 80
27			NNE	83 / 80
28			NE	82 / 80
29			E	83 / 80
30			E	82 / 79
31			(calm)	83 / 80

and the other in which it is greatest), and also the manner in which the observations were recorded.*

Electrical phenomena are of frequent occurrence in the atmosphere of Malta, especially towards the termination of the hot season, and during the autumn and winter and early spring. Towards the conclusion of the summer, when clouds begin to appear in the horizon, and when probably there are great inequalities of temperature in the different strata or regions of the atmosphere, flashes of electrical light almost nightly occur, often producing very beautiful appearances, similar to the summer lightning of our own country. Violent thunder-storms are not uncommon ; they take place but rarely in summer, more frequently in autumn and winter, are always accompanied with heavy rain, and in the cool season most commonly with hail. The two following Tables, placed side by side, show the frequency of thunder-storms and of hail-showers in Malta, during the period of Sir Howard Elphinstone's observations, from whose register they are formed.

* Rain in Sir Howard Elphinstone's register is denoted by a dot ⋅ ; sunshine by ☼ ; part sunshine, ☼ ♋ ; the upper ray before noon ; the lower ray after noon.

The winds were taken from the register published in the *Malta Gazette*, the position not being favourable for observing them correctly.

Months.	Number of days in each Month in which thunder-storms.			Number of days in each Month in which hail-showers.		
	1832.	1833.	1834.	1832.	1833.	1834.
January, . . .		1	...	...	2	1
February, . .		3	...	...	3	...
March, . . .		1	1	...	1	2
April, . . .		...	...	...	...	1
May, . . .	...	...	3	...	...	...
June, . . .	...	1	...	...	...	...
July, . . .	..	...	...	...	...	...
August, . . .	...	1	1	...	...	...
September, . .	...	2	6	...	...	...
October, . . .	3	3	1	...	...	...
November, . .	3	...	...	...	...	...
December, . .	...	1	...	4	....	

That there is a connexion between the formation of hail and a disturbed electrical state of the atmosphere, is now generally admitted, but how they are associated is obscure. This is well established, that whenever there is a thunder-storm there is a sudden and great reduction of temperature; and whenever there is hail, if the atmosphere is tested, proof is obtained of disturbed electrical equilibrium. In summer, and the beginning of autumn, when the temperature of the atmosphere is comparatively high, the water which falls in the thunder-storm is rarely frozen,—almost as rarely as within the tropics,—seeming to indicate that the region of the storm is not very elevated.

The severest hail-storm I ever witnessed in the Mediterranean, or, indeed, in any other part of the globe, occurred at Malta, at three o'clock A.M., on the 11th February 1832, the accompaniment of a violent thunder-storm. Hail and rain fell together, and the temperature of the former was sufficiently low to freeze the latter on the ground. This I infer from finding many of the hailstones agglutinated together, by an icy cement. Seven hours after the fall, I saw many hailstones as large as walnuts. They were commonly spherical,—some were hemi-spherical; they were generally opaque in the middle, and transparent towards the circumference. The opacity was owing to minute air-bubbles. I filled an eight-ounce bottle with hailstones, poured in water to expel, as much as possible, free atmospheric air, and then inverted it in water. The minute quantity of gas disengaged during the melting of the hail, by the test of phosphorus, did not appear to differ from common air; it did not contain more oxygen, nor was it inflammable.* So great was the quantity of hail which fell at this time, that it was collected for use. At noon, I saw a porter bringing in a heavy load of it into Valetta, from Floriana; and two days after there were vestiges of it in the shade in gardens adjoining the town. The destruction of glass by the storm was very great. Fortunately, its limits were narrow; its breadth did not exceed three or four miles: the wind was S.W., and in that direction it crossed the island.

Relative to the climate of Gozo, in connexion with that of Malta, a very few remarks may suffice. It has

* Particular attention was paid to this point, in consequence of an hypothesis, which has been more than once advanced, that hydrogen gas accumulates in the upper regions of the atmosphere.

the character, and I believe deservedly, of being excellent. The general surface of the island being more elevated than that of Malta, it is sensibly cooler, especially in the hottest weather ; and, as the Sirocco wind passes over Malta before it reaches Gozo, it is drier in the latter, and far less oppressive. In other respects, the climate of the two islands, as might be expected, has a close resemblance.

CHAPTER X.

ON THE SOILS, AND ON THE STATE OF AGRICULTURE
AND HORTICULTURE IN THE IONIAN ISLANDS.

Principal Varieties of Soils, and their Capacities. Present rude State
of Agriculture. Circumstances which may have conduced to it.
Tables of Produce. Implements of Husbandry. Culture of
Wheat—Maize—the Common Vine. Wine-making, and Varieties of Wine. Currant-Vine, and its Fruit. Culture of the Olive
and the Making of Oil. Cotton. The Potato. Tobacco. Rice.
Question of the Effect of Rice-Fields on the Salubrity of the Air.
Culture of Vegetables and Fruit-Trees. Modes of Propagating
the Latter. Caprification. Pasture Lands. Flocks. Pastoral
Life. Musical Instruments. Field Labour. Wages of Labour-
ers. Land Tenures. Remarks on the Neglect of Manuring and
Planting. Proportion of Cultivated and Waste Land. Examples
in Zante and Cerigo.

THE soils of the Ionian Islands may be conveniently,
and with tolerable precision, divided into three kinds,
according to their nature and composition ; 1st, those
consisting principally of calcareous marl ; 2d, of red
clay ; and 3d, of sand.

The marl-soil is very abundant ; it occurs where-
ever the gray clay or marl formation exists, from which
it is derived, partly by the action of atmospheric influences, and partly by the labour of man. The sub-

stratum and soil differ principally in consistence. The former is dense and compact in mass; the latter loose, soft, and very friable, more or less penetrated by air. There is a difference, too, in colour. The substratum is of a bluish or grayish hue; the soil is of a fawn colour, or light brown. The colour of both is owing to oxide of iron; of the substratum, to protoxide; of the soil, to the peroxide,—the one being converted into the other by absorption of oxygen on exposure to the atmosphere. There is another difference; the substratum is almost entirely destitute of vegetable matter; the soil contains a certain proportion, which is variable according to circumstances, but rarely exceeding two or three per cent., and, I believe, more frequently not one per cent. A specimen of this kind of soil which I examined in Zante, taken from a currant-vineyard in the plain, just at the foot of the Castle-hill, consisted of

21 Carbonate of lime, with a trace of sulphate of lime and of carbonate of magnesia.
72 Aluminous and silicious earths; the latter in the form of a very fine sand.
4 Hygrometric water, expelled by a temperature of 212°.
3 Vegetable matter and water, destroyed and expelled by ignition.

100

The red clay soil, next to marl, is most abundant. It is chiefly confined to the hilly and mountainous regions, and almost invariably lies over limestone. It has in perfection the characters of a clay soil, and consists principally of alumine and silica, the former predominating; it is coloured by peroxide of iron. Though incumbent on limestone, probably owing to the long-continued action of rain-water, it is frequently destitute of calcareous earth;* and when this earth does occur in it, it is not in the form of intimate mixture, as in the instance of marl, but of scattered fragments of limestone rock. The proportion of vegetable matter it contains is exceedingly small; it is not easy to determine the exact quantity, but I believe it is less than one per cent.

The sandy soils are less common than the two preceding. They may be subdivided into three kinds, calcareous, silicious, and mixed. Calcareous sand is rarely met with; where it does occur, it is generally near the sea-shore, and probably is merely drifted sea-sand. In this state it hardly deserves the name of soil, nor is fit for the purpose of supporting vegetation, unless vines be excepted, which I have seen growing on the sand-banks bounding the plain of Zante towards Kieri Bay. Silicious sand is less rare, but fortunately not abundant. Where it occurs it is commonly superficial, and it is probably, in most instances, a deposit brought from a distance by the carrying power of a flood. The mixed or compound sandy soils, consisting of calcareous and silicious sand and marl, are more frequent; they are generally in

---

* I have noticed the same absence of carbonate of lime, and probably owing to the cause assigned above, in shallow clay soils, in the county of Kent, where incumbent on chalk.

the vicinity of strata of freestone and of marl, from which, by disintegration, they are derived. And they are exceedingly various; sometimes one ingredient predominating, sometimes another.

The capacities or capabilities of these soils are not easily defined, much depending on situation, and much on the means of cultivation employed.

The marl soils generally occurring in low situations, and being very absorbent and retentive of moisture, and drying readily at the surface, seem to be well fitted for plants and crops requiring moisture during the active process of vegetation, and dryness at the time of ripening of the seed or fruit; such as maize and the currant-vine. The currant-vine is principally cultivated in the marl soils of Zante, Cephalonia, and Ithaca; maize in the same soils in Corfu, Santa Maura, and Cerigo.

The red clay soils generally occurring in higher and drier situations, lying shallow on rocks, and amongst rocks, are best fitted for those plants which require little moisture, and can bear a long period of drought, not only with impunity, but in some respects with advantage, such as the vine and the olive. The former (for the purpose of making wine), is chiefly cultivated in the rocky districts of Cephalonia, Santa Maura, and Ithaca, and in Zante on the declivity of the mountains bordering the plain. The olive has the preference in Paxo,—indeed, that island is almost an entire olive grove. It has also the preference in Fanno and Cerigo.

Occasionally the situation of the red clay soils is different, as in Santa Maura, and in the mountainous region of Zante, and in some parts of Cephalonia. I allude to the basin-like hollows already described, and to surfaces of small extent, comparatively plain, the former subject to be flooded, and the latter well adapted to the plough. In these localities in Santa Maura, grain is commonly grown, especially maize. In Cephalonia, the currant-vine is principally planted. In Zante, the culture is divided between maize, wheat and barley, and the currant-vine and the common vine. The choice is made according to supposed circumstances of fitness. If the ground is liable to be deeply flooded, and to continue so till advanced spring, it is only fit for maize. If only during the depth of winter, it is well adapted for the currant-vine. If not exposed to be flooded at all, and standing high and cold, it is considered suitable to wheat and barley, and to the vine, if sheltered and warm.

The compound sandy soils, both from their nature and situation, are the least exclusive. Little selection is shown in respect to them; they are marked by diversity of cultivation. Corfu, where light soils abound, consisting of various mixtures of calcareous sand and marl, offers innumerable instances of this. There the olive grove, the orange grove, the vineyard, the corn-field, garden, and waste, are often to be seen at one view, and blended in the landscape; and indeed to this circumstance of variety, much of the beauty of the scenery of that very charming island is owing.

The unmixed sandy soils, whether calcareous or silicious, are the reverse of the preceding; they are generally totally neglected by the natives, and left waste. The heath flourishes in the silicious soil of Corfu, and almost invariably marks its presence. Probably, in an improved system of agriculture, the vine will take its place.

The state of agriculture in the Ionian Islands at present is little advanced; it is merely a rude art, founded on traditional knowledge, a series of processes handed down from father to son, unenlightened by the methods of science.

The backwardness of this important branch of industry, in a country admirably adapted for agriculture, whether we consider its soils or its climate, is owing, no doubt, to a variety of causes;—partly, and perhaps mainly, to former bad government, and the enacting of laws and regulations arresting improvement, with the corrupt administration of justice and insecurity of property; partly to the tenures by which lands were held; partly to the neglected education of the mass of the people; and partly, perhaps, even to some of the observances connected with their religion. Some instances may be useful in illustration.

According to an old Venetian law (only very recently abrogated), the cutting down of an olive-tree was a capital crime; owing to which, and to undue encouragement given to the planting of this tree,* large tracts of country in Corfu were covered with forests of olive-trees, and some of the richest and best soils were thus occupied. Requiring little cultivation and attention, the olive was further injurious by engendering habits of idleness. Its rich, though uncertain produce was looked to as a main support; little corn was grown, little wine was made, and agriculture generally was neglected. Whilst the trees were in full bearing, and carefully cultivated,—whilst Venice had almost a monopoly of the market, and the price of oil was high,—then the plantations were a source of vast profit; the proprietors were wealthy, and the island was comparatively flourishing, certain proofs of which are afforded in the vestiges which remain,—villas, and gardens, and paved ways, in different parts of the island, now more or less neglected and in decay or ruin, the consequence of the diminished value of the olive groves, arising out of the diminished produce and deteriorated price.

Another injurious law, in its bearing on agriculture, was the old one of entail and primogeniture, only lately repealed, by which landed property was secured in a family in the male line of descent, and could in no way be sold. The consequences were, that the

* Whoever planted and reared one hundred olive-trees was entitled to a reward of twelve Venetian sequins (about six pounds). It was first offered about three hundred years ago, when the value of gold was double what it is at present. At that time there were few olive-trees in the island, and the produce was very valuable.

enterprising farmer (if such there were) could not effect a purchase in land, and the proprietor, if in debt (as was too commonly his case), was without funds to expend on profitable culture, and the largeness of the estates added to the evil. The bad effects on agriculture, from the corrupt administration of justice and consequent insecurity of property, have been incalculably great,—of almost incredible amount. Some idea of the evils which have been thus produced may be formed from the subjoined note, an extract from a letter written by an officer intimately acquainted with the state of the country, and especially of Santa Maura, where, there is reason to believe, extraordinary license prevailed, and the evils in question were felt much more severely than in either of the other islands, and this only a few years ago, when Lord Nugent was Lord High Commissioner.*

---

* Commenting on the very backward state of these islands, in reference to causes, and to give an example, he says:—" I select Santa Maura as being the fourth in rank, and the third in point of size, and as an island which latterly came more under my own observation. To begin with the *administration of justice:* its insufficiency to afford protection is evident from the frightful extent of crime. Leaving out the number of *accusations* that are brought forward, as also those that are withheld, either from want of legal proof or the machinations of unprincipled lawyers and their accomplices, the criminal convictions amount to between fifty and sixty annually; and the correctional ones, extending to imprisonment with irons and forced labour, to between three and four hundred. Let this statement be compared to that of any other country, and the amount will be found appalling, on considering that it arises from a population of only 18,000.

The Metairie system, very commonly prevailing, may be considered as another check on agricultural

" The most frequent offences, and those which engender a vast number of crimes, are those of trespass and damage maliciously done to property and produce of neighbours, added to nocturnal thefts. Owing to the absence of religious feeling, of moral principle, and to the impunity so easily procured, by means of perjury, every vindictive feeling, however trifling may have been the exciting cause, is promptly indulged in. The means resorted to are chiefly turning in flocks to graze on and ruin their enemy's vines and crops, cutting rings of bark off his olive-trees, thus insuring their speedy decay ; setting fire to corn and flax ; cutting, maiming, and blinding his cattle, with unheard-of barbarity, &c. &c. The sufferer can generally point out the aggressor ; but where there is, both among high and low so general a disregard of truth, the dread of being unable to substantiate the charge, with the unavoidable expense and loss of time, and the certainty that the offender will, if he have any property, be defended by a powerful noble, in many cases deter the injured person from seeking *legal* redress : and, smothering for a time his revenge, he at length gives loose to it by perpetrating a crime far exceeding in enormity that which gave rise to it. Thus, though a vast amount of crime is punished, the chances of escape are great, and all that thus escapes stimulates to fresh crime. This process is so notorious that I shall not dwell upon it, but merely repeat that the subject demands the most serious consideration, it being the *immediate cause,* by producing a sense of *insecurity,* of the languor with which a race of naturally hardy, active, and industrious peasant-cultivators carry on their operations in agriculture, and of the indifference with which they regard all suggestions for their improvement. In this state of things knowledge to them is perfectly *useless.* I never, in any part of the world, knew a defenceless cultivator anxious to increase his stock while marauders are in his vicinity, and it requires more than human courage to plant trees which will in all probability be destroyed. This is sufficient to account for the melancholy fact that on a surface of 160 square miles, with a population of only 18,000 souls, where almost every peasant is a landed proprietor, with a soil and climate of the finest, the exports for five successive years only averaged about L. 20,000

improvement, and especially in connexion with the
Colonia system, which, according to Sir Charles Napier,

annually, or less, while they import *more* than *half* their grain, besides the salt provisions with which they eke out their subsistence,
with many articles, including even onions and garlic, which their own
soil would almost furnish spontaneously.

" The code of laws which has been in preparation for the last fifteen
years having been partially introduced a short time since, it is to be
hoped that some amelioration *may* ensue. I yet expect but little from
a just definition of crimes and punishments (however necessary), compared to the importance that attaches to the selection of the judges
and registrars, to the degree of power with which they may be invested, to the nature of the law of evidence, and that of the rules and
forms which regulate the proceedings. In short, judges and registrars,
to whom no suspicion of partiality attaches, and a simple but ener-
getic code of procedure, with diminished expense and loss of time, are
of vital importance, and so closely connected with every measure for
the civilization of the people, that the attention of the government
cannot be too closely drawn to it.

" Perjury is an evil so widely spread, that it ought in the new code to
be especially considered. In Santa Maura, the *purchase* and *loan* of
false oaths are spoken of as a notorious fact; and I believe that the
same may be asserted of various other islands. The ordinary means
conceded to judges being manifestly inadequate to its suppression, I
fear that it cannot well be reached unless through the medium of
special tribunals, endowed with extraordinary powers. The terror
inspired by salutary severity, added to the infusion of moral principle, by means of education, would undoubtedly, in a *generation* or
two, produce the desired effects. As to immediate eradication, by
human means alone, I hold it to be impossible, yet think much might
be done if sufficient power were granted not to punish with severity,
but to facilitate conviction. I know of no people who more readily
than the Greeks abandon a bad practice, where there is a probability
of detection. If it be thought that such powers could not, com-
patibly with constitutional principles, be entrusted to a tribunal,
I cannot imagine how this dreadful evil is to be reached, and must
continue to wonder why sworn testimony is allowed such tremendous
weight, when it is known to be without the slightest foundation in

" fills the tribunals with trials and the country with thieves, besides being a constant source of bad blood between the landlord and tenant." The division of

truth. I have been assured by judges that they frequently decide *contrary to their conviction*, and the fiscal advocate of Santa Maura has assured me that he has seen the lawyers paying witnesses for false testimony, in the vicinity of the tribunals. How can improvement be hoped for, while every man, however respectable in character and station, is liable to be the victim of false swearing, and whose only chance for defence and redress, is by having recourse to the same revolting crime? What must be the situation of a conscientious man so circumstanced?

" I do not enter into the administration of the civil law, that subject being foreign to my pursuits, and far above my abilities; but some guess may be made at the state of it, when you everywhere hear complaints of the enormous rate of interest exacted for loans on *landed security*, to the amount of twenty, thirty, and even fifty per cent., including premiums, &c. What does this indicate but the difficulty of obtaining repayment, even after encountering a ruinous law-suit, which almost always attends the recovery of a loan?

" Education at Santa Maura is at a very low ebb, compared to what it ought to be. There are, as in each of the other islands—

" 1. A central primary school where boys are taught on the Lancasterian system. It also serves as a normal school for the education of masters for the village schools; about forty or fifty boys attend. 2. A secondary school, where the English and learned languages are taught, with mathematics, logic, rhetoric, &c. Thirty or forty scholars attend.

" These two schools are supported at the expense of government. The first at the annual cost of about L.40, the second at the cost of L.320 yearly. There are two private schools in the town, with about seventy or eighty boys attending, and eleven village schools, where 200 or 300 boys are educated, by the contributions of individuals. There is a female school, with twenty-five girls, supported by private subscription. When Lord Nugent first arrived, he saw it with 116 girls, with every probability of increase of numbers, but it rapidly fell off, owing to causes connected with the general administration."

the produce of the land between the farmer and the landlord may ensure a certain degree of cultivation, but it holds out little encouragement to the outlay of capital, and the exertion of skill and industry.* And the almost endless division of property which the old Colonia system permitted, was almost equally fatal to industry and enterprise in farming. The *systeme hypothecaire*, too, of credit (that in which the creditor has a claim on the rents of real property of the debtor) appears to have had a no less injurious effect,— indeed Baron Theotoki, who describes its effects at some length, in his work on Corfu (*Details sur Corfu*), published in 1826, considers them even worse than those of the Colonia system, in throwing lands out of cultivation, and in producing beggary and ruin.

The ordinances of the Greek Church have been

---

* The Metairie, or Metayer system, judiciously conducted, as it appears to be in many parts of Europe, especially in Switzerland and Tuscany, may be highly advantageous, conducive to the formation of a well-conditioned and intelligent agricultural population. Mr Laing, in his able work, " Notes of a Traveller," has stated many interesting particulars illustrating the good effects of the system well directed; its abuses he has not pointed at ;—it is these by which it is most marked in the Ionian Islands. Whether, however, the condition of the peasantry would be improved by the abolition of the system is very questionable. The well-being of any class seems to depend on a variety of circumstances, the influence of which it is often difficult to estimate, admitting of modifications not less considerable than the diet of individuals compatible with a healthy condition. Small farms answer in Switzerland; they are little successful in Westmoreland. In Westmoreland crime against the person is almost unknown ; suicide is common. It may be as difficult to account, in a satisfactory manner, for the one fact as for the other.

noticed as a check to advancement in agriculture. When it is mentioned that in the calendar of this church there are sixty feste, or holidays, which should be observed by the people, and four periods of Lent, altogether amounting to 130 days, independent of the ordinary weekly fast-days, it may easily be conceived how this effect may be produced,—in one instance, that of the feste,—by encouraging idleness ; in the other instance, that of their lents, by discouraging constant and regular production. The numerous holidays necessarily produce habits unfavourable to industry and steady exertion,—everywhere their tendency would be such, and in a warm climate, *à fortiori ;*— and besides the regular holidays, there are many more saints' days, under the pretence of keeping which, those who are so inclined may make themselves doubly idle. The effects of the long lents are very manifest in the markets. No markets are worse supplied with butchers' meat ; good meat not being constantly in request, means are not taken to insure a supply of it ; little attention is paid to cattle,— little to pasture and to the growing of forage. With these neglects others are connected detrimental to the interests of agriculture,—as inattention to animal manures, and indeed to manuring in general,—and inattention to succession of crops.

I have alluded to the neglected education of the people as one of the general causes of the backward state of agriculture in the Ionian Islands. In consequence of want of instruction, they are prejudiced and narrow-minded; satisfied with their imperfect methods; averse to new trials; and completely out of the way of improvement. Some exception to this remark, may perhaps be made in favour of the southern islands, where the currant-vine has been successfully cultivated, and has given rise to some enterprise, to which I shall have occasion to revert.

It would be tedious to dwell further on this subject. The time, I trust, is come when, under a better government, and increasing encouragement, a change will be effected, and the state of agriculture will progressively improve, and continue doing so, till these islands become some of the most productive in the world. This, at least, is the hope that should be indulged,—the object aimed at.

I shall now proceed, and briefly give such particulars as I have been able to collect respecting the system of agriculture at present in use, with some other collateral information. These details will fully illustrate the imperfections alluded to.

I shall prefix a return of the produce of agriculture and the state of stock, in the Ionian Islands, for the years 1834 and 1835, obtained from official records in the Colonial Office.

CROPS, STOCK, AND PRODUCE OF EACH OF THE IONIAN ISLANDS IN 1834.

CROPS.
Number of Acres of Land under each kind of Crop.

Islands.	Wheat.	Indian Corn, Calambocchio, Barley, and Wheat.	Oats.	Currants.	Olive Oil.	Wines.	Cotton.	Flax.	Pulse.	Pasture.	Total in Crop.	Total Uncultivated.
Corfu,	4,005	13,508	2,963	...	75,700	13,900	69	843	1,020	17,422	112,008	33,272
Cephalonia,	682	6,963	635	6,242	4,323	12,232	473	351	1,033	640	32,934	189,786
Zante,	7,182	966	492	6,440	16,766	13,600	327	134	64	1,474	45,971	53,869
Santa Maura,	1,234	3,249	380	8	8,143	4,127	111	75	212	5,494	17,539	97,661
Ithaca,	49	263	5	190	212	756	1	97	38	1,626	1,611	3,286
Cerigo,	453	8,466	...	...	513	1,365	54	109	1,595	5,285	12,555	61,686
Paxo,	...	...	...	...	11,000	406	...	...	...	...	11,406	5,234
Total,	13,605	33,415	4,475	12,880	116,657	46,386	1,035	1,609	3,962	31,941	234,024	444,793

STOCK.
Number of each kind.

Islands.	Horses.	Horned Cattle.	Sheep.	Goats.
Corfu,	4,104	2,541	18,085	16,707
Cephalonia,	3,753	1,416	26,493	5,797
Zante,	3,152	944	14,025	23,795
Santa Maura,	2,223	1,786	16,101	12,001
Ithaca,	643	89	11,513	8,206
Cerigo,	840	3,082	4,653	16,275
Paxo,	270	2	938	4,160
Total,	15,275	9,660	92,002	87,627

PRODUCE.
Nature and Quantity of each kind.

Islands.	Wheat, Bushels.	Indian Corn, Barley, &c., Bushels.	Oats, Bushels.	Currants, Lbs.	Oil, Barrels.	Wine, Barrels.	Cotton, Lbs.	Flax, Lbs.	Pulse, Bushels.	Salt, Bushels.
Corfu,	189,205	47,526	4,583	...	236,016	88,964	2,002	21,089	5,598	...
Cephalonia,	5,797	47,661	4,751	...	420	45,730	25,788	16,282	7,091	...
Zante,	23,795	1,155	630	9,457,400	1,682	63,730	6,220	3,645	767	...
Santa Maura,	12,001	31,594	3,694	7,300,000	...	62,292	6,515	23,418	2,761	...
Ithaca,	989	6,979	286	4,000	...	9,045	100	27,088	874	114,193
Cerigo,	2,940	42,150	...	310,000	57	36,200	4,520	3,000	2,745	...
Paxo,	...	...	...	...	15,748	861	...	...	...	...
Total,	234,727	177,065	23,944	15,071,400	253,923	306,822	45,145	94,145	19,826	114,193

CROPS, STOCK, AND PRODUCE OF EACH OF THE IONIAN ISLANDS, IN THE YEAR 1835.

CROPS.
Number of Acres of Land under each kind of Crop.

Islands.	Wheat.	India Corn, Calambocchio, Barley, and Wheat.	Oats.	Currants.	Olive Oil.	Wine.	Cotton.	Flax.	Pulse.	Pasture.	Total in Crop.	Total Uncultivated.
Corfu, . . .	6,112	11,821	3,964	...	75,700	13,900	93	826	1,868	26,973	174,384	30,896
Cephalonia, . .	682	6,963	635	6,242	4,323	12,232	473	351	1,033	640	32,934	189,786
Zante, . . .	7,182	966	492	6,440	16,766	13,600	327	134	64	1,474	45,971	53,869
Santa Maura,	1,296	3,229	347	5	8,143	4,150	125	220	249	5,276	17,764	97,436
Ithaca, . . .	66	362	12	190	212	756	1	98	63	1,626	1,760	3,137
Cerigo, . . .	453	8,466	...	...	513	1,365	54	109	1,595	5,285	12,535	61,685
Paxo, . . .	34	...	...	...	11,000	406	...	...	...	...	11,460	5,200
Total, .	15,825	31,807	5,450	12,877	116,657	46,109	1,037	1,738	4,872	41,274	296,808	442,016

STOCK.   PRODUCE.
Number of each kind.   Nature and Quantity of each kind.

Islands.	Horses.	Horned Cattle.	Sheep.	Goats.	Wheat, Bushels.	India Corn, Barley, &c. Bushels.	Oats, Bushels.	Currants, Lbs.	Oil, Barrels.	Wine, Barrels.	Cotton, Lbs.	Flax, Lbs.	Pulse, Bushels.	Salt, Bushels.
Corfu, . . .	4,067	2,950	21,098	18,475	18,498	41,531	15,752	...	...	62,332	2,370	26,493	5,482	...
Cephalonia, . .	2,405	1,348	28,200	16,920	6,400	51,960	5,344	14,400,000	12,580	77,050	34,300	21,820	7,740	...
Zante, . . .	3,400	1,160	19,000	21,400	29,750	850	200	10,560,000	35,000	63,970	7,080	7,320	990	100,000
Santa Maura,	2,452	1,855	11,541	20,132	16,812	41,861	4,498	4,050	77,907	51,124	5,650	28,322	4,037	...
Ithaca, . . .	643	111	5,064	7,299	2,421	9,288	473	52,500	4,500	8,402	408	21,281	3,026	...
Cerigo, . . .	888	3,084	16,600	3,960	3,670	48,950	...	...	465	34,010	5,250	3,830	2,970	100,000
Paxo, . . .	183	13	996	24	170	...	...	...	...	1,100	...	...	522	...
Total, .	14,038	10,521	102,499	88,210	77,721	195,440	27,267	25,489,050	70,452	297,988	45,258	109,066	24,767	100,000

1. *Of Corn Lands.*—The preceding return shows
how small is the proportion of land thus cultivated,
and how inconsiderable is its produce. In Zante,
where wheat is most grown, and where agriculture is
a little more advanced than in any of the other
islands, a return of eight-fold is considered a very
abundant one, and above the average. A return of
four or five-fold is considered nearer the average.
The following is a common rotation of crops observed
there:—

1st year,	. .	Manure and grass for hay
2d ...	. .	Corn.
3d ...	. .	Beans or cotton.
4th ...	. .	Corn.
5th ...	. .	Manure and grass.

In the other islands, in which the state of agriculture is much lower, manure little used, if at all, and
rotation of crops neglected, the produce is less. Year
after year, in Cerigo, corn is grown, the soil has no
fallow-rest, and rarely relief through the means of a
crop of a different kind.

For the cultivation of corn, the ground generally
is prepared for seed after the first rains, and the grain
is sown commonly in October and November. The
harvest is in the latter end of May and in June in the
low lands, and in the latter end of the last mentioned month and in July in the mountainous districts.

The implements of husbandry employed about this
crop are few and rude; principally the plough, the

hoe, and the harrow, in preparing the ground, and the hook in reaping the crop. The plough is very similar to that employed in most parts of India, of Asia Minor, and in the South of Europe generally, where agriculture has made little progress. In Plate II. fig. 1, a plough is represented in use in Cerigo ; it weighed only fifteen lbs., and, with the yoke, cost a dollar. It may be considered as a fair example of the ploughs in common use throughout the islands. Some of them are even more rude, and of the simplest possible construction, without even rudimentary mould-boards, and having the share merely shod with iron. They are commonly made by the farmers themselves.* The harrow is seldom used, excepting in Corfu. The specimens of it which I have seen have been the rudest bush-harrows, very like what we read of as having been employed in the wilder parts of Scotland a century ago, when the agriculture of the country was in a barbarous state. The hoe (zappa) used in conjunction with the plough, is generally applied to break the clods and level the furrows. † The

* Sir Walter Scott, in his Diary, published in his Life, describes a plough of very similar construction, which he met with in the Shetland Islands. He says, " An old fashioned Zetland plough is a real curiosity. It had but one handle or stilt, and a coulter, but no sock. It ripped the furrow, therefore, but did not throw it aside."—*Memoirs of the Life of Sir Walter Scott, Bart.*, vol. iii., p. 153. The plough now in use in Egypt and in China is, it would appear, very similar.

† The hoe in use in the different islands is more or less dissimilar in form. Examples of its varieties are represented in Plate II. As regards the kind adopted, some attention appears to have been paid

PLATE II.

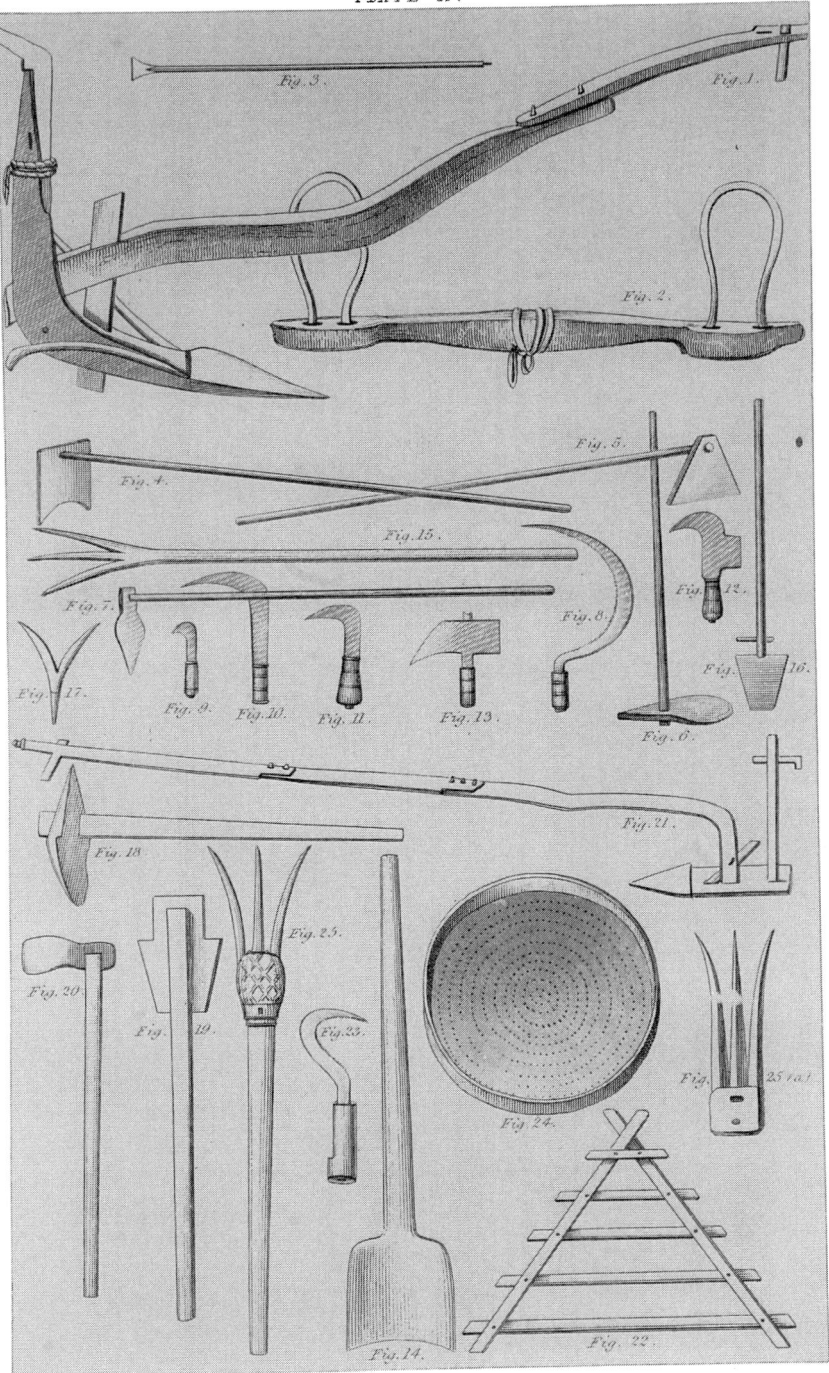

AGRICULTURAL IMPLEMENTS IN USE IN THE IONIAN ISLANDS AND MALTA.

operation of ploughing is in accordance with the instrument employed. The ground is moved only to the depth of a very few inches. Deep ploughing is impracticable, and consequently no fresh soil is ever turned up and brought into use.

In gathering in the harvest, the same carelessness and want of good methods and instruments are commonly observed. The common reaping-hook of the Ionian Islands is about the size and form of our own, but it is not always employed ; very often the pruning-knife of the vineyard is substituted for it. Of a piece with this, the operation of reaping is not a single one ; first, the corn is cut about a foot and a half from the ground, when it is tied together in bundles or sheaves, which are collected in a heap, with the heads uppermost, and are almost immediately removed to the thrashing-floor ; and next, the straw is cut close to the ground, and, with weeds included, is put apart for forage. The grain, without delay, is

to the quality of the ground and the nature of the soil. The hoe, fig. 4, is that commonly employed in the plain of Zante ; it is especially used in the currant vineyards. It costs about sixty oboli, *i. e.*, about half-a-crown. Its edge is hooked a little, on the idea that, by means of the sharp points, it is fitted to penetrate the ground the more readily. The points are also useful for breaking lumps of earth, and for digging close to the stem of the vine. The hoe, fig. 5, is that employed in the marl district of Lixuri. Fig. 6 is that in common use in Corfu, and I have not seen it in any other island ; combining the properties of the hoe and axe, it is well adapted for ground often encumbered with roots. In the mountainous and stony districts, the blade is generally narrower and more peaked, as shown in fig. 7, which is in use in Erisso, and some of the other hilly parts of Cephalonia.

beaten out, commonly in the harvest field, by men, horses, or mules, on a thrashing-floor prepared ex tempore for the purpose, where the ground is firm and dry, and the chaff is separated by winnowing, without loss of time.* The instrument employed to keep the straw under the feet of the animals, is generally a forked branch of a tree. The winnowing instrument is commonly a broad wooden shovel. † The chaff and straw are carefully preserved for the winter fodder of cattle. The value of the straw is considered equivalent to the price of the labour expended in the cultivation of the crop.

The best quality of wheat is grown on the hills and their declivities, in red clay; an inferior quality on the low grounds, and in marl. This was the remark of a gentleman of Zante, who had given his attention very much to farming. It applies, I believe, to the islands generally.

As may be seen in the preceding return, maize, or Indian corn, in Corfu, Santa Maura, and Cephalonia, is cultivated in a larger proportion than wheat. Ground under water in winter,—the deep damp soils, where water is apt to stagnate, as in plains and basin-like hollows of the mountains, are best fitted for it. The grain is sown in spring, in April and in

---

* In Corfu, if the ground is not firm, after sweeping, it is rendered so by the application of a paste formed of cow-dung, laid on in three or four successive layers, one being allowed to dry before another is used. In Cephalonia there are permanent thrashing-floors—paved circular areas—in convenient parts of the farms.

† Plate II. figs. 14, 15.

May. In these months the plough is very active in preparing the ground for its reception. The plant flowers in June. It is previously, when about a foot high, banked up with the hoe. In the beginning of July, the male flower with its leafy stem, is gathered and used as forage; cattle and horses are very fond of it. The harvest is towards the end of the hot season, chiefly in September. Where the soil is good, and the situation favourable, the produce is large, often more than a hundred-fold; there may be two or three heads on each stalk. Where the soil and situation are unfavourable, the crop is stunted, and the return is very small. Maize constitutes the principal article of the food of the labouring class in the islands just mentioned. It is used chiefly in the form of cakes. The grain is softened by boiling, beaten into a paste, and baked. The leafy envelope of the heads is used for matresses; it makes an excellent bed, admirably fitted for a warm climate, free from all unpleasant smell, perfectly clean, and, without being soft, sufficiently elastic.

2. *Of Vineyards.*—These form a very important part of the cultivation of the Ionian Islands. They may be divided principally into two kinds, one in which the produce is applied to the making of wine, the other in which the fruit is dried. The term vineyard is commonly restricted to the first. The second, from the fruit, are better known by the name of currant-grounds or plantations.

The common vine, in its numerous varieties, is cultivated, more or less, in all the islands; not one is an exception;—even Paxo has vineyards, from which wine is made sufficient in quantity for the use of the inhabitants, for about three months out of the twelve.

The mode of cultivating the common vine is much the same in all the islands, and appears to be well understood. The vines are pruned in February and March; about the same time, or a little later, the earth round them is dug with the hoe, and raised in heaps, which are levelled in May; in June the extremities of the young shoots are broken off; the vintage commonly begins in September;—in Corfu, the 19th of September is fixed by custom for its commencement. The vineyards are not commonly manured, nor are the vines supported by stakes. The latter the proprietors cannot afford to use; the low value of the produce does not warrant the expense. They are kept low, and are generally treated very much in the same manner as in France. In proportion to the poverty and dryness of the soil, the greater is the rigour with which the pruning-knife is used. In some rocky situations, as in the district of Erisso, in Cephalonia, where the vine is planted in the crevices of rocks, and the rock, it is said, is even hollowed out to receive it, only one or two of last year's branches are spared, and of these the greater part is removed,—only two or three buds or eyes are allowed to remain. This severity is exercised on principle, and from long experience of its beneficial effects. An intelligent Zantiote, with whom I conversed on the subject, remarked, that it is the property of the vine to extend its branches much more rapidly than its roots; and, in consequence, unless severe pruning is used, the branches will exceed in proportion the roots, and the plant will be weakly and unproductive; and he added, that, as the fruit-bearing branches are strictly annuals, and derived from buds of the last year, older wood is merely an encumbrance. He had been in England, and he expressed surprise at the manner in which the vine is commonly treated there, allowed to be overloaded with old wood; and he mentioned, too, the surprise and astonishment which he excited by pruning his landlady's vine in the neighbourhood of London, according to the Zantiote rigorous method. The poor vine, curtailed of its numerous branches, was considered ruined. In the autumn, however, ample compensation was given in a vintage of unexampled abundance,—the barren vine was made fruitful. The cuttings of the vine, and the early shoots, which are broken off, are carefully collected. The latter are given to the cattle; and even the dry branches are similarly used. I have often seen a bundle of dry vine twigs thrown before a horse, for a baiting, which the poor animal, not being able to get any thing better, contrived to masticate.

The art of making wine, in the Ionian Islands, is not so well understood as the cultivation of the vine.

Nowhere has it been scientifically and carefully studied. The process is commonly conducted in a rude and careless manner, and the result is never certain as to the quality of wine which will be obtained. The grapes are gathered by women and children, and carried in baskets to the press. If the grapes are black, and their skins thick, as they usually are, they are allowed to remain heaped together six or seven days to soften; they are next subjected to the pressure of the feet of men, and next to the more powerful pressure of a screw. The must obtained is fermented for a few days with the addition of about a fourth of the husks of the black grape to heighten the colour. It is then drawn off, and allowed to remain and complete its fermentation in casks. In the instance of white grapes, their skins being sufficiently tender, they do not require to be further softened, and they are subjected to the press without delay. Often and most commonly, the black and white are mixed. The process, of which the outline is thus given, is that followed in Zante. It is much the same in the other islands;—the variations are inconsiderable. In most of the islands, the greater part of the must is brought into the towns in pig-skins, from whence it is transferred to casks for the completion of the fermentation. In Santa Maura, the must is fermented in pear-shaped vats of masonry, lined with mortar.

The wines of the Ionian Islands generally deposit cream of tartar (super-tartrate of potash) on standing, after the completion of the fermentation. The porters

who clean the casks which have been used for keeping the wine, collect it, scraping it from the inside;
they dry it in the sun, and expose it to a gentle heat.
Made up in conical masses, of three or four pounds
each, the salt is exported to Venice, where it is puri-
fied. The coopers, in refitting the casks, also collect
a saline matter of the same nature as the preceding,
adhering to the inside, in the form of small hard
masses, which are sold to the gold and silver smiths,
and used by them in their work. The quantity of
cream of tartar, year after year, successively yielded
by the wine of the *same* vineyard, is very remarkable;
one is at a loss to conjecture from whence the alkali
entering into the saline compound is derived. I was
not able to learn that, after a certain number of years,
the cream of tartar ceases to appear; it is the more
extraordinary, since the soils of these islands do not
afford nitre.

The best wines of the Ionian Islands are those of
Ithaca and Cephalonia, and of the hilly and mountainous parts of Zante. They are all sufficiently strong,
and would bear exportation; and, were they allowed
to have age, I believe they would be approved in this
country, especially the red wine of Ithaca, the best
white wine of Cephalonia, and the verdea of Zante.
The last mentioned wine is at present made only in
small quantities, and with great care; and it is chiefly
given in presents by the rich proprietors. It is a
highly-flavoured wine, of a greenish hue; it will keep
for a great length of time, and continue improving

It is a good instance of what may be effected with care.*

Unfortunately, in these islands hitherto little or no encouragement has been given to the making of good wine; quantity is attended to rather than quality—a rapid sale rather than a just remunerating profit. Much of the wine that is sold is cheaper than small beer; much of it is sold quite new; little is kept a year; none is exported, excepting from one island to another. There are no capitalists,—no regular wine-merchants; each proprietor is his own merchant; his cellar is commonly the ground-floor of his town-house; having little room,—no apparatus,—apprehensive that the wine will spoil if kept,—he sells it as soon as possible, either by wholesale or retail. If the former, the doors of the cellar are thrown open,—two or three forms are provided,—and a flag of white paper, or of paper stained red, according to the quality of wine, is hung out on a stick. Should the wine be approved, the cellar is crowded with customers, and suddenly becomes a scene of merriment, uproar, and gambling, —filled with people talking loud, singing, or playing at cards, or the noisy, vulgar, and classical game of Moro, the *micare cum digitis* of the Romans.

Were just encouragement given, could substantial wine-merchants be induced to settle in the Ionian

---

* Verdea is made from choice white grapes, not subjected to the pressure of the feet or of the press; the must is obtained merely by the pressure of the grapes on each other heaped together.

Islands, who would bring both capital and a knowledge of the best methods of preparing wines,—there can be little doubt that excellent wines might be made, capable of competing with the best growths of the south of Europe, and perhaps even of France. Owing to the diversity of soil, connected with difference of geological structure, and diversity of climate, connected with different degrees of elevation amongst the hills and mountains, a great variety of wines, even at present, are made, and the number might be increased. The cooler regions produce the lighter wines, which approach the French in being more highly flavoured; the lower and warmer hilly regions produce stronger ones, more resembling the Spanish and Sicilian. The fruit, probably, is sufficiently good; the methods of preparing the wine seem chiefly to require amendment, and that, not only in relation to fermentation, but still more as regards the after processes, to which at present no attention is paid,—processes such as those to which we owe in great part the goodness of sherry, of Madeira, and, I may add, of Marsala, which last, in its first stage, as brought by the farmer to the merchant, is very like the better quality of the new white wine of Cephalonia.

The currant-vine is far less generally cultivated than the common vine; it is chiefly confined to Zante, Cephalonia, and Ithaca. The attempts to extend the cultivation of it to the other islands have been partial, on a very limited scale, and attended with doubtful success. This, I believe, is not owing, as has been asserted, to any unfitness of soil in the other islands, for their soils are very analogous, but rather to some difference of climate, especially about the time of the ripening and gathering and drying the fruit,—consisting in a greater liability to rain, a heavy fall of which is ruinous to the crop, and which in the currant-islands, during the period of the gathering, is dreaded as a great calamity. In confirmation I may remark that, equally in Zante, Cephalonia, and Ithaca, the currant-vine is planted in different soils, and in different situations,—in gray marl and in red clay,— in the plains, and amongst the mountains,—where nothing is in common excepting the long dry season. A certain soil and situation, however, is considered most favourable for its cultivation, especially the calcareous marls, which are easily worked, have great depth, are easily penetrated by the roots, and are retentive of moisture,—and low situations, where water can be easily introduced and irrigation effected. The marl of the plain of Zante contains a little sulphate of lime, and I have detected sulphate of lime in the currants of that district. It is a question, whether the compound in a minute proportion may not be beneficial, and whether the excellence of the soil may not in part depend on its presence.

The produce being valuable, the profit to the cultivator often great, much attention has been paid to the currant-plantations,—capital has been expended on them,—skill exercised, and with great success.

I shall mention briefly the manner in which they are managed in Zante, where, perhaps, the currant-vine has been brought to its greatest perfection; and I shall add a few particulars respecting the gathering of the fruit and the preparing it for exportation.

As abundance of water and irrigation are essential to the fertility of the currant-vine, measures are required to be taken to secure this; and accordingly the plantation is enclosed by mounds of earth and ditches (the ground thrown up in making the latter form the mounds), provided with sluices, by which the admission, or exclusion, and the quantity, of water can be regulated. Before the heavy rains, in October and November, the ditches and mounds are put in order. Both the broad hoe and the spade are used for the purpose,* and for this purpose almost alone is the spade employed. The mound is often planted with the aloe, which, in rows, growing luxuriantly, and attaining a great size, has a very stately and striking appearance, and is useful as well as ornamental. It makes, by means of its large, strong, prickly leaves, an admirable fence.

The vines are planted in rows, with perfect regularity, three or four feet asunder. A new plantation is formed, either by laying shoots, or by grafting the currant-vine on the common vine. The best shoots for propagation are obtained by cutting the parent trunk very low, below ground; after this operation

* Plate II., figs. 4, 16.

the shoots which spring up are very vigorous.* They are cut off in December, covered with light mould and planted in spring; six or seven years elapse before they come into bearing. The process of grafting has, of late years, been much in use, since the value of the fruit of the one has exceeded that of the fermented juice of the other, and especially in Cephalonia. It has, moreover, this advantage, that the grafted vine becomes productive in a much shorter time; in three or four years it is in full bearing. The operation of grafting is thus conducted:—a pit is dug, exposing the trunk of the common vine about a foot or a foot and a half below the surface; the vine is amputated as low as this; and two or three perpendicular incisions are made in the stalk with a chisel near the bark, into which the last year shoots of the currant-vine are inserted, of such a length as to have two or three eyes or buds above the surface; then some moist marl is applied to the engrafted part, wrapped in leaves, and bound with rushes, and the earth is thrown into the pit. The season for grafting is, of course, spring, when the sap is ascending.

The pruning of the currant-vine is an operation said to require much judgment, not as regards time, for that is fixed by custom, but in relation to the quantity of wood to be removed,—the quality and even position of the branches to be left. It is not completed

* The same holds good of the common vine.

at once, but at intervals. In December the vines are subjected to the process of cleaning; the dead, weakly, and unpromising branches are removed; only a certain number of the more vigorous branches are left—the shoots of the preceding spring—selected on account of their proper position in regard to each other, and the indications afforded in their buds or eyes of their fruit-bearing powers. In February, about the latter end of the month, the knife is again applied, and the remaining branches are curtailed, so as to insure active vegetation. Every eye is considered equivalent to a fruit-bearing branch;* and no more are left than it is supposed can be amply nourished; three or four is the usual number left.†

The cuttings of the currant-plantations are principally carried into the city and sold for fire-wood. It is calculated that what they sell for will almost defray the expense of the pruning.

* Each bud or eye throws out three branches, one large, and one on each side, which are small; the middle branch is the fruit-bearing one; the lateral branches are barren unless the principal one is cut off.

† Mr Manoti, a very intelligent Zantiote gentleman, and enlightened proprietor and cultivator, to whom I am indebted for many of the above particulars respecting the currant-vine, told me that he once made trial of pruning his currant-vines in December and April, instead of in February. Those pruned in December yielded very few grapes, which were large; those in April a great plenty, but very small. He satisfied himself by the trial that February (the adopted month) is the best for the operation. This he mentioned incidentally, with the remark, alluding to the want of disposition on the part of his countrymen to investigate, that, if he had related his results to his neighbour, he would have laughed at him, and asked, who ever thought of cutting the Uva-passa in December or in April?

Different forms of pruning-knife are used; some of them are represented in Plate II. Fig. 13 is most commonly used in the vineyards of Zante, both of the common vine and currant-vine. Fig. 12, besides being used in the vineyard, is applied to other purposes,—as for cutting grass, straw, &c. The price of each is about half-a-crown; they are manufactured in Zante, and are made of well-tempered steel. In fig. 13 there is a slight projection of the blade opposite the handle, to give it some resemblance, in form, to the cross, from a superstitious notion of the virtues of this form.

I have alluded to the irrigation of the currant-grounds, and the means employed for this purpose. Where there is a command of water, they are flooded from the latter end of October or beginning of November till the latter end of December, when the sluices are opened, and the excess of water is allowed to run off. The after irrigation is merely to keep the ground moist.

About the same time that the vine receives its last pruning, the earth is moved about its roots; it is scooped out round the stalk, and piled in small heaps at a little distance, thus favouring both the watering of the plant and the warming of the roots, and the exposure of the soil to the influence of the air. In April the ground is moved a second time, and that deeply; and then the surface is levelled. Occasionally, manure is used; it is far, however, from a general practice. It is said to increase the quantity of fruit, but to injure the quality. The new soil, brought down from the hills by the rains, is considered the natural and most appropriate manure.

The currant-vine is allowed to grow without check; the ends of its shoots are not broken, like those of the common vine: and the luxuriancy of its annual shoots, in favourable circumstances, is extraordinary. They are always supported by stakes, which are imported, at a cost of about fifteen dollars a thousand.

Great care is paid at all seasons to the currant-plantations, especially in spring, when vegetation is commencing; the opening buds and young shoots are so tender as to be very susceptible of injury. This is well illustrated by a common saying,—that, after the 10th of March (old style), not even a dog without a tail should be allowed to enter a vineyard. If the bud is broke, the embryo branch is destroyed.

The currant-vine is one of the earliest of the vines. Its fruit is often sufficiently ripe for the use of the table in the last week of July; it is then of a purplish hue, not too luscious, as when thoroughly ripe, but very agreeably sweet and subacid. The period of the vintage in the plain of Zante is commonly in the middle of August. This is a very interesting and important period to the Zantiote. The rich proprietors now take up their abode in their country villas to superintend the crop, on which they principally depend. Every plantation is now carefully watched; a watch-place, constructed of interlaced branches of trees (as it commonly is), covered with leaves or thatch, elevated on poles, situated conveniently, is tenanted nightly by a watchman, armed with a loaded gun and aided in his duty by one or more dogs, who act the part of patroles, and give warning, by their barking, of the approach of any footstep. The value of the fruit, and the manner in which it is exposed at this time, render such protection necessary.

As soon as the fruit is fully ripe, when it is almost black, it is gathered and carried to the drying-ground, an area in the vineyard, to which the watch-house is close, prepared by the removal of weeds, and by covering the clean, firm, and dry surface with a paste of cow-dung.* Here the fruit is exposed to the sun and air, and is frequently turned, till quite dry. It is separated from the stalk, put into hair-bags, and carried on pack-horses and mules into the city, where it is deposited in magazines prepared expressly for its reception.† Previous to being shipped for exporta-

---

* We are apt to associate an idea of want of cleanliness with any process in which cow-dung is used; but erroneously. The Hindus use it expressly for the purpose of cleanliness; they smear their floors with a paste of it. When dry, it presents a smooth, firm surface, quite free from any unpleasant smell, and entirely excluding insects, so that one can spread one's mat on it and rest in perfect security from their attacks. Consisting principally of vegetable fibre in a finely divided state, the indigestible woody fibre, mixed with a small quantity of bile and other viscid animal juices, it is a substance possessing many good qualities, and is applicable to many useful purposes.

† In Sir Charles Napier's work on the Ionian Islands, there are some curious and instructive details relative to the system of storing currants, which, in spite of their length, I am tempted to extract, chiefly on account of their importance in relation to the abuses ex-

tion, it is transferred to casks, in which it is tightly packed, being trodden down by the feet of men.

posed.   The store-rooms, in which the currants are deposited, are called " *Seraglie.*"   " These are rooms, or rather boxes, lined with boards, and the fruit is packed close, and neither light nor air admitted.   The gentlemen who possess these, receive the currants of the growers, who pay a per-centage for the use of the ' Seraglia.'   Here we come to the first fraud played upon the peasant, informing the reader that I cannot tell him all, for I do not know half the frauds practised; and also informing the said reader that there are good and bad ' Seraglianti,' as these proprietors of Seraglie are called : I only describe a bad one.   Now, to proceed, which I do in a dramatic form, as the simplest.   We will call our poor proprietor (who is also a labourer, or a tenant of the Seragliante), Gerasimo, and a third character is the confidential servant of the Seragliante.

Scene I.—*A Room, with a hole in the floor-door, down which the fruit is thrown into the Seraglia ; the door is open from the chamber into the apartment where the Seragliante sits; the servant waiting with a steel-yard.*

Enters Gerasimo, *with his Currants.*

Servant.—Well, Gerasimo, you have a heavy weight of fruit there?
Gerasimo.—Yes, sir, Virgin fruit, not touched by the rain.

(His sons, who have helped him, are sent out by the servant).

Servant.—How much have you?

[Seragliante *sits behind the door, looking through the chinks unseen.*

Gerasimo.—A thousand pounds.
Servant.—What! a thousand pounds there? Impossible!
Gerasimo.—Yes, sir ; there are just a thousand without the bags.
Servant.—Well, come, let us see.

(Weighs them and finds there are about a thousand).

O you rascal !

It is at the critical season of the drying of the currants that rain is most dreaded by the natives of

(Pressing the yard with his elbow, as he shoves the weight closer to the point of suspension).

Look, knave, look! six hundred marked on the yard!

GERASIMO.—Ah! sir, you know I can't read; but there are a thousand pounds, as I hope for mercy on myself and my children.

SERVANT.—I lie, then, do I? What is it to me how much your currants weigh : I act for my master. However, I won't be called a villain by you. There are six hundred ; so it's of no use to argue.

(Empties the currants into the hole, and gives Gerasimo a receipt for six hundred pounds).

GERASIMO.—I can't take that; there are a thousand; and I must have a receipt for the whole.

SERVANT.—You are a scoundrel, and may settle with the master yourself. There, my lord, here is Gerasimo disputes weight.

(Enters Seragliante, with great dignity, from behind the door, where he has been watching, for fear his man and Gerasimo might come to a private understanding).

SERAGLIANTE.—Well, Gerasimo, what is the matter?

GERASIMO.—My lord, I brought one thousand pounds, and your servant says there are but six hundred.

SERVANT.—Yes, my lord, six hundred exactly! but he can't read, and he says I cheated him.

SERAGLIANTE.—What, scoundrel! accuse my servant! a person whom I have known all my life, and who is the honestest man in Argostoli? Take your fruit away: you are a villain.

GERASIMO.—It's down in the Seraglia; and there are a thousand pounds, my lord.

SERAGLIANTE.—I am sorry that it is down; however, there is your receipt for six hundred, so go away, and let me have no more insolence. Hark ye! my friend, you owe me ten dollars, advanced this year, to get your fruit in: if you are not off with your receipt, pay me the money this minute, and you may take your six hundred pounds back. My servant and I are witnesses that it weighed so much. There is interest on the ten dollars due to me; so, if you like to pay

the southern islands. They now watch the heavens with anxious eyes; the appearance of a cloud fills

me, do so, or go to jail; and, if any Seragliante takes your fruit, I shall consider it a personal insult, and so I shall tell him.

(*Here Gerasimo is silent, takes his receipt, and is going away*).

SERVANT.—My lord, as he is a good man, and to show your generosity, and that I have no malice for his abuse of me, let me give him credit for fifty more.

SERAGLIANTE.—Well, do so; it's lucky for you, Gerasimo, to have so good a master. Some Seragliante would have had you before the tribunals for defamation; and a month's imprisonment would have taught you better manners to your superiors;—go away.

(*Exit Gerasimo*).

Such is scene the first. If Gerasimo had taken away his six hundred and fifty pounds, and sacrificed the other three hundred and fifty, his debt of ten dollars would have been made into thirty or forty, and the new Seragliante would have made a deduction of three hundred and fifty pounds more.

SCENE II.—GERASIMO *returns*.

GERASIMO.—My lord, I hope you will advance me a trifle on the currants. You know I have not a shilling to buy bread for my family.

SERAGLIANTE.—Humph! Money is scarce, Gerasimo; you have 10 per cent. to pay for the hire of the Seraglia; ten dollars you owe me already, with interest at 20 per cent. thereon. I cannot lend you any under. I can make 48 per cent. this minute on my money.

GERASIMO, (*sighing*)—My lord, you are too hard; but what can I do? I consent to 15 per cent.

SERAGLIANTE.—No, Gerasimo; twenty, or no money.

GERASIMO.—Well, be it so; your lordship will take work and fowls, as well as money, I hope.

SERAGLIANTE.—Oh, yes; make out a receipt for him.

SERVANT.—Yes, sir.

(*Makes out an acknowledgment for more than is lent, which Gerasimo puts his mark to, and goes away, followed by the servant, to get a tip for his good offices in the added fifty pounds*).

But this is only a part of what the peasant loses; for, when the cur-

them with dread; for even a single shower injures greatly the value of the fruit if it fall on it in drying; and heavy rains prove ruinous to the crop, rendering it totally unfit for the market, depriving it of all its value.

3. *Of the Olive.*—The soils, and what, perhaps, is more important, the climate, of the Ionian Islands are peculiarly favourable to this plant; nowhere that I am aware of in the world does it flourish more, or is more productive, or yields, with care, better fruit. Where the soil is good, as it commonly is in Corfu, the olive attains a great size,—that of a forest-tree,— and there literally, there are forests of olive-trees, exhibiting picturesque beauties not easily forgotten by those who have had the pleasure of riding under their cool shade in the summer noon-day, or in the evening, when lighted by the slanting rays of the

rants are sold, the prices fluctuate, and Gerasimo's unhappy six hundred and fifty pounds invariably fetch the lowest price; or, if any fruit remain unsold, that fruit is Gerasimo's six hundred and fifty pounds; so that he is defrauded in the weight, in the sale, and in the money advanced. Another fraud is thus practised:—A merchant and a Seragliante make their written agreement for a false price; and this is entered at the custom-house, but privately, the merchant pays *more* than the sum stated in the written legal agreement, the proprietor receiving only the sum mentioned in the letter. I do *not* say all the Seragliante do this, but all *can* do it, and that most *do*, is well known." Farther details are given by this author relative to the Seraglia abuses, with his suggestions for correcting them, which are well deserving the attention of the government.

setting sun. The sketch, Plate III., from a drawing
of Lieutenant-Colonel Irton's, will give some idea
of olive woodland scenery; the town of Corfu, surmounted by the citadel, the *aeriæ arces* of Virgil,
with the Acarnanian mountains beyond, is seen in
the distance.

The olive is not, like the currant-vine, confined
to certain islands; it is, more or less, universally
cultivated, partly to supply the wants of the natives, who make great use of its oil, and of its fruit
variously preserved, and partly for the purpose of
exportation.

The cultivation which the olive-tree receives varies
in the different islands and on different estates,
according to the intelligence, activity, and means of
the proprietor. When I was in the Ionian Islands, the
greatest neglect of cultivation prevailed in Corfu;
extensive tracts of olive-plantations were there almost
entirely neglected,—neither pruned, nor manured, nor
dug about; setting idle habits aside, the main cause,
partly owing to the low price of oil, and partly in
connexion with this low price, to the poverty of the
owners. In Cephalonia, and Ithaca, and Cerigo,
and, more especially, in Paxo and Fanno, the olive-
plantations had more attention paid to them. When
duly cultivated, the earth round the trees is broken
up annually,—excavated so as to form a pit, into
which, by a channel, water is directed; and manure
is applied, according to the quality of the ground,
every third, fourth, or fifth year, excepting the soil be

very rich, when it may be dispensed with. In Corfu
and Zante the best pasture is under the shade of the
olive-groves. In the former island, where cultivation
is neglected, the fern grows luxuriantly, and often the
myrtle, forming a fragrant underwood. In Paxo the
little corn that is raised is grown in the olive-grounds,
which, in that steep and rugged island, are chiefly in
the form of terraces, carefully and laboriously walled
up. You may there see frequently a single tree thus
fortified : without the walled terrace the soil would
be washed away by the rains, and the tree would be
impoverished by the want both of soil and water. The
olive-tree requires to be pruned ; the axe is used for
the purpose of removing the dead and superfluous
branches. The loppings are valuable for fuel ; scarcely
any other fuel is used in Paxo.

The olive-tree comes into flower in the month of
April; its fruit is of slow growth ; it ripens at the
same season as the orange, in the depth of winter. In
January the greater part of the fruit is collected.   In
most of the islands it is left to ripen and fall, and is
collected from the ground ; in Zante, contrary to the
old Roman law referred to by Pliny,* the trees are
beaten with long sticks, and the fruit is struck off
and gathered below in a table-cloth placed to catch
them. The best oil is that of Paxo and Fanno,
where it is expressed from the ripe fruit as soon as
they fall, collected from the ground, previously freed

---

* Oleam ne stringito neve verberato.—Hist. lib. xv. cap. 3.

from weeds, and swept clean. The oil of Corfu is coarser, little care being taken in the gathering of the fruit, either as regards time or cleanliness; indeed the fruit, from too long keeping, is generally in a state of partial decomposition before it is subjected to the mill. In Zante the oil is of an intermediate quality; the olives are collected before they are ripe,—are salted, and so preserved,—and are subjected to the press at the time when it is most convenient.

The process for extracting the oil is generally the same. The olives, after having been steeped in warm water, for the purpose of correcting their dryness, which is specially necessary in Corfu, are crushed in the mill, which is a heavy circular disc-like stone, revolving perpendicularly on another circular stone or platform of masonry, slightly grooved or inclining inwards. It is worked by a horse or mule, attached by harness to one end of the projecting axle of the mill-stone; its other end being secured in a strong perpendicular pivot, which revolves with the stone. The olives are kept as much as possible in the mill-course by the attendant, by means of a wooden shovel.*

---

* In Cerigo a ruder and simpler method even is employed; it is thus described by Mr Robert Jameson, prefaced with the remark that it is curious, from its apparent antiquity:—" The olives are placed on a nearly flat stone, and another heavy one, of a square shape, is rolled backwards and forwards on them, so as to press the fruit; when thus bruised, the mass is put into a large bag (made of the fibres of a sco-perta), which is closed and thrown into a vessel containing hot water, and allowed to remain there till heated; it is then taken out and

During the olive harvest the loud creakings of the mills, and the blue volumes of smoke, widely heard and seen, proceeding from the numerous scattered magazines, denote strongly the occasion, and impart a pleasing animation to these otherwise solitary regions. From the mill the crushed olives are transferred, in coarse bags, to a simple screw-press, which is often loaded with a heavy weight, and turned by levers, attached by a cord to the screws, moved in a very rude and laborious manner by men, and with a trifling effect compared with the great muscular exertion and impetus of body applied. (*Vide* Plate IV.) After the oil has been expressed, what remains, consisting of the broken seed and pulp still retaining a minute quantity of oil, and on that account well adapted for fuel, is used for heating ovens, and is even exported for that purpose to Malta.

The olive-plantations of the Ionian Islands yield

placed in a shallow trough with a plugged hole on the one side. The trough is elevated about two feet above the chamber floor; a man treads on the bag thus filled, from which the oil is expressed along with the warm water: as soon as the trough is nearly full, the plug is withdrawn, when both the substances escape into a vessel placed beneath, having, near its bottom, a plugged orifice. By the time this vessel is filled the greatest part of the oil has separated from the water and floats on its surface, from its specific gravity being much less; therefore, when the orifice near the bottom is opened, the water escapes, mixed with only a small quantity of oil, into a hole dug in the ground outside of the chamber, where this oil also, when the mechanical mixture ceases, is collected by skimming it off by means of a branch or bunch of straw. In this manner a man, assisted by a woman and child, will make a barrel or more a-day."

very little fruit, excepting every other year.* In Provence it is said that there is an annual crop. The difference has been attributed to the fruit of Provence being gathered earlier than that of the Ionian Islands, in November, before it is ripe, but with how much truth I cannot say. The olive is a tree of great delicacy; both its blossom and its fruit are easily injured by climate, requiring different qualities of atmosphere at different stages. The consequence is unavoidable, that the crop often suffers; a very abundant year is uncommon; and of late, since less attention has been paid to cultivation, what used to be considered as an average crop, is of rare occurrence.

The olive-tree is of great longevity. In Paxo trees were pointed out to me three hundred years old, and they did not bear the marks of very advanced age; they produced less fruit than younger plants, but of equally good quality. In old age no tree is more venerable, or picturesque, or more characteristic of the powers of vegetation and of the eternal youth of the living plant, existing in its bark and leaves and the corresponding parts of its roots. It is not uncommon to see an aged olive, hollowed out by decay, a mere shell,—that shell a sound bark,—the branches supported by props,—vegetating vigorously, and bearing fruit.

The varieties of olive are numerous; they are pro-

* This is shown in the preceding returns of produce of two consecutive years; in 1835 Corfu yielded no oil; in 1834, 236,016 barrels.

pagated in several different ways. The three following are most used. 1*st*, By shoots from the parent
tree, having roots. 2*dly*, By cuttings of branches
(each about a foot long), which are placed horizontally in a bed of earth, and covered entirely with soil,
to the depth of five or six inches. They are thus
placed in January ; in March they are taken up; their
ends are dipped in a mixture of cow-dung and earth,
of the consistence of paste, and are then planted, and
at such depth in the soil as to be three or four inches
beneath its surface. As the spring advances, the cuttings vegetate, take root, and throw up small shoots.
Most of the cuttings thus treated live and thrive.
This is the most common way of propagating the
olive-tree, especially on a large scale. 3*dly*, By
cuttings of large branches, five or six feet long The
large end is split a little way by a slight stroke of a
hatchet; a stone is placed in the fissure, and a few
stones are thrown into the hole dug to receive the
cuttings. The varieties are obtained from seed, as is
the case with the majority of our cultivated fruit-
trees ; and according to the same analogy, the majority of the seedlings, even from the seed of the best
varieties, have the character of the wild plant, and
are of little use, excepting for the purpose of grafting
—a process which, in the Ionian Islands, is little
applied to the olive-tree.

The wood of the olive-tree has some valuable properties ; it possesses much hardness, great durability,
and considerable beauty of appearance; it is finely

veined, and takes a fine polish, and, in consequence, it is well adapted for the cabinet-maker. As fire-wood it is excellent, as every one can vouch who has spent a winter in the Mediterranean, and enjoyed the comfort of an olive-wood fire. Occasionally a resin exudes from the trunk of the olive-tree, which is not a little prized on account of its fragrant smell in burning.

The olive and the olive oil constitute two of the principal articles of food amongst the natives, and the quantity consumed by them is great, when their means are equal to their inclinations. Each person, on an average, it is supposed, uses from four to six ounces daily. It is used with wild herbs as a sallad, with bread as a substitute for butter, and in other ways. The fruit is used variously preserved, both green and ripe; the former in salt and water, after a slight maceration to extract the bitter principle; the latter in vinegar and oil, as well as in brine. The ripe fruit has the preference, and is much more largely consumed than the green. It is commonly eaten with bread; as a relish, a Sardinia is occasionally added.

4.—On the other articles of produce a few remarks will suffice, as, from the small quantities in which they are grown at present, they are comparatively unimportant—such as cotton, tobacco, flax, &c. In Zante a crop of cotton is so little profitable, that I was assured by an intelligent cultivator, that were it not beneficial to the soil in preparation for wheat, it would not repay the cost incurred in raising it. The value of the potato, too, he considered too low for it to be profitably cultivated. It is not at present used by the natives; at least it was not when I was in the Ionian Islands, and it is to be hoped never will be, as a principal article of food. Perhaps a limited cultivation of it may be advantageous and profitable in situations and soils peculiarly favourable to its growth, and in the vicinity of the principal stations for the supply of the English inhabitants.* Tobacco at present is very little grown in Corfu. It is chiefly cultivated in conjunction with maize; the two in alternate rows. Rice, it is said, was once grown in the Val di Roppa, in Corfu, but of late years, I believe, it has been discontinued. Probably, in an improved system of husbandry, both these last mentioned articles will have more attention paid to them, especially rice, for the growth of which there are very many situations in the larger islands, especially in Corfu and Zante, admirably adapted;—marshy grounds, now-perhaps sources of malaria, at all events unprofitable,—which, by the cultivation of this excellent grain, might be made highly productive, with the advantage, at the same

---

* Recently, I am informed, an attempt has been made to introduce the cultivation of the potato into Corfu. Sir Howard Douglas, when Lord High Commissioner, supplied the small farmers with seed-potatoes, provided they brought a certificate from the primate of their village that they had prepared a certain quantity of ground for their reception. This offer, it is said, was in many instances accepted ; and though in some abused, it has had the desired effect of encouraging the growing of the root.

time, of improving the air in the neighbourhood.* There is a generally prevailing prejudice against rice-grounds in the south of Europe, especially in Lombardy, connected with the idea of their insalubrity,— an idea which I believe is erroneous. The situations may be unwholesome; the error seems to be in attributing to the crop what is owing to the situation. The subject is candidly and ably discussed in a little tract on the cultivation of rice by Professor Giovanni Beroli.† The conclusion at which he arrives is, that the low

---

* Probably the upland rice, which does not require irrigation, might be successfully cultivated in many parts of the Ionian Islands, especially in Corfu. In Ceylon and Sumatra it is pretty extensively grown, and much valued. An able judge, the late Sir Stamford Raffles, was of opinion that it might be introduced, even advantageously, into England. In a letter to the Reverend Dr Cartwright, the distinguished inventor of the power-loom, contained in an interesting MS. memoir of his life, which I hope soon to see published, are the following remarks on this grain, written in 1820 at Fort Marlbro:—
" So little seems to be known in Europe respecting the culture of dry rice, and as it is not impossible this important grain may be introduced into the British Isles, I take the liberty of sending you a small quantity for seed. It is grown on the hills and generally on lands recently cleared from primitive forest. The ground is not ploughed, but on the approach of the rainy season small holes are made with a stick, and two grains of seed thrown in. The rice is then left to itself until reaped. It is the principal cultivation of Sumatra, particularly in the mountains, where the soil is richer, and the climate colder than below. The soil is generally enriched by the ashes of the newly-cleared forest, burnt on the spot. I also send you a specimen of the rice. It is considered full twenty per cent. better than the lowland or irrigated rice, and bears a proportionate high price. It is far more nutritious, and less likely to perish."

† Del Riso Trattato Economico-Rustico del Professore Giovanni Beroli. Milano. 1825.

grounds would be more unwholesome were they not so cultivated; that even grass-meadow would be more unwholesome, and marsh very much more so. Rice-grounds require irrigation; and the effect of irrigation,—of flowing water, in contradistinction to stagnant water, invariably appears to be beneficial. In Ceylon, under an almost vertical sun, the rice-grounds are not considered productive of malaria; it is not where paddy-fields are most widely spread that the severe remittent fever prevails, but, on the contrary, where not a grain of rice is grown, viz., on the uncultivated wilds,—in the low plains, once cultivated and populous, now deserted by man, and the abode only of wild animals. It seems to be a happy and beneficial arrangement of Providence that the cultivation of the soil, whatever may be its kind, without any exception, should be, both directly and indirectly, advantageous to man; that we cannot improve the soil, and render it better fitted for profitable vegetation, without at the same time ameliorating the qualities of the atmosphere.*

5. *Of Garden-Grounds.*—This species of cultivation is of very limited extent in the Ionian Islands, very

---

* In the *Morning Chronicle* of the 26th May 1837, it is said,— "From a letter, addressed by one of the French missionaries in China to a member of the Academy of Sciences, it appears that, contrary to all experience elsewhere, the cultivation of rice is managed in that country without injury to the health of the labourer. This exemption is ascribed to the regimen observed, which seems to consist chiefly in copious potations of tea and the liberal use of the warm bath!!"

much more restricted than might be expected, considering the long and severe lents of the Greek Church. It may be divided into two kinds,—one the cultivation of vegetables,—the other of fruit-trees. The first is very trifling indeed. In the neighbourhood of the principal towns, particularly the town of Corfu, the kitchen-gardens are cultivated with some care, but chiefly by Italians and Maltese; and a considerable variety of vegetables are grown, chiefly for the use of the English. The natives are mostly satisfied with the artichoke and garlic, the cabbage and onion. These they seldom grow in their own grounds; they more frequently purchase them when they go to town.*

* The want of gardens is particularly remarkable in Santa Maura. An officer, whose remarks I have already quoted on this subject, writes, in 1835,—" If a thousand gardens were formed to-day in Santa Maura, it is possible that in a single week not one of them would exist, unless most extraordinary precautions were taken for their defence and preservation. Hence the peasants say that, under the Venetians, when they were allowed to bear arms, and murder each other with impunity, every man had a chance of being able to defend his own property, and that, consequently, gardens were attached to all the houses in town and country. Gardens are now almost unknown in the interior. I met with one attempt, in a few square yards of soil, under the window of a dwelling in one of the villages, being surrounded with a high stone-wall, and possessing a few heads of garlic. On congratulating the owner, who was the primate or chief officer of the village,—' Alas, sir, he replied, ' if I were not to watch, night and day, the very soil would be taken from it.' This speaks but ill for the administration of the laws, which are intended to defend the peasants' property ; and I believe to their insufficiency alone may be ascribed the singular exhibition offered by the peasants, who invariably come in from the remote villages, twenty miles off, to purchase their onions and greens from the chief town."

The lower classes are dependent chiefly on the fields for their vegetables. They use a variety of wild plants, which are gathered in spring by the women, to whom the occupation appears to be equally an amusement and a duty. They make the selection knowingly, and are acquainted partially with the qualities of the herbs which they gather.

The cultivation of fruit-trees is more generally attended to, and is considered of much more importance. The principal fruits are the orange, lemon, fig, almond, grape, pomegranate, and apricot, for which the climate is peculiarly favourable. Next may be mentioned the cherry, plum, pear, service, medlar, and apple ; to which the climate, on account of its temperature, seems less congenial,—these fruits, in comparative quality, being inferior to the same kinds, the produce of more northern and cooler regions. Of the small fruits, of which there is so great a variety in our own country, and of such excellent qualities, the strawberry is the only one known in the Ionian Islands or cultivated to any extent. Of the tropical fruits, very few are to be met with, and none can be said to have succeeded. The plantain, in low, sheltered situations, grows and bears fruit, and ripens, and occasionally its fruit is tolerably good ; but its ripening is uncertain, and not to be depended on. The date-palm, too, occasionally bears fruit, but of a poor and insipid kind. The tree is cultivated principally for the sake of its leaves, which are used in the ceremonies of the Greek as well as of the

Roman Church on Easter or Palm-Sunday. Preparatively, the leaves are tied up; they are blanched, by the exclusion of light, of a delicate white; ingeniously cut, they make pretty ornaments, and are regularly sold for the purpose; and so also is the flower of the palm.

In the horticulture of the Ionian Islands, in common with that of the south of Europe, there are two things deserving of attention and imitation; one the watering of the fruit-trees at stated periods;* the other, the moving the earth about their roots, and the raising it in heaps, as in the instance of vineyards, to

---

* The effect of watering is remarkably displayed in the vine. I may mention a particular instance, of which I kept a note, on account of the extraordinary growth of the plant in a short time, and its productiveness. The vine covered an extensive verandah; its trunk was as thick as a man's thigh, and its branches were in proportion, and it abounded in fine fruit, in different stages of ripening, according to the degree of exposure to the sun. And yet this vine had been only four years planted. It is true it was then of some size, but small in comparison with that which it had attained. This rapid growth the proprietor attributed to two things,—to the manner of planting it, and the manner of watering it. A pit, he said, was dug about four feet deep and six long, in which the vine was laid in a mixture of four different kinds of earth, viz., lime, terra rossa (red clay), gypsum, and marl, which were beaten down firmly, and every day watered, and that without interruption, up to the time he spoke. All the year round, a jar of water was daily administered. This vine was at Ipsa, in Corfu, and a party, of which I was one, dined under its shade.

So essential is water to horticulture, that you may be sure, where you see a garden, that there, there is a well or fountain, and almost invariably, where there is a spring of water there, there is a garden;— the one seems to be the habitual companion of the other,—and, in a hot climate, the connexion is every way agreeable,—it is a spot of natural beauty and refreshment.

be exposed to atmospheric influences: and I may add a third circumstance, which is the regular pruning of the trees.

In the modes of propagating fruit-trees some ingenuity is displayed. I shall mention a few of them, which have been in use from time immemorial.

The method of grafting the currant-vine has been already noticed; that method is also applied to fruit-trees generally, with this difference, that the operation is performed above ground. There is another method of grafting practised, which is very neat, but which is applicable only to very young or small trees, or to the branches. The graft and the trunk or branch receiving it must be of the same size; each is cut obliquely, so as to be in exact apposition; then two or three perpendicular incisions are made in each, and they are joined, as it were, by dove-tailing. A flat surface of wax is applied round the graft to make it tight and strong, and some clay, &c., over this. When united, the graft and trunk can scarcely be distinguished. This method is applied to young apple and pear-trees; and by the florist to the jessamine and rose, to propagate the garden jessamine and the rarer varieties of the latter flower.*

Grafting by inoculation is much used, in the instance of the orange and lemon, the pomegranate and fig-tree. A square portion of bark is detached from

* The garden-jessamine is propagated with difficulty by shoots, whilst the wild is propagated with the greatest ease, and therefore the latter is used for receiving the graft of the former.

a large branch or trunk, with the exception of one side, by which, as by a hinge, it is turned back. Then a piece of the same size and figure, with a bud in it (the older the better), is taken from the tree to be propagated, and applied to the wound, so that the cut edges may be as nearly as possible in apposition. Next the bark folded back is drawn forward, and is used as a cover for the new piece. Lastly, some clay is applied, and it is bound up lightly with some leaves, &c., which are removed at the end of about a week, when, if successful, union of the two barks should have taken place.

There is an ingenious and very successful mode of multiplying orange and lemon-trees in use, which probably admits of application to fruit-trees and to shrubs generally. From a branch, conveniently situated, a portion of bark, about an inch wide, is peeled off. The part is bound with flax; then put into a box (which may be made extempore, about a foot square, or smaller), filled with earth, and watered daily, or as often as may be required to keep the soil moist. At the end of six months, if a lemon-tree; or of ten or twelve, if an orange, the branch may be cut off from the parent trunk: two or three days previously the earth should not be watered, that it may be pretty dry and firm for removal. The box must be carefully taken to pieces, and the branch immediately planted. The part of the branch so treated has thrown out a vast number of roots, both above and below the decorticated portion; the lower roots decay and fall off, whilst the upper remain and increase, and support the detached branch, whether it be in leaf or flower, or bearing fruit.

There is a method practised of transplanting trees with little injury to them, which may be deserving of mention ; I heard of it in Zante, where horticulture is more attended to than in any other of the Ionian Islands. A circular pit is made at a proper distance from the tree to be removed, according to the size of its trunk, and of a proper depth, according to the depth to which its roots extend,—the object being to leave the root insulated and the earth containing the root undisturbed. Then a frame, formed of thin pieces of wood, fastened together by means of cords, is wrapped round the cylinder of earth containing the root, and is firmly bound ; some earth is then placed above, and beat down ; then the tree is gently thrown over, and a piece of sacking is placed over the bottom of the root, and made fast by a cord. Thus prepared, the tree may be removed and transplanted with safety, even when in fruit. The same care is, of course, requisite in introducing it into the new site as in removing it from its old, not to injure the roots, on which the success of the operation mainly depends. By the method of propagation last mentioned, and this of transplantation, a garden may be formed in a very short space of time, and stocked with the best fruits.

Some artifices are commonly practised in the Ionian Islands, for the purpose of rendering trees fruitful, which are not a little curious. I shall mention only two. To the branch of the service-tree, when in flower, it is thought necessary to fasten stones for the purpose of securing fruit. It is said, that unless this be done, the flowers are abortive. Perhaps the effect (if true) is owing to the ligature, by means of which the stone is commonly tied, obstructing in part the free flow of the sap. The other process is that which is well known in the Levant under the name of caprification, and which for many years has excited the attention of the curious. It consists in attaching the fruit of the wild fig-tree to a certain variety of the cultivated, when the fruit of the latter is forming. This insures their maturation; the omission of it as certainly, it is said, is followed by the falling off of the immature fruit. The effect is connected, in the first instance, with the decay of the suspended wild figs, and the production, from eggs deposited in them, of a vast number of minute insects (*Cynips psenes*); and, in the second, with the puncturing, by these insects, of the immature fruit to lay their eggs in them. According to M. Bernard of Marseilles, who appears to have carefully studied the subject, the puncture and the depositing of the eggs act merely in the way of irritation; and he has succeeded in imitating the effect by puncturing the fruit with an awl, and introducing a drop of oil into the wound to prevent a too rapid cicitrization.* In Malta I made a

* It would appear that the touching of the young fig merely with oil has much the same effect. Carlo Giacinto, in his work on the

somewhat analogous experiment,—but the result was not successful; it was by introducing pins and small thorns into the fruit. M. De Candolle states that, through the influence of caprification in accelerating the ripening of the fig, two crops of fruit may be obtained in the same season. This I have never witnessed, either in the Ionian Islands or in Malta. According to the same deservedly high authority, the fruit obtained by means of caprification is of a somewhat deteriorated quality, " comme nous le voyons dans nos poires et nos pommes *verreuses*."* This is not the opinion received where I have made inquiry on the subject;—the fruit is supposed to be improved, not deteriorated in quality, and my experience was in accordance. One season, for the sake of trial, I forbid the usual practice of suspending the wild figs, in a garden which I had in Malta, in which were several fine fig-trees that usually bore abundant and excellent fruit of the white kind. That season the crop almost entirely failed; the young figs dropped off before they had attained a quarter of their full size; and of those which remained on and ripened, at least a moiety were of inferior quality. Perhaps the subject is deserving of still further inquiry. Whoever has an

Agriculture of Malta, thus notices this practice:—" Che dovrà dirsi di quella industriosa operatione degli ortolani, i quali e per anticiparc la maturità dei fichi, o far si, che nessuno ne resti immaturo sull' albero, invece di ricercane il caprifico, toccano l' umbilico di ciascun frutto con un poco d'olio di oliva, e ottengono il bramato inténto ?" —P. 162.

* Physiologie Végétale, tome ii., p. 580.

opportunity, and should direct his attention to it, cannot fail to be interested and amused, even in watching the development of this apparently mysterious fruit, and the changes which take place in it, especially during the short period of maturation, when a firm, insipid, or disagreeably tasted mass, enveloped in a rind abounding in acrid milky juice, is almost suddenly converted into a luscious, saccharine, and mucilaginous soft fruit, abounding in sugar and gum.

6. *Of Pasture Lands and Flocks.*—The pastures of the Ionian Islands are chiefly uncultivated, and, in very many instances, unenclosed, and subject to be trespassed on by the flocks of those who are destitute of land, and who make a practice of using the land of others without payment and without acknowledgment. In Corfu, where there is the greatest extent of pasture, their situations are various. A large portion lies under the shade of olive-groves; certain portions are mountainous; and others, of some extent, are hilly. Of the last mentioned, a good example offers in the northern extremity of the island —now almost a wilderness, without resident inhabitants, the haunt of the jackall, the occasional resort of the shepherd and his flocks, especially in early spring, when the little glades and hillocks which are not overrun with shrubbery afford good pasturage. In Santa Maura the character of the pastures is equally mixed. In Zante and in Cephalonia

they are chiefly confined to the mountainous regions. In none of the islands are there any grass meadows* —in none of them is any kind of forage sown ; the little hay that is made is from grasses self-sown, many of them of excellent quality, and indigenous—peculiarly belonging to calcareous soils.

In the preceding return is given the number of animals, of different kinds, depending on these pastures for subsistence. The flocks of sheep and goats constitute a large proportion of them, and the most important. It is from them exclusively that milk is obtained and cheese made. Lamb and kid are the principal butcher-meat used by the natives ; beef is not in request amongst them ; nor cows' milk ; the bullock is chiefly kept for the plough.

The occupation of shepherd is an acknowledged one in the Ionian Islands. It is chiefly followed by Albanians, especially in Corfu, to whom the pastoral life seems natural, and their habits and habiliments appropriate. As in the south of Europe generally, and in the east, they go before their flocks—leading, not driving them. They live very much in the open air when alone, satisfied with the covering and shelter of their shaggy capote ;—when they have their families with them, satisfied with a cabin of the rudest construction.

---

* I speak of them as I left them in the year 1828. Since then, I am informed that the old salines, in the neighbourhood of the town of Corfu, have been drained and cultivated, and have produced rich crops of clover.

In spring, particularly in the month of April, when the pastures are rich, and the shepherds are busily employed in cheese-making—it is not a little interesting, in a country excursion, to fall in with a flock, and witness the primitive processes and usages employed· I remember once having this pleasure in a wild part of the north-west extremity of Corfu—that already alluded to. It was on a fine green hill, above the little port of San Stefano. There was a shepherd's establishment complete—a · hut, made of a wicker frame, covered with barley-straw—and a bed of straw in the interior, for the shepherd and his family's use. Outside, close to the entrance, was a pole fixed in the ground, from which coarse worsted bags were suspended, that held and drained the new-made curd. A fire was hard by, on which stood a pan or crock of milk simmering, and by the side of it a wooden strainer to separate the curd. Near the shepherd's hut was a small one for the lambs and kids ; and at a little distance a screen—a wicker-frame lined with straw, for sheltering the flock at night from the wind.

In the rocky districts, where there are caverns, they are often resorted to by shepherds and their flocks, and they present scenes even more rude and primitive than that just noticed. I may give as an instance one which I witnessed in Cephalonia, in visiting the cavern Dracondispilo, already mentioned. About a quarter of a mile from the sea-cliff in which the cavern is situated, another cavern was pointed

out to us, in coarse conglomerate-rock, as the abode,
at the time, of two shepherds, and the nightly abode
of their flocks, amounting to three or four hundred
sheep and goats. In front of the cavern, for folding
the flocks at night, there was an enclosure, formed of
rude stone-walls. Within the cavern, there were
two or three small penns, the floors of which were
covered with fleece, where the lambs and kids apart
were confined during the inclement weather of winter, without their dams, who by day were abroad
grazing on the hills. It was late in the afternoon
when we passed, yet the young ones made no noise,
and appeared to be much at their ease, although
they had not sucked since the early morning, and had
no other food.* Over a small penn in which were
some young kids requiring great care and warmth (it
was in January) a herdsman had his bed, which
was a layer of dry grass, strewed on a wicker-
frame, on which was spread his shaggy capote, and
another bed, similarly constructed, was made in a
recess of the rock.†

* This is a good instance of the high nourishing power of milk, and
of the many hours that it may be presumed are required for its digestion
—a fact perhaps deserving of the attention of too sedulous nurses,
especially of hired ones, having nothing serious to do but to suckle.

† Turning to the Odyssey, after the above was written, I find a singular resemblance of circumstances between this shepherd's cave in
Cephalonia and the manner of penning the flock at present, and
that so minutely and powerfully described by the poet in the ninth
book, where, in the extraordinary scene and incidents of the Cyclops'
Cave (passing over the incongruity of the shepherd being a cannibal),
he gives a picture of early pastoral life. It is expressly mentioned

I may here add, that, in Corfu, the usage prevails of not allowing the lambs and kids, after birth, to have the first milk. As soon as they are born, they are taken from their dams, and are not allowed to suck till the following day. The first milk is drawn off by the shepherds. The practice is not confined to the flock; it extends to the human race. During the first twenty-four hours, the new born infant is not permitted to have the mother's breast. It is drawn by a stranger child, and a stranger mother first suckles the child, unless the mother's breast is small and the secretion of milk scanty, when the mother and child are not interfered with. The usage is founded on the erroneous notion that the new milk is injurious to the new-born. The same notion once prevailed, and may still keep its ground in the north of Europe, notwithstanding the efforts of enlightened physicians to explode it, and to show that the following natural instinct is not injurious, but the interfering with it; the new milk, from its peculiarities, its aperient qualities, being specially fitted to act on the bowels; and, whilst it nourishes, remove accumulated meconium from

that, whilst the flocks pastured abroad by day, the kids and lambs were confined in penns in the cave, and apart according to their ages, and also that there was an enclosure outside the cavern, " the cavern-yard." Taking the whole account of the proceedings of Polyphemus, as a shepherd, and comparing them with those of the Greek shepherd of the present day, I think it must be admitted that, during the lapse of more than 2000 years, no material change has taken place in the pastoral habits and methods, even in the making of a cheese.

the intestines of the infant. It would be strange indeed, if nature erred on such an occasion. *

The cheese made in the Ionian Islands is not sufficient for home consumption. It is an article in great request, and large quantities of the poorer kinds are imported. Some of the home-made cheeses are good, especially in Cephalonia, in the rich pastures of the Black Mountain. Curd as well as cheese is a favourite article of food amongst the Greeks. It is made by adding a little rennet in powder to milk warm from the goats, and immediately stirring it for a half hour or hour, without interruption. If allowed to cool, and to rest, the rennet has no effect. The powdered rennet used is a lamb's stomach, reduced to powder, by pounding, after having been well dried in smoke. It will keep twelve months without losing its efficacy.

The shepherds of these islands, as shepherds commonly are, are the chief native musicians. Three instruments are in use amongst them, of which figures are given in Plate IV. The clossoscambuno or bagpipe (fig. 7) is composed of a skin bag, of a reed mouth-piece, and of a reed pipe, with ten stops, terminating in a horn top. Within the pipe are two small reeds, with slits through which the air passes. This instrument is played very much in the same manner as the Scotch highland pipe; its sounds are very similar, and the airs played on it are not unlike. It i

* In Marher's admirable Prælectiones on Boerhaave, there are some excellent remarks on this subject.

not in very common use; I heard it only once, and in Ithaca, in a lonely glen, below the hill of Aito, where its wild and rude music was not unappropriate.

The pipe (fig. 6) has four stops; its mouth-piece is formed of an oaten straw, with a rest for the lip to press against in the act of playing, to prevent the closing of the fine slit. It is very similar both in construction and sounds, to the Ceylon kandyan pipe, the mouth-piece of which, instead of an oaten straw, is formed of the leaf of the talipot palm; it is probably the same instrument that was used by the ancient shepherds noticed in the line of Virgil:—

"Silvestrem tenui musam meditaris avena."

A simpler form of pipe (fig. 5), and most primitive, is of reed, with six stops on one side, one on the opposite side, and one in the extremity, in the diaphragm of the reed. It is played not like a fife, but a flagelet, the extremity A, which is fully open, being compressed by the lips. This is the favourite instrument of the shepherd-boy; and, rude as its music is, heard in a suitable place, it is not unpleasing to unfastidious ears. Besides these, the country people use drums, which have also the oriental character, and very closely resemble the tom-toms of India, both in form, the manner of beating time, and their effect. Their sounds have often deceived me; and, when listening to them, I have fancied myself for a moment in the interior of Ceylon.

7. *Of Field Labour, and the Wages of Labourers.*
—The price of field labour in the Ionian Islands is comparatively high. Fifteen-pence a-day may be considered as about the common rate of payment in Zante, Cephalonia, and Corfu. When I was in Zante, in the autumn of 1824, an enlightened proprietor and cultivator informed me that he paid his labourers each this amount, and four obole more (about two-pence),* in lieu of an allowance for one meal, of a certain portion of cheese, salt-fish, and wine, to which they consider themselves entitled. They begin to work at sunrise, and finish at sunset. They have three or four meals a-day—something, perhaps, before they start in the morning, breakfast at ten o'clock, dinner at two, and supper in the evening after the labour of the day. Each man may save about twenty obole a-day, his food costing about twelve or fourteen (six for bread, and six or eight for wine, caveare, &c.)† The same gentleman gave but a bad account of this class of his countrymen; he described them as unprincipled, endeavouring to get as much as possible from their employers, and to work

---

* This was in 1824, when an hundred obole were equivalent to a dollar, at the valuation of four shillings and two-pence sterling. Since then, according to the money tariff, established in May 1828, the value of the obolo is one-tenth of a penny.

† In Cephalonia, I was informed that the day-labourer, all the year round, can make thirty obole a-day, and live on five obole, on bread and wine, working hard. This was the allowance, it was stated, of the prisoners employed at hard labour, who generally have very good health.

as little as possible; that unless narrowly watched, they will do little;* will come late to the field, and go away early. The majority of them are small proprietors, and are apt to reserve their strength to work on their own ground, to which late and early they apply themselves very industriously.

The wages of the ploughman are still higher: he provides the plough and oxen, and is paid at the rate of a dollar and a half a-day, besides which he is allowed three meals. Very few farmers keep their own ploughs; they commonly prefer having them on the above terms. Some proprietors of land, who cultivate their own grounds, purchase bullocks, and transfer them to a ploughman on certain conditions; first, the ploughman, on receiving each bullock, pays the landlord three dollars; next, he engages to deliver to the latter one hundred and eighty pounds of corn yearly for each, equivalent to about three dollars; and lastly, he is bound, whenever required, to plough for the proprietor, without the power of offering any excuse. The landlord pays him at the usual rate; he also runs the risk of the loss of the bullocks, either by accident or disease. This information I obtained in Zante, where there may be seven or eight hundred ploughs in use; nearly the same practice, I believe, is followed in the other islands. In Zante,

---

* Even the manner in which they employ the hoe, he said, required vigilant watching. The idle workmen slur over their work, and save themselves labour, by applying the hoe very obliquely, paring with it rather than digging.

oxen are worked about twelve years, that is, till they
are about fifteen years old. They are then fattened
and killed for the market. Though old, the meat is
better than the beef in general, as they are better fed
than the animals ordinarily imported from the continent, and as they are commonly slaughtered in winter,
when the pasturage is rich. The bullock is divided
between the landlord and the ploughman, who kept
it. The age of plough-oxen is expressed in a peculiar
manner; speaking of them, it is not the usage to
say they are so many years old, but that they are so
many loaves old.

8. *Of the·Tenures of Lands.*—I have alluded some
pages back to the Colonia and Metairie system.
The former includes the latter. The former word
may be translated lease, and is of two kinds, " *Colonia perpetua,*" and " *Colonia semplice.*" In the first
instance, the land (it is invariably waste) is granted
for perpetuity, on the condition of planting it, and
bringing it into cultivation. The colono becomes
proprietor of one-fourth of the land, and has to pay
to the lord half, or some other proportion, of the produce of the remaining three-fourths.* In the second

* " In very early times, when the population of the Ionian Islands
was smaller than at present, the proprietors were glad to let their
lands on perpetual leases, on condition of receiving a trifling ground-
rent, and a proportion of the produce. The proportion varied from a
tenth to a third, according to the eligibility of the property, or the
increase of population. The laws on the subject of the colonia are
much involved; the whole system is subject to numerous abuses,

instance, that of *Colonia semplice*, the grant is merely temporary; the lease-holder takes the land, and pays in kind—the proportion of the produce the proprietor receives being regulated by circumstances, as the quality of the soil, the state of the plantations, &c., varying from three-fifths to one-third.

9. *Of Manures.*—One of the most remarkable defects in the farming of the Ionian Islands, is the little use that is made of manure. I have already mentioned, that Zante was the only island where it was habitually employed; and there its use was chiefly confined to the plain, and the vicinity of the town, and to one description of manure, viz. stable-dung; and even that was so little valued, that it might be had without payment, merely for the trouble of carrying it away. In Corfu, such was the neglect of manure, that the sea, not the land, was the depository of the rich dirt of the city. Heaps of dirt, fit to act as good manure, were thrown back by the waves, on the shore close to the city, where, instead of the beneficial effect which they might have had, properly applied, they were offensive, and probably by their effluvia injurious to health. Sir Frederick Adam, the then Lord High Commissioner, had an experimental farm, for the purpose of giving instruction in agriculture by example, in which the natives had an oppor-

and properties have become numerously subdivided and neglected."— *Note to a Speech of Lord Nugent, on the 23d February 1835, to the Senate of the United States of the Ionian Islands.*

tunity of witnessing the efficacy of manure. Old habits in agriculture appear to be peculiarly tenacious. When I left Corfu, in 1828, the example, I believe, had little effect. It was only by the exertions of an active police, that accumulations of filth could be prevented in the streets, which, were its value known as manure, would have become to the town an article of no inconsiderable profit.* The use of manure is a beautiful instance, out of the very many by which we are surrounded, of co-aptation for good, the neglect of its use as striking an instance of the contrary. In this country, we have the best example of the former; of the latter hardly an idea can be formed by those who have never been abroad, and in a Greek or Turkish town, in the bye-streets of which every thing that is abominable is thrown, and where the sense of smell, and of sight, are equally offended by impurities, whilst the neighbouring hungry fields are exhausted and starved, being deprived of their natural food.

In treating of the geology of these islands, it was shown how they abound in mineral manures, as calcareous marl, gypsum, and limestone, capable of affording the best lime. Marl in many places is found in the vicinity of poor, almost barren land, consisting chiefly of silicious sand and pebbles; occasionally a layer of the latter is immediately incumbent on a

* Now, I am informed, the farmers in the immediate neighbourhood of the town of Corfu, are beginning to use manure, and purchase stable-dung.

stratum of the former; by mixing the two a fertile soil might be produced. Simple and easy as this is, it has been neglected;—neither marl, nor lime, nor gypsum has yet been applied, that I am aware of, to agricultural purposes.

The keeping and feeding of cattle, which, in connexion with the forming of manure, is so important a part of a good agricultural system, has hitherto received little attention. The difficulty of procuring good butcher-meat has already been alluded to;—a few years ago, at certain seasons of the year, especially during the periods of Lent, it was difficult indeed to procure any. Only twelve years since, when I was in Corfu, provisions were almost as regularly expected by the English packet as letters and newspapers, such as butter, hams, tongues, cheese; and a round of beef from Ancona was esteemed a prize, and spoken of as an event. At that time a good market-place was constructed. A few years before, when it did not exist, I have heard officers say that the providing of a mess-dinner in Corfu was very little easier than in the field. During the whole period of service of the 90th regiment in these islands, from about 1820 to 1830, their mess, which was an excellent one, was almost independent of the market; the mess-man fed his own mutton, and imported a large proportion of the articles used at the table—and not from choice but necessity; the greater part of the time the regiment was stationed in Zante.

10. *Of Woods and Forests.*—In consequence of
the profusion of olive-trees, and the abundance of
shrubs in most of the islands, they appear to be well
wooded. Considering merely picturesque effect and
natural beauty of scenery, there is nothing perhaps to
be desired; but if usefulness is attended to, the defi-
ciencies in regard to timber will be found to be great.
This is strongly expressed in some remarks on the
subject which occur in the speech of the late Lord
High Commissioner Sir Howard Douglas to the
Legislative Assembly in 1837. " These states,"
he observes, " labour under another great disability
which admits not of any immediate natural remedy,
but which, nevertheless, demands the serious consideration of the government—I mean the total want
of every thing in the shape of timber for construction,
from the slender twig which trains the vine, to the
plank required for the internal and external transport of your produce and the beam which supports
your roofs. It appears by the return, which will be
submitted to you, that no less than L.30,000 are
annually abstracted from these states in procuring
from abroad these great essentials, whilst extensive
tracts, upon which forests formerly stood, are waste,
and many others might be equally available for planting." The Black Mountain, in Cephalonia, is the
most remarkable of the tracts thus alluded to. It
was once covered with pine-forests—the greater part
of which was destroyed by fire, rather less than half
a century ago, during the period of anarchy which

for a short time prevailed after the fall of the Venetian power. This was not only a great loss in itself, but is believed to have been also injurious in its consequences.*

That the soil of the Ionian Islands is fitted for the growth of timber-trees does not admit of question. The trees, of various kinds, scattered through the islands, afford demonstrative proof of this. The pine flourishes on the higher mountains ; the common oak and the evergreen oak on the hills, and the Valonea oak† on the hills and plains. Where, as in these islands, there is such a variety of soil and climate, according to different elevations, there is no difficulty in supposing that the majority of the fruit-trees of Europe might find suitable situations, and, if thought desirable, be grown with success. To insure, however, success, many precautions would be requisite, and special protection would be required from the wasteful and destructive depredations of cattle, and especially of goats. On this point, and on some others of interest, I shall give below, in a note, the valuable remarks of Sir Charles Napier, than whom no Englishman, perhaps, is better acquainted with the Ionian Islands ;—they were made

* See Note, p. 76.

† The Valonea, or Velani oak (*Quercus œgilops*), is a tree of great value, as well as of much beauty; I have heard of the produce of one tree alone selling for L.15. From seven to eight thousand tons of Valonea (the cup of the acorn) are annually consumed in this country in tanning and dyeing. At present it is imported chiefly from Turkey ; and the supply, it is said, is not equal to the demand.

incidentally, when treating of the roads of Cephalonia, in his Memoir on the subject, published in 1824.*

* " With regard to trees and hedges, this climate is so dry that they do no injury to a road, and ought to be planted every where ; but in Cephalonia it is quite impossible to preserve trees, as the goats destroy them all, and are rapidly annihilating the public forest on the Black Mountain, which forest would be a source of great wealth to the island, if protected, but thousands of goats prevent the growth of every thing like a plantation, and, what is worse, are the cause of more litigation, ill-blood, crime, and idleness, than any other source of mischief in the island. Neither vineyards, fields, nor gardens, can escape the devastations of these animals, as it is impossible to make any sufficient fence to exclude them. The reason the peasant likes goats are— *First,* they cost him nothing to feed, as in the day-time he drives them to the mountains, and at night into his neighbours' cultivated grounds, who cannot catch them ; nor is it easy to prove whose goat does the damage ; for in a country where the peasants all live in villages, and the landlords in the capital, no look-out is kept at night. Even were they to live among their fields, it would be still very hard to prove whose goat did the mischief, for the goat-herd is not so silly as to be seen ; he trusts to his goat for getting both into and out of the scrape, which they do with equal ease.

" *Secondly,* The peasant likes goats, because the milk, cheese, and flesh maintain him, with scarcely any labour ; he therefore spends his time in festivals and gambling. From the want of population the price of labour is high ; and he can always earn in three days as much as will keep him for a week with the aid of his goats.

" *Thirdly,* The peasant prefers the goat to sheep, not only because it is more active in trespassing, but also because it is more hardy ; it lives upon less and coarser food, and gets it among the rocks, where the sheep cannot climb. Goats mount up trees to the top, and eat the leaves ; in short, a goat is the most accomplished thief in existence ; and although it is digressing from the subject, I will say that no measure of government would do so much good to this island, or be more welcome, than a tax upon goats, which would gradually clear it of this curse ; and, instead of them, introduce sheep, which are less mischievous, and more easily fenced out.

11. *Of Waste Lands.*—The following return, designed to show the different descriptions of land in

" It is not to be supposed that the whole of the peasants keep goats,
and that gentlemen alone possess the land, and suffer. This is by no
means the case. It is, generally speaking, the idle part of the community that keep goats, while the small portion of land that they possess is left unattended to, and their industrious neighbour, who turns
his ground to account, suffers from the trespass. Almost all the peasants of Cephalonia possess some land themselves, or have the ' right
of labour' on the property of some more wealthy neighbour; that is
to say, the peasant has the right to cultivate the ground, and the produce is divided, in certain proportions, between him and the proprietor
of the land. Now, all these men who cultivate the soil, whether rich
or poor, suffer from the goats; indeed, the trespass is more injurious to
the poor man than to the rich, the destruction of a vineyard being
ruin to the first, and only a partial loss to the last."—*Memoir on the
Roads of Cephalonia,* 1824, p. 20.

A gentleman, whose opinion has been given in note, p. 320, on the
evil effects of corrupt administration of justice in Santa Maura, thus
describes the mischief produced by the depredations of goats in that
island :—" Another serious impediment to improvement arises from
the ravages of an enormous quantity of goats, upwards of 20,000 being
allowed to range the island under but slight restraint, and whose
depredations effectually prevent all attempts at improvements in
planting the hills and wastes, and the formation of orchards, gardens,
&c. Their inevitable incursions lead to innumerable actions for trespass, to feuds and heartburnings, which can scarcely be made evident
to an English auditor." He adds,—" I am the more struck with the
importance of this evil, from having, when at Cerigo, witnessed the
same destruction attending every attempt at improvement, and which
induced me to call the attention of the proprietors of vineyards and
olive-plantations to it. At length, after I had excited general discussion for the space of four or five years, and that a large majority agreed
with me, I, through the constitutional authorities, proposed the revival
of an old municipal law, which prohibited the pasturing of goats within
a certain distance of olive-plantations, vineyards, &c.

" The effects of this regulation were gratifying beyond all calcula-

the Ionian Islands, was drawn up in 1833, and is an
official document:—

Islands.	Acres in Pasture.	Acres in Crop.	Acres of Uncultivated Land.
Corfu, ...	7,422	112,008	33,272
Cephalonia, . . .	1,644	32,934	189,786
Zante, ...	1,474	45,972	53,868
Santa Maura, . . .	6,225	17,643	97,557
Ithaca, ...	1,626	5,442	22,718
Cerigo, ...	5,285	12,741	61,499
Paxo, ...	...	11,406	5,234
Total, . . .	23,676	238,146	463,934

From which it appears that the proportion of land
lying waste considerably exceeds, in the total, that
which has been cultivated,—is nearly twice as great;
and the disproportion of the two would be even
greater were the neglected olive-forests of Corfu not
included in the acres in crop. Of all the islands,
Cerigo, next to Santa Maura, affords the most striking
example of defective cultivation, as well as of scanty
population,* arising from neglect, combined with ignorance, and from poverty; the defective cultivation the
result of the one, and the scanty population of the
other. In that island even an orange-tree has not been
planted, or was not when I visited it in the summer of

tion; and very many spirited proprietors commenced planting, to such
an extent, that I am convinced *protection* only would call forth what
alone is wanting to enrich their possessions,—that is, *industry*, in place
of the Asiatic languor which (robust and clever, and alive to their own
interest as the Ionian peasant proprietors are) at present pervades all
their agricultural operations."

* About seventy-five to the square mile.

1827, although the climate is perfectly fitted to bring this fruit to perfection. In that island. as in Corfu and Santa Maura, and the north-east coast of Cephalonia, it is not merely the rugged and rocky surfaces which lie waste, but even tracts of good soil. The district of Calamo, in Cerigo, is a striking example. It is a marl district, gently hilly and undulating—abounding in water, capable of high cultivation, and of supporting many thousands of inhabitants, if duly cultivated. Now it is uninhabited—without a single house; and cultivated to a very limited extent, and that by labourers, who visit it occasionally for the purpose, coming from the nearest villages.

Zante, of all the Ionian Islands, is the richest, best cultivated, and most productive; and yet it is very much below the limit of its capacity. For the purpose of illustration it may be worth while to glance at the statistics of the two great divisions of this island —the mountainous, and the plain with the adjoining hills including the city.

The population of the mountainous district—the area of which is but little less than that of the plain and the adjoining hills—in 1824 was estimated at 4,116 souls; that of the plain and adjoining hills at 15,793 ; and that of the city (not including foreigners) at 15,176.

The produce and number of animals in the two divisions were as follow :—

Mountainous.		Plain, or Hilly.
150,500 lbs. Currants, ...		6,950,500
2,635 Oil, every second year (Venetian barrels),* .		47,365
9,123 Wine yearly (Venetian barrels), . . .		49,377
17,380 Corn, &c. [Bacili],†		23,087
167 Horses, ...		1032
300 Mules, ...		638
167 Asses, ...		839
6,992 Sheep, ...		4,717
14,211 Goats, ...		2610
717 Bullocks, ...		1,077‡

How striking is the contrast between the two districts, both in population and productiveness! And, notwithstanding, at least a third of the plain is lying waste, in the state of marsh, exhaling unwholesome effluvia, yet capable of being rendered hardly less rich by draining and culture than the finest parts at present in cultivation. The mountainous rocky district, by nature poor, is of far more limited capacity, and has more nearly reached its limit.

The state of agriculture in Malta, to which I shall now pass, will afford even more striking examples of the effects of cultivation in relation to productiveness and population.

* The Venetian barrel = 18⅓ English gallons.

† One bacile of land = 400 passi; one passo (Venetian square foot) = 5 feet English.

‡ I am indebted for the above to Mr Chiranda, of the Commissariat Department, late Collector of the Customs in Zante.

[389]

CHAPTER XI.

ON THE SOILS, AND STATE OF AGRICULTURE AND HORTICULTURE IN MALTA.

Description of the principal varieties of Soil. Manner of bringing Ground into Cultivation, and forming " *Campi artificiali.*" Proofs of extraordinary labour. Points of difference between the Agriculture of Malta and of the Ionian Islands. Superiority of the former, and the circumstances conducive to it. Principal Productions. Tables in illustration. Rotation of Crops. Manner of cultivating Cotton. Wheat. Table showing the quantity grown and imported, and the price of Bread. Sulla. Particulars relative to farms, rent, labour, and labourers. Implements of Husbandry. Manner of using Manure. Horticulture. Its imperfect state. Hints for its Improvement. Brief notice of the Soils and Agriculture of Gozo, and of the condition of its Agricultural Population.

1. THE soils of Malta are very similar to those of the Ionian Islands; and I may add, of Sicily, and of Calabria, and of a considerable part of Italy. They are principally of three different kinds; and, like those of the Ionian Islands, are each associated with a particular kind of rock or substratum. The three kinds referred to are red clay, gray or fawn-coloured marl, and a " terra bianca," or white soil, composed principally of carbonate of lime. Of each kind there are many varie-

ties, differing in tints of colour and somewhat in composition, and occasionally passing one into another,
either from artificial mixture, or from the operation of
natural causes of an obscure kind.   The red clay, as
in the Ionian Islands, is almost invariably found connected with the limestone stratum,—that stratum
which prevails on the hills and higher grounds, and
of which the most rugged and barren parts of the
island are formed.   It is almost invariably mixed
with minute particles of calcareous rock; every specimen of it which I have examined, has effervesced
with an acid.   It is a soil of excellent quality, but
unfortunately scanty.   It is found chiefly in crevices
and cavities of the rocks, from whence it is transferred
to the surface, in the operation of making fields
" *campi artificiali*" which will presently be described.

The calcareous marl soil occurs wherever the marl
formation appears, from whence it is derived, and
from which, in composition and qualities, it differs
very little.   A specimen of the marl of Malta, which
I examined, was found to consist of

24 Carbonate of Lime.
69 Clay (a mixture of alumine chiefly, and very fine silicious
  sand).
 1 peroxide of iron, with a trace of magnesia.
 6 Hygrometric water, expelled by a temperature of 212°.
───
100

The third species of soil, which is not so easily defined as the two preceding, and which, after the
natives, I have called " terra bianca," a term which

is also applied to marl, is commonly associated with and incumbent on the softer freestone, and is probably derived from it by disintegration. One specimen of it which I examined was found to be composed of

91.0 Carbonate of lime.
7.0 Earthy matter, not soluble in acid, chiefly composed of alumine and fine silicious sand, coloured by peroxide of iron.
1.5 Vegetable matter.
.5 Hygrometric water.
———
100.0

2. I have alluded to the " campi artificiali" of Malta. A large proportion of the cultivated land of the island may be so considered, land which has not been reclaimed from waste, but actually formed by dint of art and human industry of the most laborious kind. With the exception of a small extent of surface, the probability is, that originally the whole island of Malta was an almost naked rock, and that it owes its present condition of cultivation to the uninterrupted labours of man through a long series of ages, commencing in a very remote antiquity. Even before the commencement of the Christian era it was extremely fertile.

" Fertilis est Melite, sterili vicina Cosyræ,
    Insula, quam Libyci verberat unda freti :"*

and then, perhaps, as now, it might have been the

* Ovid. Fast. lib. iii.

boast of the inhabitants, that not a spot capable of cultivation was uncultivated.*

The appearance of all the hilly cultivated districts is very characteristic of the origin and mode of formation alluded to. Every field is a terrace, a level surface of two or three feet of soil, resting on rock, and enclosed by stone walls; and every declivity that is cultivated is a succession of such terraces; and they are often so small and narrow as to convey the idea of steps rather than of fields. The manner of forming their terraces, their "campi artificiali," as they are called by an ingenious native writer on the agriculture of Malta, Professor Carlo Giacinto, is sufficiently simple, though very laborious. The rugged parts of the rock are cut away and broken up; the surface of the rock is furrowed, at intervals, an inch or two deep; the fissures and cavities are filled up with small fragments; the soil collected, whether in fissures or cavities, or brought from some little distance, is laid on regularly, to the depth of one or two feet; and, finally, a wall is built, five or six feet high, of the larger stones. This enclosure is not only useful to prevent the trespassing of animals, and the washing away of the soil, but also, and in a higher degree, as a defence from the winds. When describing these walls, and the facility of forming them by the abundance of stone on the spot, the author just

* In the distant fabulous time alluded to by the poet, the ruler of the island is noticed as wealthy, and unwarlike " arma perosus :"
" Hospes opum dives rex ibi Battus erat."

referred to, in an amiable and grateful state of feeling, exclaims, " Oh quanto perciò è amirabile la divina providenza! Non si forma un campo, che non si trovano sul luogo le pietre per alzarli d'intorno il muro di tanta necessità per proteggerlo." It may be added, that the rock is furrowed for the purpose of admitting water into its substance, and that occasionally, when the surface of the rock, after a lapse of time, from the deposition of calcareous matter, and the formation of a crust on it, has become impervious to water, the operation of furrowing or grooving is repeated. In a former part of this work, I have stated that the soft freestone is capable of absorbing and retaining about one-sixth its weight of water, like a sponge, which in a dry air it slowly gives off. This is a most important property, in relation to agriculture and fertility, and more deserving of exciting a feeling of admiration than the inevitable presence, and the fitness of the rock, when broken up, for the construction of protecting walls.

Probably on no spot of the same dimensions has the power of man, his skill and patient industry, been more exerted than in Malta, as exemplified in the extension of its cultivated grounds; and yet, notwithstanding, as large a proportion still remains uncultivated. The circumstance of this extended cultivation is well adapted to convey an idea of the vast sum of labour applied, in conjunction with the fact, that the population has gone on increasing in as high a ratio, and equally pressing on the produce.

In the early part of the sixteenth century, before the island was taken possession of by the Knights of St John,* on its being ceded to them by the emperor Charles V., according to the statement of the commissioners employed by the grand master, L'Isle Adam, to examine and report on the state of the island, Malta poorly supported 12,000 inhabitants, which is at the rate of about thirteen to the square mile, and these were chiefly dependent for corn on Sicily. From the year 1525, when the report of the commissioners was made, let us pass to 1833; according to official returns, the total population of Malta, in that year, including foreigners, was 105,477, and exclusive of foreigners, 1,110 to the square mile!

Whether the extent of cultivation of land, or rather the formation of productive land in these islands, has reached its maximum, it is not easy to determine, that depending on contingent circumstances; but the probability is, that it has not, that the operation of making " campi artificiali" will be continued, and that, in process of time, nothing but the naked surface of hard limestone rock will remain uncovered with soil, and barren.

Whether the condition of the people will at the same time improve, is a still more difficult problem to solve. That they will increase in number more rapidly than the cultivation of the island and means of support will increase, I fear, can hardly be doubted ; and, consequently, unless new energies can be im-

---

* Vertot, History of the Knights of Malta, vol. iii., p. 286.

parted, and new resources made available, there seems on this score little foundation for hope.

3. The agriculture of Malta will very well bear comparison with that of the Ionian Islands: the differences between them are great, and they are generally in favour of the former.

As regards the collateral circumstances of the tenures and lettings of land, Malta has greatly the advantage: the Metairie and Colonia systems are there unknown; land is let very much in the same manner as in England, on lease, for different periods, or from year to year; and rent is paid in money, not in kind.* No tax is imposed on land; and the farmer is equally free from tithe and poor-rate. As regards the cultivation itself, the chief points of difference are,—in the abundant use of manure,—in keeping the good land which will bear it constantly in crop,—and in working the ground deeply, on the principle of the spade husbandry, or its representative the hoe, rather than of the plough, and in weeding most carefully.

* The crown land, for instance, is let on short leases from one to eight years, on long leases from nine to ninety-nine, and on leases for three generations. The terms of the holding or grant are frequently inscribed on stone in a conspicuous place. The following is an instance, copied from the arched way leading to the farm-yard of a tenement, formerly belonging to and attached to the Inquisitor's Palace:—

SS.ma Inquisitionis Militen.
Concess. ad emphutensim
Josepho Muscat
pro annis nonaginta novem
die 1 Julii 1792.
Per acta civilia eiusdem
SSmæ inquisitionis.

Of the Ionian Islands, the principal productions are fruits, wine, and oil, the produce of the vineyard and olive-grove. In Malta, the most important crops are grain and cotton. And it is on the cultivation of these, in connexion with an active convertible system of husbandry, that the superiority of the Maltese farmer is chiefly displayed.

The following returns, made to Government for the year 1833, show, 1st, the manner in which the cultivated land is applied; 2dly, the amount of produce; and 3dly, the number of animals maintained; all of which, with the exception of the sheep and goats, are stable and stall-fed, and are the chief source of manure; the goats and sheep are allowed to range amongst the rocks, and they subsist chiefly on the scanty herbage which they find there.

I.—NATURE OF THE CROPS AND NUMBER OF ACRES OF LAND IN EACH.

Islands.	Wheat.	Meechiato.	Barley.	Beans and Pulse.	Cotton.	Forage.	Sesamum.	Cummin seed.	Pasture.	Garden Vegetables.
Malta, . .	8,205	4,307	5,749	3,319	8,414	5,518	207	1,028	2,001	3,479
Gozo, . .	542	2,890	62	1,518	3,139	2,216	9	..	786	1,638

II.—NATURE OF THE PRODUCE AND QUANTITY OF EACH.

Islands.	Wheat.	Meechiato.	Barley.	Beans.	Cotton.	Forage.	Sesamum.	Cummin seed.	Garden Produce.
	Bush.	Bush.	Bush.	Bush.	Lbs.	Soma, or load of 10 bundles.	Bush.	Lbs.	
Malta.	72,399	52,581	57,245	30,566	2,192,554	100,474	731	975,140	26,430,753
Gozo.	6,559	43,607	708	23,719	1,449,375	32,876	82	..	1,593,725

III.—DESCRIPTION AND NUMBER OF STOCK.

Islands.	Horses, Mules, and Asses.	Horned Cattle.	Sheep.	Goats.
Malta, ...	3,299	5,342	8,123	3,364
Gozo, ...	1,300	601	3,662	779

The rotation of crops observed in Malta somewhat varies, partly according to the judgment of the farmer, but even more according to the nature of the soil. Where the soil is good, it is expected to produce six or seven crops in the course of four years, which is the short lease period; for instance, two crops of cotton, two of green barley, one of wheat and one of sulla; besides intermediate minor crops of certain vegetables.

Let us follow the farmer in his operations during this period of four years, considering him as a new tenant, and entering, as is usual, on his engagement in the middle of August.

1st, In the end of September, or the beginning of October, he sows barley, which is plucked up in its green state, in January or February, as fodder for cattle.

Next, after the middle of April, he sows cotton, and at the same time with it, as not supposed to be injuriously interfering, sesamo, and perhaps some radish and melons.

2d, In October, the field being free, the cotton crop having been gathered, and the plant rooted up, excepting it be kept standing for a second or third year, as it occasionally is in very good ground, he sows anew barley for winter forage; or, in lieu of barley, either peas for the market in winter, or beans, garlick, or radishes; or in February or March, either cabbage or fennel.

In May, the field is hoed for the cultivation of the cotton, the minor crops mentioned, whichever may have been grown, having been removed, that the cotton plant, whether fresh from seed or of a former year, may have full possession of the ground, as is considered requisite.

3*d*, After the gathering of cotton, if the roots are pulled up, in the middle of November he sows wheat and barley together (called by the Maltese Mischiato*); or wheat alone, which is ready for cutting in the end of May.

4*th*, In August, at the beginning of the fourth year, he sows sulla, which springs up after the first rains, and is in a fit state to be cut in the middle of April, and is laid up dry for winter forage.

Another order of rotation is the following, supposing in this instance, as in the former, the same field to be in continued cultivation.

1*st*, The field taken in August is left fallow till about the 12th of March; melons then are planted in it, of various kinds, up to about the 11th of May.

---

* The barley mixed with the wheat is considered advantageous in giving support to the latter, and tending to prevent its being laid. The two kinds of grain are dexterously separated by sifting.

The cabbage, turnip, and lettuce, are planted amongst the melons, and the planting of the cabbage is continued up to the latter end of October.

2*d*, After the middle of April cotton is sown.

3*d*, In August, sulla; or in November, barley, is sown between the cotton stalks, to be cut unripe in March or April, before the active vegetation of the old cotton plants commences.

4*th*, and lastly, After the cotton has been gathered, and the ground cleared of its roots, barley or wheat, or a mixture of the two, is sown for a concluding crop

Besides these, there are other rotations of crops, depending on a variety of circumstances, which it is not easy to point out. I shall notice only a few, to give some idea of them.

Some farmers, after cotton of the preceding year, in February and March sow Amino dolce, called *Anacio* (*Pimpinella anisum*, Lin.), or Comino acre (*Cuminum cyminum*, Lin.) The growing of these aromatic seeds is considered very profitable to the farmer, but very injurious to the land, and, in consequence, their cultivation is limited. Neither cotton nor wheat can be advantageously cultivated after them. Some years ago, proprietors of land made it even a condition in the leases, that cummin should never be cultivated, and especially prohibited it the last year. It is a Maltese proverb, that one year of cummin is worse for the land than a hundred other years. In some parts of the island, where the soil is deep, and water not scarce, Indian corn is occasionally grown after the grain or sulla, and preparatory to cotton. Of late years, in certain parts considered favourable for the potato, this root has been cultivated to a considerable extent, and profitably. It is usually planted in September or October, and is ripe in January.

Occasionally in new ground, wheat is the first crop cultivated; sown in January, it is pulled up when ripe in May; and then the ground is ploughed and harrowed, and beaten and well irrigated, in preparation for the succeeding crop of cotton. In some soils too shallow for cotton, a species of wheat, called *Tommonia dura*, is sown in December; or that which is simply called Tommonia in February, either alone or mixed with barley; or *Scorpiurus muricata* is sown, commonly called *Widna*, for the cattle, especially for the sheep. This information I give, as also much of the preceding, from the work already mentioned of Carlo Giacinto.* According to the same author, in such ground, sulla is occasionally grown; not, however, for the purpose of forage, but for procuring good *seed* for the raising of forage in better grounds; the Maltese farmer being well aware that the produce of seed may be large and good, whilst that of the leaves is stunted and indifferent.

4. Relative to the more important crops,—cotton, and grain, and sulla,—for the sake of illustrating the

---

* Saggio di Agricultura per le Isole di Malta, e Gozo. Del P. Carlo Giacinto, Professore di Botanica, &c. Malta, 1811.

Maltese agriculture, it may be worth while to enter into more minute particulars.

The cotton-plant, in all its circumstances, relations, and properties, is peculiarly interesting and fitted to excite attention. Produced during the hottest season of the year, planted at the commencement of the dry season, gathered before its termination,—and during the greater part of the time green and refreshing to the eye, and tempering the heat, yielding a fibre admirably adapted for clothing and for protection both against cold and heat, and a seed containing much nourishment; and of which cattle are very fond, it is a precious gift to countries having a climate like that of Malta, where a long drought prevails in the summer and autumnal months, and where the temperature is too high for animals bearing the finer wools, and the heat too great to use them in dress, excepting during a short period of the year.

From time immemorial there is reason to believe that cotton has been cultivated here, and has been an article of manufacture even, and of export. Anciently the *vestis Melitensis* was celebrated; and it seems most probable that it was made of this material.* It is

* The opinion expressed above is that which prevails in Malta; there is no tradition relative to the introduction of the cotton-plant into the island. As it would appear from Pliny that this plant in his time was cultivated in Upper Egypt, it is not improbable that it may then also have been grown in Malta, the climate and soil of which

alluded to by Cicero, in his oration against Verres :—
" *Insula est Melita, in qua est eodem nomine opidum,
quò iste nunquam accessit ; quod tamen isti textrinum
per triennium ad muliebrem vestem conficiendam
fuit.*"

The cotton now cultivated in Malta is of three
kinds—the brown, or Nankin cotton, *Gossypium re-
ligiosum*, Lin. ; the Indian, white cotton,—or as it
is called, from the colour of its seeds, green cotton,
Gossypium hirsutum ; and, lastly, that kind which is
peculiarly called the Malta cotton, a variety of the
*Gossypium herbacum.** Each kind has some properties to recommend it, either in connexion with its
cultivation or produce.

The brown cotton is most esteemed, and is of the
highest value, both on account of its colour, which is
not destroyed by washing, and the fineness of its fibre.
It requires, for its successful cultivation, a good soil.
In such a soil, well prepared and watered, the plant

---

are so well adapted to it. The circumstance that linen, and not cotton,
was in use in Egypt, in the preparation of mummies, as has recently
been proved by a pretty extensive microscopical examination of mummy
cloth, may seem unfavourable to this inference ; but the argument it
affords is not conclusive. The embalmers might have given the preference to linen bandages over cotton, on account of the greater strength
and durability of the former, and its other superior qualities ; or the
continued preference (supposing a choice) might have been the result
of ancient usage and indisposition to change, as we witness at present
amongst ourselves in the instance of the funeral shroud, required to
be of woollen.—*Vide* " *History of the Cotton Manufacture in Great
Britain,*" *&c.* By E. Baines, jun., Esq., chap. ii., and Appendix.

  * Saggio d'Agricoltura, p. 62.

grows to the height of a man. The colour of the cotton is very apt to degenerate. To have it in perfection, it is necessary to use seed, the produce of land which has not been watered. The seed of well watered plants produce what is called the bastard cotton, which is of a light flesh-colour. Even the cotton of plants raised from seed of the first description, it is said, is apt to be impaired in colour if grown a second year; but that the cotton may be restored by exposing the pod entire to the sun and dew for about thirty days.*

The Indian cotton is of fine fibre, and white. It, too, requires a good soil for its successful cultivation; irrigated, it is most productive; but it may be cultivated with profit even without irrigation.

The Malta cotton may be cultivated, where the other two species do not thrive, in soils not of the best quality. Its fibre is shorter and coarser, and the cloth made from it has more pile, and is said to receive and retain better the colours of the dyer.†

---

* Carlo Giacinto, op. cit. p. 62. The above, as stated by the author, appears to me of questionable accuracy. When I have so exposed the brown cotton it has become white.

† When Giacinto wrote, in 1811, the current price of these three different kinds of cotton, per quintal, was as follows:—Malta cotton, 30 scudi; Indian, 32; and the brown, from 45 to 55—not separated from the seed.

The seed in his time sold for from six to eight scudi the quintal. As food for cattle, it is generally given mixed with the small straw, or with the chaff of wheat or barley.

The manner of cultivating these different varieties of cotton is very similar. Nowhere, probably, is its cultivation better understood or better observed. As fundamental in the system of agriculture of Malta, which it truly is, I shall give such information as I have happened to collect respecting it, even at the risk of being tedious.

The preparation of the ground commences in August, when it is broken up, manured, and levelled. If barley is sown preparatory to the cotton, as already mentioned, it is pulled up in the early spring for use as forage. The early cotton is sown in April or May : the ground is previously ploughed; the seed is either scattered over it by the hand and covered in by the use of a rude harrow, or dropt into small pits made to receive it. When the plant appears, the land is hoed two or three times; and when two or three inches high, the tops of the shoots are nipped off, to prevent a too luxuriant growth of stalk and leaves. It flowers in July; and in September or October the pod is ripe for gathering.

The following detail, for which I was indebted to the late Sir Frederick Ponsonby, who obtained it from a gentleman of Gozo, accurately conversant with its agriculture, which is almost identical with that of Malta, will, at the same time, show the successive operations required in the progress of this crop (exclusive of any intermediate one), and the expense attending its cultivation :—

	Scudi.	Tari.	s.	d.
" 1. All land ought to be well broken and manured, at least every eighth year; * and the proportion of expense for such on two tumoli of land (something more than half an English acre), may be calculated at about	4	0	= 6	8
" 2. In October and November, it requires sapping (hoeing), when four persons are employed for one day, at four tari each, . . .	1	4	2	6
" 3. In April it must be ploughed, when two men are required for half a-day, ...	0	10	1	6
" 4. In the same month, shortly after, two men are required for one day to level the ground, .	0	8	1	2
" 5. In May a man is employed for one day to dig small pits in the superficies of the ground, wherein to lay the seeds, ...	0	4	0	6¾
" 6. Four pesi of seed, the price of which is .	1	0	1	8
" 7. In the same month, a boy and woman are employed for one day to sow, . . .	0	2	0	3¼
" 8. Ditto, ten boys and women are employed to carry water and to water the seed, one day, . .	2	6	4	2
" 9. Ditto, a man for one day to draw water from the well or tank, ...	0	4	0	7
" 10. In June, the plants having appeared, the superfluous ones must be taken from the pits, leaving in each only four or five; for which purpose two women are required one day, . . .	0	6	0	10
" 11. Shortly after the preceding operation, the ground is superficially sapped by four men, one day, .	1	4	2	2¾
" 12. In July, the plants are topped and clipped, to prevent the overgrowing of the stalk and leaves, which is performed by women, . . .	0	8	1	2
" 13. In September the cotton is gathered (generally by women and children), for which ten tari the quintal is paid; and supposing the produce to be two quintals, the expense would be . .	1	8	2	10

* Every fourth or fifth year is preferred in Malta by the most successful cultivators.

Scudi. Tari. *s. d.*

' 1 4. The cotton is generally kept six weeks; the
expense of keeping it in the loft is two tari per
week, ... 0 1 = 21 8

" 15. The expense of separating the cotton from the
pod and seed by the wheel,* is one scudo per
quintal, ... 2 0 3 4

" It is calculated that the above two quintals will
give about 12 pesi, or 60 rotoli, of cotton-wool.

" When the cotton is sown without the operations
set forth in Nos. 4, 5, 7, 8, 9 (is broadcast), the expense attendant thereon is saved ; but in such case
the ground must be twice ploughed, and six, instead
of four pesi of seed must be sown. This latter method is most usually practised; but great disadvan-
tage arises should not the sowing be followed by a
sufficiency of rain, when loss of labour and expense
is the consequence ;" and it is then necessary to have
recourse to the first mentioned plan, viz., the making
of separate holes for the reception of the seed, and of
watering them separately after the putting in of
the seed.

The amount of expense of cultivating two tumoli
of land with cotton, according to the preceding details,
is L.1, 11s. 1¾d. Let us suppose the rent of the
two tumoli to be L.3. Further, let us suppose that
the produce of cotton-wool of the two tumoli is
12 pesi ; and that the farmer sells it at the rate of

---

* The wheel is a small hand one, of rude construction; the seed is
pressed out and separated from the cotton by one cylinder revolving
on another. The same simple rude implement is in use in Turkey
and in the Levant generally.

8s. 4d. the peso, the amount of the crop (exclusive of the seed and stalks) will be L.5 (and this is considered a fair average price for cotton). Thus it appears, deducting the rent and expense of cultivation from the value of the produce, that the difference in favour of the farmer is only the small sum of 8s. 10¼d.

Several kinds of corn are cultivated in Malta, but, with the exception of two, in a very limited manner, viz., hard-wheat (*Triticum turgidum*), and common barley (*Hordeum vulgare*). As has been already observed, they are very commonly grown together, under the name of Meschiato. The time of sowing is the latter end of November; the reaping-time, the latter end of May and the beginning of June. The expense attending the cultivation of grain after cotton is not considerable; one ploughing before sowing the seed, and one immediately after, to cover it, are sufficient. When the corn appears above ground the ground should be hoed, the weeds plucked up, and the young plants, if necessary, equalized by transplanting. The produce of grain is various, according to the quality of the land. In poor, shallow soils, it is from seven to nine-fold; in good soils from twenty to thirty; and even according to Giacinto considerably higher— from forty to fifty-fold for wheat, and from twenty-nine to thirty-eight-fold for barley.* The poor soils

* According to information given to Sir Frederick Ponsonby, the average produce of good land is from twenty to twenty-four-fold of wheat, about the same of meschiato, and from twenty to thirty of barley;—the higher numbers represent the produce of the very good lands.

are in small proportion to the good. They are partly so little productive because it is not considered worth while to cultivate them carefully, or run the risk of expending much labour on them, or of incurring much expense; they are not even manured. The corn is pulled up in Malta, not cut; the grain is procured from it very much in the same manner as in the Ionian Islands.

The growing of wheat or barley two years running on the same ground is prohibited, being considered too exhausting. The farmer grows grain principally for the use of his family; bread is a principal part of the diet of all classes of the inhabitants; and of the working class it is almost the exclusive food. The straw, especially of the barley, is reserved for forage, particularly for mules and horses; and, excepting sulla, is the only dry forage in use. The quantity of grain grown at present is about sufficient for four months' consumption, and in Gozo for eight months. It is not easy to obtain information to be depended on on this subject, and I have heard the quantity of produce of both these islands very differently stated. The preceding estimates were those of Sir Frederick Ponsonby, who was at much pains to arrive at the truth, and possessed the very best means of obtaining it.

The following return shows the quantity of grain produced, the quantity of foreign grain consumed, and the price of bread per lb., from 1820 to 1834, derived from official documents collected by the distinguished officer just mentioned.

Year.	Grain grown in Malta.		Foreign Wheat Consumed.	Bread, per lb. avoirdupois.
	Wheat. Salms.*	Meschiato,† Salms.	Salms.	d.
1828, . .	19,069	23,948	49,854	1 6-12ths.
1829, . .	15,843	25,040	54,960	1 5-12ths.
1830, . .	17,757	21,195	49,904	1 2-12ths.
1831, . .	5,682	15,538	65,459	· 1 5-12ths.
1832, . .	9,986	29,914	53,612	1 3-12ths.
1833, . .	9,983	12,787	59,588	1 2-12ths.
1834, . .	15,711	26,539	55,150	1 3-12ths.

The quantity of grain grown in Malta is variable—the same soil being equally applicable to grain and to cotton ; and consequently, when the market price of cotton is high, the greater is the encouragement to raise it, and the greater is the quantity cultivated, and *vice versa.*

The price of bread, given in the preceding return, is that of white bread ;—the common brown bread, that which is used by the labouring class, seldom, I believe, exceeds a penny a pound. Notwithstanding that it is heavily taxed,‡ Sir Frederick Ponsonby was

* The Maltese salm is equal to about seven and seven-eighths bushels imperial measure.

† One-third wheat, and two-thirds barley.

‡ A large proportion of the revenue of Malta has hitherto been derived from a tax on bread made of foreign wheat. The average revenue of Malta is L.100,000 per annum—derived as follows:—

From Rent of Crown Property,	. .	L.28,000
Tax on Foreign Corn,	. .	30,000
Customs and Port Dues,	. .	14,000
Excise, . .	. .	16,000
Quarantine Dues,	. . .	5,000

of opinion, and his opinion was founded on returns, that the price of bread in Malta was cheaper than in any other part of the Mediterranean ; seeming to prove how safely a country may be dependent on other countries for the greater part of the supply of the first necessary of life.

Frequent mention has already been made of sulla (*Hedissarum coronaria*), a very important article in the agriculture of Malta. It is cultivated in the same manner as barley when intended for forage. The ground is ploughed once preparatory to its sowing, which is at the height of the hot season, in August, a considerable time before any rain is expected. The opinion entertained, founded on experience, is, that exposure of the seed to a high temperature is favourable to its germination.* It springs up after the first rains, and in good land attains the height of two or three feet. It is in flower in the latter end of April and the beginning of May, when it is cut and dried for use during the remainder of the year. From the field, as soon as dry, it is generally transferred to the terraced roofs of the farm-houses, where it is kept rudely stacked, and is safe from pilferers. The salm

Judicial Fees,	.	.	.	.	L.4,000
Minor Taxes,	.	.	.	.	3,000

The duty on foreign grain has been regulated according to the price, from 12s. per salm on wheat, to 1s.; the former when it is under 25s. per salm, the latter when at 63s.

* As the seed is covered with a strong pellicle, probably in the drying from exposure, it becomes fissured, and may thus conduce to its vegetation. Occasionally, the seed lies dormant one or two years.

of land (four English acres and four-fifteenths) of good quality, requires about four salm of seed, and affords, on an average, 192 loads of sulla. The luxuriancy of this crop is very great, as is indicated by the produce; nowhere does it flourish more than in Malta; and when it is in full bloom, its large flowers of the richest red, it makes a very brilliant and pleasing appearance.; Malta then exhibits in perfection the *ver purpureum*.

A large proportion of the sulla grown is sent into the city, and sold for the use of riding-horses. It is more employed in the fattening of cattle than in their ordinary keep. It is too expensive for the latter purpose. They are fed principally on broken straw and chaff, and on leaves of various kinds, as of the fig, vine, reed, and prickly pear. With these helps, without any natural pastures, the Maltese farmer has no difficulty in keeping a comparatively large stock.

The return in p. 397, shows the large number of cattle and of beasts of burden in Malta. The latter are principally used in draught. In 1811, when P. Carlo Giacinto published his work on the agriculture of Malta, there were, according to him, more than twelve hundred carts in the island, and nine hundred public calêsses, besides private ones.* Since that

---

* Malta, then, as has been already observed, was in a forced unnatural state of prosperity. Owing to the war and the prohibitory decrees of Napoleon, it had become a vast entrepôt of British commerce, and not only for the Mediterranean countries, but even for a great part of Europe, by means of the contraband system then perfectly

time, the number of calêsses has diminished; the number of carts has remained much the same. In 1835, there were 264 licensed calêsses in Malta, and fourteen in Gozo; and 1137 licensed carts in the former, and twenty-five in the latter, besides about 800 carts, solely employed on farms and not taxed.

5. No mention hitherto has been made either of the size of the farms, or of the general value of land, or of the rate of rent, or of the condition either of the farmer or labourer. In connexion with the state of agriculture, I shall advert to each of these points separately, however briefly.

As might be anticipated, considering the proportional dense population of the island, and the system of cultivation followed, the farms are never large; they are often extremely small; the largest seldom exceed thirty acres; the smaller tenements are often less than an acre. These last (provided they command a supply of water) are commonly called gardens.*

organized, by which our merchants set at nought all the efforts of Napoleon to paralyse the power of this country by the exclusion of our merchandise.

* The superficies of the island of Malta is estimated (somewhat vaguely) at ninety-four square miles. The cultivated land is estimated at 50,000 acres, of which 24,000 are private property; 14,000 crown lands; and 12,000 church lands. The government property is divided into 550 separate tenements, let at short leases, from one to eight years; long leases from nine to ninety-nine years; and on leases for three generations. The revenue of government, from this source, is about L.8000.

Further, as might be anticipated, the price of land is high, and the rent which it produces great. The price of the best land is from five to six hundred scudi the tumolo; of inferior quality, from two to one hundred ; or per English acre, the price of the very best is L.189, and of the worst L.31, reckoning the tumulo as equivalent to about $\frac{26}{100}$ of the English acre, or a little more than one quarter.

The rent of land now varies from about fifteen scudi the tumolo, to ten, and even five and two scudi, according to the quality of the soil; that is, from about L.4, 10s. an acre, to thirteen shillings. Land in small allotments, as garden tenements, well supplied with water, brings even double the first mentioned rent. In 1811, when the island was most prosperous, the price of land did not differ much from its present value, but its rent was very much higher. Then, according to P. Carlo Giacinto, a tumolo of land, the selling price of which was 240 dollars, or L.50, produced a yearly rent of twenty-five scudi, or L.2,1s., which is at the rate of about L.8 an acre; and garden land, the higher rent of fifteen dollars a tumolo, or L.3, 2s., equivalent to about L.12 an acre.

But the different degrees of value of land, according to the quality of soil, the nature of the subsoil, and the supply of water, is perhaps best exemplified in the instance of land applied to the growing of cotton. According to P. Carlo Giacinto, at the time he wrote, viz., in 1811 (and it is equally true now relatively), a tumolo of good land, rather exceeding

in depth two feet and a half of red earth, well prepared by the proprietor for cultivation,* provided
with a small cistern of water, for occasional use, as
for watering the cotton-seed, and the intermediate
crops of vegetables, would let for twenty-five scudi
per annum, for the short term of four years, and its
crop of Malta cotton, which requires little irrigation,
would yield a produce of a quintal and a half of cotton in the pod.

Similar land, in every respect, but with the advantage of running water for irrigation, would let for the
same rent, viz., twenty-five scudi the tumolo, for any
term of years the proprietor pleases, and without his
being put to any expense in preparing the ground;
and it should yield above two quintals of either brown
or Indian cotton, independent of vegetables.

If there is no supply of water for irrigation, or if
the depth of earth did not exceed one foot, it would
bring little more than eight scudi of rent a-year to
the proprietor, when let for a term of eight years; or,
if well prepared by him, from twelve to fourteen
scudi, for the short term of four years, and would yield
only about half a quintal of Malta cotton, the only
kind which it will bear.

Farther, if, in addition to shallowness of soil, the
rocky substratum is hard and close, preventing the
penetration of the rain-water in winter, and exhaling
little or no moisture in summer, then, though well

* By deep hoeing and manuring, at an expense to the proprietor,
in 1811, of about thirty scudi.

prepared by the proprietor, it would not let for above ten scudi per annum, the cotton crop being precarious, and the produce comparatively small.

According to the same authority, land, consisting of white earth or marl, will let rather more advantageously than that of red earth just noticed; or, which is equivalent, will bring the same rent with a less depth of soil and convenience of water.*

The condition of the farmer can hardly be considered as prosperous. All his industry and thrift are required to pay his high rent, and support himself and family, living in a very frugal way. By means of his cotton crop, and cattle chiefly, he pays the rent, and keeps up his stock. On the grain he grows, he and his family chiefly subsist, and the surplus enables him to pay servants and labourers, and his profits are derived principally from the minor crops and other little helps, as poultry, &c., and consequently he has the most powerful motive to exert himself, and turn his land, by uninterrupted cultivation, to the best account.

* He supposes that it has a superiority over the red earth, in being more argillaceous and retentive of water. This is very doubtful, considering the composition of the two soils. To me it appears more probable that the apparent advantage of the marl is in part connected with the circumstance that it usually rests on a softer and more porous substratum than the red earth. Be this as it may, the fact which he mentions of the difference between the cotton grown in the marl and red clay is curious,—how, in the former, the seed is smaller, and the cotton heavier, so that a peso or five rotoli of cotton in the pod, grown in marl, will give one rotolo and three quarters of cotton-wool, whilst the same weight of cotton in the pod grown in the red clay, will afford only one rotolo and a quarter.

The condition of the labourer is very poor indeed, and reduced. When Giacinto wrote, he received rather more than the third of a dollar a-day, or eighteen-pence; now, he receives only four tari, which are equal to sixpence halfpenny, and he is obliged to furnish his own tools.

His day's work is sufficiently laborious. I shall give a sketch of it, from Giacinto's graphic description, including his manner of living.

He begins with observing:—"That it almost exceeds belief how the Maltese peasants bear the excessive heat of the climate, especially in summer. They may be seen exposed to the sun, through the whole day, in the middle of a field, at their hard work, unrefreshed even by the shade of a tree. At sunrise, their day's work commences. At eight o'clock, they rest a half an hour, and take their breakfast. At eleven they rest again until one, when they dine. Both their breakfast and dinner are of the most frugal kind, consisting very often merely of barley-bread, with a few small onions or radishes, failing which, they use a few salted olives, a little oil, a sardinia, or some other relish (*altra cosa salata*). After dinner they take their siesta, either under some slight shade, if they can find it, or under cover of the stone-wall of the field, the head covered, the rest of the body exposed to the scorching rays of the sun. At one o'clock, after this rest, they return to their labour with the greatest energy and vigour, and continue at it till the setting of the sun, when in the churches universally the bell sounds,—that which they call the first *Ave Maria*,—their signal to leave off work, and which they do accordingly immediately. They then hasten home and take their supper, consisting of pottage with maccaroni and bread. And when they can afford it, both at dinner and supper, they take occasionally a little wine. All the year round, their course of life is the same, with the exception that, in winter, they rest at dinner a shorter time, only from eleven o'clock till noon." To this indefatigable activity and steadiness of the peasantry, the author attributes the marvels that have been effected in the extension of cultivation.*

6. The instruments of husbandry in use in Malta are few and simple, and differ but little from those employed in the Ionian Islands. They are comprehended in those required for the soil, as the hoe, the plough, and the leveller; and those required in gathering in the harvest and obtaining the grain, as the sickle, fork, shovel, and sieve. Figures of these implements are given in Plate II.

Of these implements, the hoe (figs. 18, 19, 20) is the most important; it holds the place of our spade. Its form and size are various, according to the situation, purpose, and kind of soil for which it is required.

The plough (fig. 21), light and single-handed, is commonly employed after the hoe for equalizing the

* Op. Cit., p. 26.

surface; in fact, in performing the part of the harrow with us; whilst the Maltese harrow (fig. 22), or rather levelling frame (if it may be so called), is used after the seed is sown, partly for smoothing the ground, but chiefly for the purpose of pressing in the seed and covering it with soil.

The hook (fig. 23), used by the reapers in the corn-fields, is serrated, but not sharp. It is not employed in cutting, but for gathering the corn together after it has been pulled up by the roots. Without delay the corn is transferred to the thrashing-floor, where the rude fork (fig. 25) is useful for putting the corn in the track of the animals employed to beat out the grain. With as little delay as possible, the grain is separated from the chaff; and this is effected chiefly by the wooden spade (fig. 14), and the sieve (fig. 24); by the one, the chaff is got rid of with the aid of the wind; by the other, the barley and wheat of the meschiato are separated from each other.

7. The perfect knowledge and the free use of manure is one of the most important features of Maltese farming;* and therefore it may not be amiss again to refer to it, in conjunction with the man-

---

* The manure used is principally stable and farm-yard dung; no composts, no mineral, fossil, or saline manures, have yet been employed. Some of the saline kind, especially the alkaline nitrates, may be very deserving of trial, considering how long most of the soil of Malta has been under crop, and its little depth.

ner of breaking up the ground, and of employing
irrigation.

The operation is commonly performed in one of
two ways: either the ground is trenched or merely
dug up; one or other method having the preference,
according to the quality of the soil. In the first
instance, trench after trench is dug, and a layer of
manure introduced and covered with soil, till the
whole field has been thus treated. The trenches are
made about a foot deep, and about six inches of
earth is laid on the manure. After the depositing of
the manure, and the filling up of the trenches as
they are successively made, the ground is ploughed
for the purpose of equalizing its surface and making
seed-fallows: the plough does not penetrate more than
two or three inches in depth. Or, the whole field is
first trenched, and the earth that has been thrown up
is left for some time exposed to the air, before the
manure is introduced. When the second method is
used, the manure is laid on the surface of the land,
preparatory to its being broken up. This is effected
with the strong hoe, or more frequently with the
pick, and in the act a great part of the manure is
buried. In this state it is left till the rains commence, that the manure may be well washed in. The
large clods are then broken with hoes, and the ground
levelled.

Irrigation is another favourable feature in the agriculture of Malta; and its efficacy as a means of im-
parting fertility to the land is as well understood and

appreciated as that of manure. The process of irrigation in use is sufficiently simple. The field to be subjected to it is divided into a sufficient number of small square compartments, formed of little embankments, the earth being thrown up with the hoe, and a channel left between each. A larger channel, dug through the middle of the field, receives the water and conducts it to the smaller ones in succession; from whence it is admitted into the enclosure. The workman, as it approaches, moves aside a little of the mould forming the embankment of the compartment, and having allowed a sufficient quantity of water to enter, closes it again; and so on, till every compartment of the field has had its due supply. Then, when the earth is saturated, the little embankments are thrown down, and the surface is levelled and beaten, preparatory to the sowing of the seed. Such a preparation, where there is abundance of water, as in the neighbourhood of the aqueduct, is occasionally used for cotton, but more frequently for vegetables.

8. The desiderata in agriculture in Malta are comparatively few, and relate rather to implements than methods. The defectiveness of the former is obvious, especially in the instance of the plough. Their improvement, however much needed, it is to be feared can hardly be expected, considering the limited resources of the farmer—his want of capital, his want of instruction and knowledge. So long as the population of Malta continues excessive, and labour unduly

cheap—and the labouring class and the small farmers poor and ignorant, agriculture can hardly be otherwise than stationary. Reflecting on the present circumstances of the island, the feeling of surprise is that it has advanced so far, and that its condition is so respectable.

Comparing the state of the agriculture of Malta with the condition of the people, it is instructive to find, at the same time melancholy to observe, what little relation there is between them. And reasoning on the prosperity of the one and the poverty of the other, the great productiveness of the land, and the small profits of the farmer and the miserable wages of the labourer, it is impossible to avoid the conclusion, that the highest degree of cultivation of the land is not incompatible with great wretchedness of the population, should the latter be, as in the case of Malta, in excess.

Malta, compared with the Ionian Islands, seems to afford a demonstrative proof that wages—the wages of the agricultural labourer as well as of the artificer —are not regulated by the price of bread, or of food generally, but by the demand for labour. In both, the larger proportion of corn consumed is imported; the price of bread in both is about the same, but the wages are very different. In the Ionian Islands they are rather more than twice as high as in Malta; the one thinly peopled, the other densely; in the one an excess of land for cultivation, in the other a deficiency. And, that the demand, *cæteris paribus*, fixes the price of labour, seems farther to be proved by the fact already mentioned in page 416, that, in the time of Malta's great commercial prosperity, when there was ample occupation for the people, the wages were very much higher.

9. In gardening, the Maltese, with a few exceptions, are comparatively backward. The exceptions exist chiefly in the cultivation of certain fruit-trees, for which the climate is peculiarly favourable—as the orange, the lemon, the fig, and the vine. The method of managing these is thoroughly understood; their fruit is excellent and abundant: and of each there are several varieties. And another exception may be made, in the instance of the ordinary vegetables—as the cabbage, cauliflower, brocoli, spinach, onion, tomata; and, amongst the small fruits, the strawberry.

Their backwardness in regard to horticulture is chiefly remarkable in the careless manner in which they cultivate almost all other fruit-trees, exclusive of those already mentioned, and especially the apple, pear, plum, cherry, pomegranate, and a few more—as the peach, apricot, nectarine. No pains have been taken about these; the varieties of them are generally bad; little attention is given to their management, and, consequently, their fruit is of the lowest character, and of little value. And even in the growing of vegetables, there is much remissness and carelessness, excepting in the vicinity of Valetta, the immediate market of which acts as a strong stimulus to exertion. At the distance of a few miles from the town, in admirable situations, with good soil, abundance of water—circumstances altogether most favourable—it is melancholy to witness the state of poverty of the gardens, and the corresponding poverty of their proprietors ; the latter without intelligence and without enterprise—satisfied, if they can merely support existence.

Nowhere, perhaps, is there greater room for improvement in horticulture than in Malta, and nowhere, probably, would intelligent gardeners, with some little capital and a thorough knowledge of their art, be better rewarded. The climate is perfect for all the fruits of the south of Europe, and it is compatible even with a few tropical species. Those fruits that have been cultivated with care are excellent— such as are grown in the gardens of St Antonio, and in one or two other gardens which have been for some time in the possession of English gentlemen, who have been at pains to introduce choice varieties. And, as regards vegetables, in the favourable situations above mentioned, there might be, throughout the year, a constant succession of different kinds; and by the importation of seed, almost any vegetable of the north of Europe, almost all our spring and summer vegetables, might be raised, in any, or in every season.

Were an intelligent activity exercised in this branch of industry, a vast improvement probably might be effected, much wealth might be added to the island,

and much misery relieved. Now, it is boasted, that not a spot of ground admitting of cultivation is allowed to lie waste; were horticulture extended and improved, then it would be truly the case: the vine, the fig-tree, the olive, the prickly pear, the pomegranate, the caruba, might be planted amongst the rocks, and a new character might be given to the hills; even the climate might perhaps be ameliorated, and the excessive heat of its summer moderated. Formerly, there is reason to believe that Malta was not so destitute of wood as at present. It is the opinion of some writers, that the olive-tree, which is now comparatively scarce, was once widely grown, and that olive oil was made not only in sufficient quantity for the use of the inhabitants, but even for exportation. Professor Carlo Giacinto is of this belief, and in advocating the forming of new plantations of this tree, he indulges in hopes similar to those above expressed. In one place he says:— " Non si vedrebbero più nude, e a prima vista quasi deserte, ma si vestirebbero di quel preziosò manto, che ne formerebbe ben tosto la più brillante amenità."* And in another, he remarks that, "whatever may be the true cause that the olive has not been cultivated in Malta for many years, he is satisfied that there are proprietors who would willingly act with the Government to renew its cultivation, and that it might soon be spread and extended even in

* Op. Cit., p. 214.

situations then lying waste." And he adds, " that
the plantations might be so regulated as not to interfere with the lands destined for cotton, or for grain,
or for any other annual produce; so disposed, that
the country might be well wooded, but not in excess,
and the other crops defended from the winds." And
besides this advantage, he counted on another, " the
incalculable one of having rain in more frequent
and copious showers."

The same writer advocates the planting of the
vine very generally, with a view to the covering of
the innumerable stone-walls by which the fields are
enclosed. He anticipates, without injury to the ordinary crops, a good produce of wine. And, even
leaving the fruits and the wine out of consideration,
he is of opinion, and perhaps justly, that the growing
of the vine, in the manner proposed by him, would
prove advantageous in other respects, partly in the
produce of leaves for the use of cattle, and of the
cuttings of the branches for fire-wood; and partly in
defending the cotton crop from the parching heat
radiated and reflected at present from the naked
walls of stone. In one instance which I recollect,
the suggestion has been carried into effect by a native
gentleman, distinguished for ability and soundness of
views, and, I believe, with success. To the eye, the
appearance is most pleasing and grateful, and perfectly in accordance with Giacinto's expectations:—
" Di qual amenità non si vestirebbero tosto, si rico-
perte fossero li dispiacevoli muri, di Aprile a tutto

Novembre dalle foglie della Vite?" And he intro-
duces the reflection, by comparing the country, at
present divided into so many small fields by rough
walls of white stone, to the field of Ezekiel.

An attempt has been made to form plantations of
the mulberry-tree, in connexion with the breeding of
the silk-worm and the obtaining of silk. Encouragement has been afforded by Government, and considerable exertions have been made by a British Silk
Company; but, I apprehend, the result hitherto has
not answered expectations. It is true, the climate is
admirably fitted for the silk-worm, and that the silk
of Malta is of excellent quality. The difficulty is in
relation to the food of the worm : the generally shallow soil of the island is peculiarly unfitted for the
mulberry-tree;* and consequently this tree cannot
be grown to any great extent without sacrificing to
it the best land, the propriety of which is very questionable. In a limited and modified way, the breeding of the silk-worm may be of a certain service to
the Maltese peasants, as a help; but it is to be apprehended that evil, rather than good, would result
from it, were it to become very extended and a main
object.

In the year 1833, when I left Malta, an Agricultural Society was about being formed, with the good
intent of endeavouring to ameliorate the agriculture
of the island, and extend its cultivation. Judiciously

* The soil of Gozo being generally deep, is probably well fitted
for it.

conducted, such a society ought to have the best effect. It cannot fail to do good, if, proceeding in an enlightened manner, it bring the light of science to the aid of the natives, collect their experience, and recommend, and at the same time endeavour, to carry into effect only such measures of probable improvement as seem to be justified by the peculiarity of the soil and climate. Horticulture, it is to be hoped, will have their consideration and encouragement.* Were prizes offered, either by the Society or by the Government, to stimulate the exertions of the people in this branch of industry, probably, ere long, gardening would rapidly advance; especially were the prizes given not only for the best fruits, but also for the best vegetables, and that at different seasons of the year, and in different districts of the island. It is the fruits and vegetables most suitable to the soil and climate of the island, and which are capable of being naturalized, that are most deserving of encouragement, such as, if they succeed, will be of permanent benefit; and not rare exotics, the cultivation of which is difficult, owing to uncongenialness of climate, such as the plantain, the date,

* This society, I fear, has been a failure; I have not heard of any good it has done, and probably now it has ceased to exist; to be recorded merely as one of the abortive attempts to do good, of which there are so many instances in Malta and the Ionian Islands, arising in part, perhaps, from the inveterate habits of an old people, and in part from want of persevering zeal in the movers,—most of them strangers liable to be removed, and taking no permanent interest in the objects proposed.

the pine-apple, which require a higher and more equable average temperature for their successful growth; or such as the gooseberry, currant, and raspberry, the fruits of our colder regions, and the plants of which suffer as much from the summer heat of Malta, as the preceding do from the winter's cold. The plantain and the date-palm have been long introduced into Malta, but neither has made much progress in extension of cultivation, for the reasons already assigned. The plantain is grown rather as a curiosity in sheltered hot situations, for the sake of its fruit which occasionally ripens; and the palm, as in the Ionian Islands, chiefly for its leaves. Palms have borne fruit in Malta, but not, it is understood, of any value. And the person, after the experience of the past, would be considered extremely chimerical, who should attempt the formation of groves of the one, or of fields of the other, with a view to a profitable return,—as much so, perhaps, as any native of the tropics would be considered chimerical, were he to undertake the cultivation of wheat at the level of the sea under the line, or the planting of vineyards. It is a fundamental rule that each climate is fitted only for certain plants; and that the most profitable husbandry consists in growing the crops best fitted for the soil and climate; trusting to commerce for a supply of foreign produce, on the cheapest terms,—on terms vastly more advantageous than those by which they could be procured, were they expensively forced into growth on the spot.

On the soils and state of agriculture in Gozo, I shall intentionally be very brief.

The soil of Gozo generally is calcareous marl, of a fawn colour. It is commonly deep, and of an excellent quality, and admirably fitted for all agricultural purposes. There are, I believe, several varieties of it ; and all of them either rest on, or are in the neighbourhood of, the marl formation, from whence they are derived. Red clay soil is of comparatively rare occurrence. It is confined chiefly to the tops of the hills and ridges, which are formed of sandstone. It is generally shallow; and in consequence of this circumstance and its situation, and the unfavourable nature of its substratum, it is but little productive.

The returns already given, p. 396, convey a tolerable idea of the agricultural resources of Gozo.

The proportion of fertile land in Gozo is much greater than in Malta; in 1833 it was estimated at 12,800 acres, and the uncultivated at 1678, whilst its proportional population is very much less; in the same year it was only about 16,565, or 614 to the square mile.

The manner in which land is let and rent paid, is much the same in the two islands.

The system of farming, also, in the two islands, is almost identical. I am not aware of any methods adopted in the one not practised in the other, excepting, perhaps, that in Gozo more attention is paid to the mixing of varieties of soil.

The proportion of garden ground in Gozo is larger

than in Malta; the art of gardening appears to be better understood there, and the fruits of the island are of superior quality, especially the apples and pears.

Owing to the extent of cultivated land, and the great fertility of the land, I believe it is admitted that the produce of the island is more than sufficient to support the population. It might be expected, then, that the population would be flourishing, or at least in easy circumstances; but this, I am sorry to say, does not appear to be the case. It is to be feared, generally, that they are even worse off than the Maltese. Their poor condition is probably owing to their being entirely dependent on agriculture, without the aid of commerce or of manufactures; to there being very few small proprietors, very few resident proprietors; and, in brief, to their condition being somewhat analogous to that of the Irish. The principal estates belong to Maltese families resident in Valetta, where their rents are remitted, and where they are spent; and the demand for land being considerable, and the rent consequently high and the profits small, the farming population are necessarily poor. Some idea of their needy circumstances may be derived from the very small quantity of animal food consumed by the inhabitants. When I visited the island in the spring of 1834, I was assured by a person of accurate information, that only one bullock was killed weekly for the market, and that that was sufficient for the whole population, including a detachment of our troops, who used a considerable proportion of it; and the appearance of the people, their dress, houses, and villages, were in accordance, all indicative of a reduced and impoverished condition.

Another circumstance which may be adduced in proof of it, in conjunction with the admitted salubrity of the climate, is the low average of the duration of life. For ten years, viz., from 1827 to 1836, it would appear to be only 30.5 years. For this information I am indebted to Dr Charles Galland, the able Professor of Anatomy in the University of Malta, who obtained it by consulting the parish registers, in which the age of each person buried is recorded. The following numbers give the average age of the dead for each year:—

1827, ...	30¼
1828, ...	29½
1829, ...	30¼
1830, ...	19⅛
1831, ...	32
1832, ...	35¾
1833, ...	29⅔
1834, ...	34
1835, ...	35
1836, ...	29⅓

This low average Dr Galland attributes to the great mortality amongst infants * (nearly four times as great

* This appears clearly from the following Table, containing the results of Dr Galland's inquiries :—

TABLE OF 3639 DEATHS, THE MORTALITY IN GOZO, DURING TEN YEARS, FROM 1827 TO 1836 INCLUSIVE, SHOWING THE RELATIVE MORTALITY AT DIFFERENT AGES, AND IN DIFFERENT MONTHS.

Months.	0 to 1.			1 to 3.			3 to 5.			5 to 10.			10 to 15.			15 to 20.		
	M.	F.	Tot.	M.	F.	Tot.	M.	F.	Tot.	M.	F.	Tot.	M.	F.	Tot.	M.	F.	Tot.
January,	67	55	122	11	12	23	7	2	9	6	7	13	1	5	6	2	5	7
February,	48	56	104	16	9	25	1	6	7	1	1	2	..	3	3	1	5	6
March, .	53	48	101	7	9	16	2	3	5	2	2	4	1	3	4	4	1	3
April, . .	28	38	66	10	12	22	2	4	6	6	2	8	4	3	7	1	4	5
May, . .	31	25	56	12	9	21	2	7	9	6	1	7	1	4	5	1	7	8
June, . .	24	25	49	17	19	36	3	7	10	2	1	3	2	6	8	..	4	4
July, . .	40	40	80	17	17	34	5	4	9	3	3	6	5	2	7	2	4	6
August, .	50	31	81	29	38	67	9	5	14	4	7	11	7	3	10	7	2	9
September.	53	43	96	31	33	64	9	9	18	8	8	16	7	5	12	3	5	8
October,	50	62	112	31	43	74	15	20	35	13	3	16	3	3	6	6	5	11
November,	55	47	102	36	42	78	7	13	20	8	4	12	9	5	14	6	6	12
December,	59	40	99	31	31	62	5	,7	12	4	8	12	3	3	6	1	6	7
	558	510	1068	248	274	522	67	87	154	63	47	110	43	45	88	34	54	88
Monthly Mean, }	46.5	43.3	89.	20.6	22.7	43.5	5.6	7.2	12.4	5.2	3.9	9.2	3.5	3.7	7.1	2.9	4.5	7.3

Months.	20 to 30.			30 to 40.			40 to 60.			60 to 80.			80 to 100.		
	M.	F.	Tot.	M.	F.	Tot.	M.	F.	Tot.	M.	F.	Tot.	M.	F.	Tot.
January, . . .	7	7	14	2	3	5	17	9	26	41	33	74	19	15	34
February, . . .	3	1	4	2	2	4	16	19	35	27	30	57	12	18	30
March, ...	7	7	14	1	7	8	15	15	30	27	29	56	15	10	25
April, ...	3	5	8	2	5	7	13	18	31	33	32	65	7	7	14
May, ...	5	8	13	3	6	9	12	16	28,	17	33	50	6	9	15
June, ...	6	9	15	3	7	10	13	23	36	28	36	64	16	8	24
July, ...	1	6	7	4	4	8	20	13	33	26	31	57	14	8	22
August, ...	4	5	9	2	4	6	15	17	32	29	44	73	8	8	16
September, . .	3	9	12	1	3	4	10	10	20	34	33	67	14	8	22
October, . . .	6	10	16	5	4	9	8	13	21	30	38	68	7	11	18
November, . .	5	4	9	2	6	8	11	21	32	33	32	65	13	12	25
December, . .	6	5	11	7	8	15	13	13	26	28	35	63	13	17	30
	56	76	132	34	59	93	163	187	350	353	406	759	144	131	275
Monthly Mean, }	4.7	6.3	11.	2.8	4.9	7.7	13.6	15.6	29.2	29.4	33.8	63.2	12.	10.9	22.9

Mean yearly, 363.9.

Of the 3639, there were 1763 Males ; 1875 Females.

as in the population of London)—and that, indirectly, to the extreme poverty of the parents.*

I shall give from my note-book a few extracts, rough notes descriptive of the face of the country, according to the impressions made at the time, viz., on the visit already referred to in the spring of 1834.

" Went in the afternoon (May 2d) to Ramala, where Sir Frederick Ponsonby has a little shooting-box, and where we dined in the open air, under the shelter of rocks, amidst a scene of extraordinary wildness and ruin, from the falling down of great masses of cliff. Yet even here, amongst these natural ruins, cultivation was not neglected : every little spot of soil was enclosed with stone-walls, and planted with vegetables or fruit-trees. The area of some of them did not exceed a few feet.

" The country through which we passed in going from Rabato to Ramala, was not uninteresting, and in many places possessed considerable beauty, partly

* Dr Galland found that the Marriages and Births, from 1829 to 1836 inclusive, were the following :—

Years.	Marriages.	Births.
1829,	89	416
1830,	122	500
1831,	110	580
1832,	94	475
1833,	107	506
1834,	159	518
1835,	158	592
1836,	128	558
Total,	951	4,145

from its natural features of scenery, and partly owing to cultivation. The plain parts of the country, and the gentle declivities generally, were covered with crops of grain. The steep declivities of the sides of the hills presented a succession of terraces, which, rising rapidly one above another, all on a very small scale, gave the idea of the seats of an immense amphi-theatre, and the curved lines of the opposite hills strengthened the idea. These little terraces were prettily planted with fruit-trees, especially the apple and vine intermixed. They were well pruned and kept low; few even of the apple-trees were larger than gooseberry bushes. In full bloom at the time, and covering so considerable an extent of ground, they made a singular appearance, reminding me of home, and at the same time assuring me of being abroad.*

" On our way, we also passed the valley of the Bos-chetto, which in returning I visited. A great part of it is laid out in orchards, if the term may be applied to plantations of orange, and lemon, and pomegranate, and olive-trees. The first enclosure we passed

---

* Perhaps this mode of cultivating the apple (probably borrowed from the mode of cultivating the vine) might be employed in many situations in England and Scotland, with advantage, especially where the winds are strong, and the exposure bleak and cold. Kept low, and so near the ground, the trees would be better sheltered, and the fruit would ripen sooner and more perfectly. The admixture of the apple and vine, in Gozo, may be advantageous, as the fruit of each ripens in different months, the apple in June, the grape in August and September.

through was an olive-plantation in very nice order, the ground clear, the trees dug about, of comparatively large size, and carefully pruned : they were in blossom. The next enclosure was chiefly a plantation of orange and lemon-trees, with some other fruit-trees intermixed. All the trees appeared beautifully fresh and healthy; the orange-trees just out of flower, the lemon, as usual, in flower and fruit at the same time. * Owing to the shelter of the place, they had escaped the blighting effects of the winds which had lately prevailed, and spoilt the beauty of the gardens in Malta."

Another day we visited the Fungus rock, situated on the shore of the western part of the island. The following is a slight notice of the country through which we passed :—" Excepting near the shore, the whole way, a distance of several miles, the ground was tolerably level, and the bridle-path good; and, except near the shore which was rocky, all the way the country was fertile, chiefly arable land, covered with abundant ripening crops of grain. We passed a few houses and one small village. The solitary houses, the village, even the walls enclosing the fields, had a peculiar air, giving the idea of greater antiquity than in Malta. The cultivation was neat, the field-walls generally in good order; but the houses commonly were more or less ruinous, and the

---

* Within the tropics, at least in Ceylon, the orange-tree, like the lemon-tree in Malta, all the year round, is in fruit and flower, there being a constant succession of flowers.

village mean.   The people, the few we saw, were ill dressed, and squalid, and mostly meagre and ill-looking.   We did not see a single tree, excepting in the village, and there only a few of the prickly pear kind."

END OF VOLUME FIRST.

MURRAY AND GIBB, PRINTERS, 21 GEORGE STREET, EDINBURGH.